CARDIOVASCULAR DISEASE:
Risk factors
and intervention

CARDIOVASCULAR DISEASE:
Risk factors and intervention

Edited by

NEIL POULTER,
MBBS, Msc, MRCP

Senior Lecturer in Clinical Epidemiology, University College of London Medical School; and Honorary Consultant Physician and Epidemiologist, St Mary's Hospital, London

PETER SEVER,
MA, MB, BChir, PhD, FRCP

Professor of Clinical Pharmacology and Therapeutics, St Mary's Hospital Medical School, Imperial College of Science, Technology and Medicine, London

SIMON THOM,
MBBS, MD, MRCP

Senior Lecturer in Clinical Pharmacology and Therapeutics, St Mary's Hospital Medical School, Imperial College of Science, Technology and Medicine; and Honorary Consultant Physician, St Mary's Hospital, London

RADCLIFFE MEDICAL PRESS, OXFORD

© 1993 Radcliffe Medical Press Ltd
15 Kings Meadow, Ferry Hinksey Road, Oxford OX2 0DP

British Library Cataloguing in Publication Data

A catalogue record of this book is available from the British Library

ISBN 1 870905 54 7

Typeset by Acorn Bookwork, Salisbury, Wiltshire
Printed and bound in Great Britain by
Biddles Ltd, Guildford and King's Lynn

Contents

Preface

Coronary artery disease remains the major single cause of death in the UK—where one of the highest mortality rates in the world prevails. Whilst data suggesting the inadequacies of treating any cardiovascular risk factor in isolation accumulates, the relevant sub-specialties tend to operate independently. Consequently, in 1992 we arranged a large multidisciplinary meeting designed to encourage interaction amongst the specialties whilst outlining the current consensus views on the major risk factors, how best to intervene and the benefits likely to ensue. Having brought together some of the world's leading authorities on these topics for the meeting, it seemed a great opportunity to try to capture the distillate of this meeting in one source. The result is this book which was not intended to be yet another 'meeting proceedings' but provides a contemporary review of cardiovascular risk factors from aetiology to secondary prevention.

PETER SEVER
NEIL POULTER
SIMON THOM
April 1993

Foreword

Medicine's basic ethos is the relief of suffering, and traditionally this has led doctors to see their task simply as responding to patients' symptoms and existing complaints. Nowhere is the incompleteness of this view more evident than in cardiovascular diseases, where stroke, heart attack or sudden death come seemingly unannounced and where damage to brain or myocardium are largely irreversible. Slowly we have come to realize that the clinical illness is the end-stage of silent but long-established arterial disease, that warning signs are there if we look for them, and that timely action can reduce the risk both of a first attack and of recurrence.

Cardiovascular medicine has been among the leaders in this wider understanding of clinical responsibility. This has involved first a change in role-perception and then a new technology, which is still evolving. We are learning to move beyond the stage of treating the single risk factor, such as raised blood pressure or blood sugar, to the new concepts of multifactorial risk and multifactorial interventions; and doctors are also learning (albeit slowly) that the patient's recovery from an acute illness can be a signal not for discharge but for a long-term plan for prevention.

The incidence of cardiovascular diseases depends ultimately on the social, economic and political factors which shape the population's eating habits, lifestyle and environment. These are not the responsibility of the health services (although medical staff have a key role as opinion formers); but there is still much scope for individual patients, guided by their doctors, to modify their risk factors and thus greatly to improve their health prospects. This book will help clinicians to understand and exploit these exciting new developments.

GEOFFREY ROSE
Emeritus Professor of Epidemiology
London School of Hygiene and Tropical Medicine

Contributors

R AKEHURST, *York Health Economics Consortium, University of York, York*

DJP BARKER, *MRC Environmental Epidemiology Unit, Southampton General Hospital, Southampton*

E BARRETT-CONNOR, *Department of Community and Family Medicine, School of Medicine, University of California, San Diego, USA*

DG BEEVERS, *Department of Medicine, Dudley Road Hospital, Birmingham*

I BERIOT, *Laboratory of Epidemiology and Social Medicine, Brussels Free University, Belgium*

DJ BETTERIDGE, *Department of Medicine, University College and Middlesex School of Medicine, London*

RWF CAMPBELL, *Department of Academic Cardiology, Freeman Hospital, Newcastle upon Tyne*

JP COX, *The Blood Pressure Unit, Beaumont Hospital, Dublin, Eire*

MJ DAVIES, *Histopathology Department, St George's Hospital Medical School, London*

AT DIPLOCK, *Division of Biochemistry, Guy's Hospital, London*

M DRAMAIX, *Laboratory of Epidemiology and Social Medicine, Brussels Free University, Belgium*

PN DURRINGTON, *University Department of Medicine, The Royal Infirmary, Manchester*

MM EPPERLEIN, *Department of Histopathology, University College and Middlesex School of Medicine, London*

G FOWLER, *Department of Public Health and Primary Care, Radcliffe Infirmary, Oxford*

JS GARROW, *Rank Department of Human Nutrition, St Bartholomew's and Royal London Medical Colleges, London*

AE HARDMAN, *Department of Physical Education, Sports Science and Recreation Management, Loughborough University, Loughborough*

MJ KENDALL, *Department of Medicine, Queen Elizabeth Hospital, Birmingham*

K-T KHAW, *Clinical Gerontology Unit, University of Cambridge School of Clinical Medicine, Cambridge*

F KITTEL, *Laboratory of Epidemiology and Social Medicine, Brussels Free University, Belgium*

M KORNITZER, *Laboratory of Epidemiology and Social Medicine, Brussels Free University, Belgium*

A LOAIZA, *Department of Academic Cardiology, Freeman Hospital, Newcastle upon Tyne*

J LYNAS, *Department of Dietetics, Royal East Sussex Hospital, Hastings*

PM McKEIGUE, *Department of Epidemiology and Population Sciences, School of Hygiene and Tropical Medicine, London*

TW MEADE, *MRC Epidemiology and Medical Care Unit, The Medical College of St Bartholomew's Hospital, London*

AA NORONHA-DUTRA, *Department of Histopathology, University College and Middlesex School of Medicine, London*

EOIN O'BRIEN, *The Blood Pressure Unit, Beaumont Hospital, Dublin, Eire*

K O'MALLEY, *Department of Clinical Pharmacology, Royal College of Surgeons in Ireland, Dublin, Eire*

RM PITTILO, *School of Life Sciences, Kingston University, Kingston upon Thames*

NR POULTER, *Department of Epidemiology and Public Health, University College London Medical School*

MW RAMPLING, *Department of Physiology and Biophysics, St Mary's Hospital Medical School, London*

JPD RECKLESS, *Royal United Hospital, Bath*

LD RITCHIE, *Department of General Practice, University of Aberdeen*

PM ROWLES, *Department of Histopathology, University College and Middlesex School of Medicine, London*

TAB SANDERS, *Department of Nutrition and Dietetics, King's College, London*

PS SEVER, *Department of Clinical Pharmacology and Therapeutics, St Mary's Hospital Medical School, Imperial College of Science, Technology and Medicine, London*

AG SHAPER, *Department of Public Health and Primary Care, Royal Free Hospital School of Medicine, London*

RW STOUT, *Department of Geriatric Medicine, The Queen's University, Belfast*

S THOM, *Department of Clinical Pharmacology and Therapeutics, St Mary's Hospital Medical School, Imperial College of Science, Technology and Medicine, London*

GR THOMPSON, *MRC Lipoprotein Team, Hammersmith Hospital, London*

J WEIL, *Department of Public Health, Dudley Road Hospital, Birmingham*

AF WINDER, *Department of Clinical Pathology and Human Metabolism, Royal Free NHS Trust School of Medicine, London*

PH WINOCOUR, *Department of Medicine, University of Newcastle upon Tyne*

N WOOLF, *Department of Histopathology, University College and Middlesex School of Medicine, London*

The Coronary Heart Disease Epidemic: British and International Trends

NEIL POULTER

Coronary heart disease (CHD) is the largest single cause of death in the United Kingdom (UK) accounting for approximately 26% of all deaths in England in 1991 (HMSO, 1992), with even higher rates in Scotland, Wales and Northern Ireland. In 1990 there were almost 150 000 deaths due to CHD in England and Wales (OPCS, 1990) and CHD events account for 2.5% of the total National Health Service (NHS) expenditure which results in the loss of 35 million working days (HMSO, 1992).

The risk factors for CHD are generally considered to be much the same as for stroke. However, as shown in Table 1.1, the wide range in the ratio of CHD to stroke deaths around the world suggests either that risk factors for CHD are different from those for stroke or more likely that the same risk factors do not share the same importance for the two disorders and are distributed very differently worldwide. International comparisons such as those made in the Seven Countries (Keys, 1970) and Ni-Hon-San (Marmot et al., 1975) studies suggest dyslipidaemia is the major risk factor for CHD whereas hypertension is most important for stroke. Whilst much more remains to be learned of the aetiology of CHD, the major risk factors do seem apparent from national and international data. The largest prospective study, for example—that of the 356 222 men aged 35–57 years, screened for the Multiple Risk Factor Intervention Trial (MRFIT) Study (Stamler et al., 1986)—provide very good evidence that blood pressure, smoking, dyslipidaemia and glucose intolerance explain the majority of CHD cases (Table 1.2).

CHD is not evenly distributed within the UK, either in terms of geography, social class or ethnic group as shown in Table 1.3, Figure 1.1 and Table 1.4 respectively.

The regional and social class differences in CHD rates are not fully explained by differences in classic risk factors but the British Regional Heart Study identified quite marked differences in smoking rates and mean blood pressure levels in keeping with both the geographical and social class differences (Pocock et al., 1987). Serum total cholesterol did not seem to be a major predictor of the CHD rate differences observed either across the social classes or geographically. However, throughout the UK and in all five social groups, mean levels were significantly higher than the ideal level of 5.2 mmol/l (and well above the critcal threshold apparently necessary to produce atherosclerosis).

USA	4.63
New Zealand	4.19
Australia	3.61
England & Wales	3.58
Singapore	2.20
Sri Lanka	1.94
France	1.44
Hong Kong	0.91
Japan	0.46
Korea	0.08

Table 1.1: Number of ischaemic heart deaths for each cerebrovascular death (males, 1985–89).

Cause of death	Low risk[†] ($n = 11\ 098$)	Others ($n = 342\ 815$)
Coronary heart disease	2.0	14.9
Cancer	11.8	16.3
All causes	23.9	45.6

*Age adjusted
[†]Non smoker, serum total cholesterol <4.7 mmol/l
Blood pressure < 120/80 mmHg

Table 1.2: MRFIT screenees: 10.5 year mortality rates/1000* among males free of DM & PMH OF AMI.

	Men*	Women*
Scotland	119	123
Northern Ireland	118	123
North West	117	116
North	116	124
Yorkshire and Humberside	111	116
Wales	111	106
West Midlands	103	104
East Midlands	99	102
South West	91	88
South East	89	87
East Anglia	86	89

*All UK = 100

Table 1.3: CHD in the UK: 1988 SMRs by region. (Source: OPCS, 1990.)

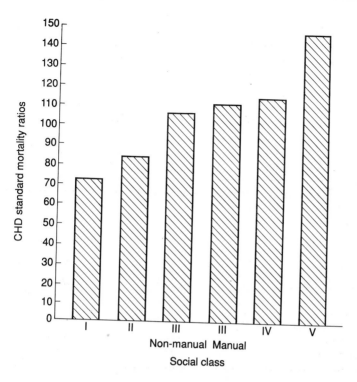

Figure 1.1: Standard mortality ratios for CHD, males aged 20–64 years in England and Wales, 1979–83. (Source: OPCS, 1986.)

It is important to note that the relationship between CHD and social class has totally reversed since the beginning of the century when the disorder began to show a rapid rise in prevalence in the UK (Marmot *et al.*, 1978*a*). This observation raises doubts about the role of stress as a major aetiological determinant of CHD rates at the population level, unless the relative levels of stress associated with different occupations have also reversed since the beginning of the century. Nevertheless, in the Whitehall Study of Civil Servants the majority of the difference in CHD rates observed across the social classes could not be explained by the standard risk factors studied (Marmot *et al.*, 1978*b*). It is proposed amongst this cohort that different levels of stress perhaps mediated through fibrinogen levels are an important determinant of the different CHD rates observed (Markowe *et al.*, 1985). Just as the emergence of CHD in the UK occurred in social class I, the same pattern is seen in the Third World as the chronic degenerative 'westernized' disorders start to replace infectious diseases. However, as shown in Table 1.5, the lifestyle trends which occur in the professional classes in the developing and the developed world are very different and are certainly in keeping with the changes in CHD rates observed.

The very large differences in CHD rates observed amongst Asian and Afro-Caribbean immigrants to UK being respectively much greater and much less

Country of birth	SMR (England and Wales = 100)	
	Men	Women
Scotland	111	119
Ireland	114	120
South Asia	136	146
Caribbean	45	76

Table 1.4: CHD mortality of immigrants aged 20–69 in 1979–83.

than the UK average rates, serve to emphasize that the 'stress' of immigration cannot be a major determinant of the CHD rates of these communties.

Once again the large differences observed do not seem to be explained by the standard risk factors, in that the Asian community generally smokes less, has a smaller body-mass index than the white UK population, and a similar total cholesterol (McKeigue *et al.*, 1991). However, a series of studies carried out in London suggest that differences in glucose intolerance, central obesity, serum triglyceride and high-density lipoprotein (HDL) cholesterol are major contributors to the different CHD mortality rates of the three ethnic groups (McKeigue *et al.*, 1991) (Table 1.6).

Scotland and Northern Ireland lead the international league table of CHD mortality rates (Figure 1.2) with England and Wales not far behind (Uemura and Pisa, 1988). However, as shown in Figure 1.3, these rates are by no means static (Pisa and Uemura, 1982) and during the last 10–15 years CHD rates have been falling in the UK amongst men and women (HMSO, 1992) (Figure 1.4).

The reasons for the falling rates in the UK are not clearly defined. However, smoking rates have been falling since the early seventies (Office of Health

	Developed	Developing
Age	↑	↑
Exercise	↑	↓
Smoking	↓	↑
Alcohol	↓	↑
Stress	?	?
Weight	↓	↑
Salt	↓	↑
Saturated fats	↓	↑

Table 1.5: Dietary and lifestyle changes among professional classes in developed and developing countries.

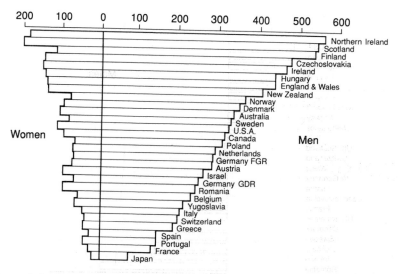

Figure 1.2: CHD mortality rates for men and women in the industrialized world, 1985.

Economics, 1990) and the poly-unsaturated to saturated fat ratio in the diet has almost doubled since 1976 (National Food Survey Committee, 1990). No national survey data are available to confirm whether the equivalent changes in serum cholesterol expected to follow these dietary changes have occurred nor are statistics available to monitor whether the prevalence of hypertension and its management has improved during the last two decades. A survey in 1990

	European $(n = 1515)$	S. Asia $(n = 1421)$	Afro-Caribbean $(n = 209)$
Median systolic blood pressure, mmHg	121	126	128
Median diastolic blood pressure, mmHg	78	82	82
BMI	25.9	25.7	26.3
Plasma TC mmol/l	6.11	5.98	5.87
Prevalence DM (%)	4.8	19.6	14.6
W/H ratio	0.94	0.98	0.94
Plasma HDL	1.25	1.16	1.37
Plasma TG	1.48	1.73	1.09
Fasting insulin mU/l	7.2	9.8	7.1

BMI = body mass index; TC = total cholesterol; DM = diabetes mellitus; W/H = waist/hip ratio; HDL = high density lipoprotein; TG = triglyceride.

Table 1.6: CHD risk factors in London males by ethnic group. (Source: McKeigue *et al.*, 1991.)

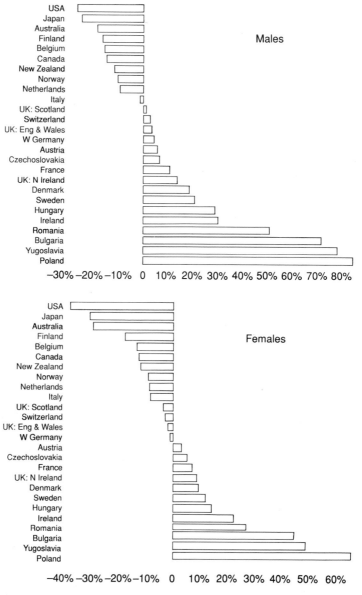

Figure 1.3: Average percentage change in mortality from ischaemic heart disease at ages 40–69 years over 1968–79 (based on the slopes on linear regressions fitted to mortality trends in six quinquennial age groups). (Source: Pisa and Uemura, 1982.)

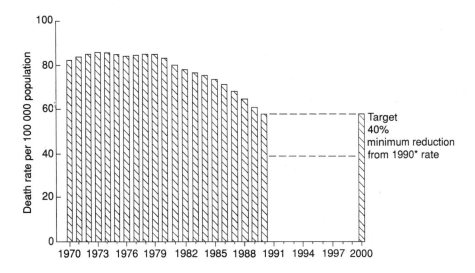

Figure 1.4: CHD rates in England, 1970–90*; and target for the year 2000 (all persons aged under 65). (Source: HMSO, 1992.)

and 1991 of 2000 hypertensives from 13 general practices in England did show that only 53% of those taking antihypertensive medication had their blood pressure levels controlled (<160 mmHg systolic and <95 mmHg diastolic) (Poulter, 1993). On the other hand, it is likely that as opportunistic screening for hypertension has become increasingly accepted, a greater percentage of hypertensives are now identified compared with 20 years ago.

Whilst the improving rates of CHD witnessed in the UK are encouraging they are much less impressive than those experienced in the USA and even Japan (Pisa and Uemura, 1982) where rates have always been very low (Figure 1.2).

In the USA, CHD rates have halved in the last 20 years. It is estimated that approximately 80% of this fall results from the improved risk factor status of the population, but it is not certain what proportion was attributable to changes in which of the risk factors, since levels of almost all of them have improved. Dietary changes include reduced consumption of cigarettes, saturated fat, salt and cholesterol and increased fibre, polyunsaturated fat and alcohol ingestion (Stamler and Stamler, 1984). Somewhat surprisingly, mean body weight has if anything risen!

The large percentage change in CHD rates in Japan seems to result from two major changes. The first is a dramatic fall in hypertension prevalence (which has followed a drastic reduction in dietary salt intake), and the second a rise in detection and treatment rates of hypertensives (Ueshima et al., 1987). As shown in Table 1.7, however, there is a disturbing trend toward increasing saturated fat intake. It will be interesting to see if the trend towards more westernized foods, particularly amongst the young in Japan, will result in a subsequent rise in CHD events when this cohort reaches middle age.

	1956	1980
Hypertension (SBP $\geq$ 180 mmHg) %	7.3*	3.4
Smoking %	83	70
BMI (g/cm^2)	2.14	2.28
CVD treatment/10^5	110	850
Polyunsaturated fat (g/d)	8.2	13.6
Alcohol (ml/head/yr)	3657	8084
Saturated fat (g/d)	5.1	12.0

*1963

Table 1.7: Coronary risk factors in Japanese males aged 30–69, 1956 and 1980.

One of the apparently rogue results amongst the international CHD mortality rates is the often-quoted low rate experienced in France (Renaud and de Lorgeril, 1992). This low rate does not seem compatible with the apparently high saturated fat intake and smoking activities of the French. Indeed, as shown in Table 1.8, whilst the levels of standard risk factors in France are preferable to those found in Scotland, the major dietary differences between these two countries seems to be in terms of the intakes of possible protective factors such as antioxidants (from fruit and vegetables), alcohol and monounsaturated fats. Further discussion of the protective role of each of these dietary constituents is to be found later in this book.

The data necessary to explain why countries (mainly from eastern Europe) have shown a dramatic increase in CHD rates (Figure 1.3) are even scarcer than those relating to the improvements seen in UK. However, such data suggest adverse changes in standard risk-factor status. For example, Figure 1.5 shows relative price increases in Hungary of various items (Kaposvari and Bales, 1988). Such changes will inevitably affect the eating habits and lifestyle habits of the population in a direction likely to produce higher levels of CHD.

Variable	Scotland	France
CHD death rate/10^5	540	120
(aged 40–69 years)	6.3	5.8
Serum cholesterol (mmol/l)	138	139
Systolic blood pressure, mmHg	52	36
Smokers %	1.35	1.35*
HDL chol. (mmol/l)	114 (12% nil)	260*
Vegetables (g/d)	70 (20% nil)	180*
Fruit (g/d)	Low	High
Monounsaturated fat intake	Low	High
Wine intake		

*Monica data

Table 1.8: Risk-factor status in Scotland and France.

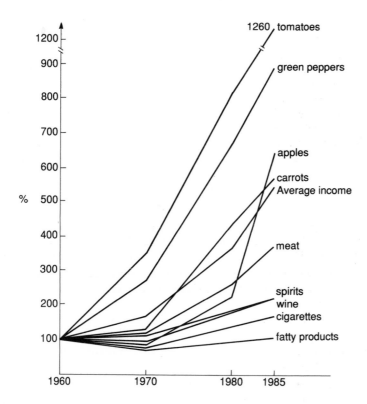

Figure 1.5: Differential price increases in Hungary.

In summary, the CHD levels in the UK which are amongst the highest in the world, are compatible with the high levels of standard risk factors—dyslipidaemia, smoking, hypertension and glucose intolerance currently prevalent in the UK.

The recent reductions in CHD event rates are on target for the 40% and 30% reduction for those under 65 years and 65–74 years respectively set out in *The health of the nation* document (HMSO, 1992). Nevertheless, the current rate of reduction is suboptimal and less than that experienced in several other countries. It seems likely that increased efforts to improve the levels of the standard risk factors in the UK will generate an improved rate of fall in CHD morbidity and mortality.

References

HMSO (1992) *The health of the nation. A strategy for health in England.* HMSO, London.

Kaposvari I and Bales LA (1988) Mag yarovszag. Feb 26.

Keys A (ed.) (1970) Coronary heart disease in seven countries. *Circulation*. Suppl. 1:1–211.

Markowe HLJ (1985) Fibrinogen: a possible link between social class and coronary heart disease. *British Medical Journal*. **291**:382–6.

Marmot MG *et al*. (1975) Epidemiologic studies of coronary heart disease and stroke in Japanese men living in Japan, Hawaii and California: prevalence of coronary and hypertensive heart disease and associated risk factors. *American Journal of Epidemiology*. **102**:514–25.

Marmot MG *et al*. (1978*a*). The changing social class distribution of heart disease. *British Medical Journal*. **2**:1109–12.

Marmot MG *et al*. (1978*b*) Employment grade and coronary heart disease in British civil servants. *Journal of Epidemiology and Community Health*. **32**:244–9.

McKeigue PM *et al*. (1991) Relation of central obesity and insulin resistance with high diabetes prevalence and cardiovascular risk in South Asians. *The Lancet*. **337**:382–6.

National Food Survey Committee (1990) *Household food consumption and expenditure 1989*. HMSO, London.

Office of Health Economics (1990) *Coronary heart disease, the need for action*. OHE, London.

OPCS (1986) *Registrar General's decennial supplement on occupational mortality (1979–83)*. HMSO, London.

OPCS (1990) *Mortality statistics, cause. Leaflet DH2 (17)*. HMSO, London.

Pisa Z and Uemura K (1982) *World Health Statistics Quarterly* **35**:11–47.

Pocock SJ *et al*. (1987) Social class differences in ischaemic heart disease in British men. *The Lancet*. **ii**:197–201.

Poulter NR (1993) In preparation.

Renaud S and de Lorgeril M (1992) Wine, alcohol, platelets, and the French paradox for coronary heart disease. *The Lancet*; **339**:1523–6.

Stamler J and Stamler R (1984) Intervention for the prevention and control of hypertension and atherosclerotic diseases: United States and international experience. *American Journal of Medicine*. **76**:13–36.

Stamler J *et al*. (1986) Is the relationship between serum cholesterol and risk of premature death from coronary heart disease continuous and graded? *Journal of the American Medical Association*. **256**:2823–8.

Uemura K and Pisa Z (1988) Trends in cardiovascular disease mortality in industrialised countries since 1950. *World Health Statistics Quarterly* **41**:155–78.

Ueshima H *et al.* (1987) Declining mortality from ischaemic heart disease and changes in coronary risk factors in Japan, 1956–1980. *American Journal of Epidemiology*. **125**:62–72.

2

Risk Factors in the United Kingdom

AG SHAPER

The underlying theme of this review is that strategies for the prevention of coronary heart disease (CHD) directed towards the whole population, and those directed towards subjects at highest risk of major CHD events, are complementary and indivisible. The population strategies are vital to the reduction of the incidence of CHD, but by the nature of the disease process they are likely to be long-term investments. The high-risk strategies are likely to have a more immediate and dramatic effect but cannot, by virtue of their selectivity, do anything to diminish the continuing epidemic of CHD. No brief overview of this kind can possibly evaluate all the known or suspected risk factors for CHD and comment on their distribution in the United Kingdom and on their complex interrelationships. Therefore this review is highly selective and is intended to illustrate some key issues.

The aetiological model

The concept of multifactorial risk has led to simplistic assumptions that any one of the many risk factors may be responsible individually for causing CHD. International studies such as the Seven Countries Study (Keys *et al.*, 1980) have led us to consider a more complex model upon which strategies for prevention may be based. Figure 2.1, showing the blood cholesterol concentrations in two communities with very different levels of CHD—South Japan and East Finland—illustrates the aetiological model.

In South Japan, where dietary patterns are associated with relatively low mean blood cholesterol levels, there is little CHD despite high rates of cigarette smoking and hypertension. In East Finland, where blood cholesterol levels are similar to those in the UK, high mean blood cholesterol concentrations are associated with high rates of CHD, and risk is increased further by the presence of cigarette smoking and hypertension. There appears to be a specific susceptibility to atherosclerosis and CHD related to the mean level of blood cholesterol in a population, with an optimum level below which CHD is uncommon and not endemic. Above the optimum level (probably around 4–5 mmol/l), susceptibility to CHD increases progressively as the level of mean blood cholesterol increases and CHD becomes endemic in the population

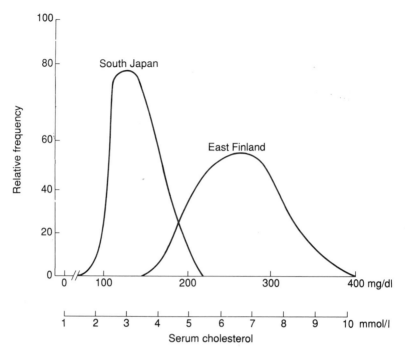

Figure 2.1: Cultural differences in serum total cholesterol distribution. (Source: Rose, 1992)

(Shaper, 1988). The degree of CHD endemicity above the optimum blood cholesterol level depends in part on the population level of blood cholesterol and in part on the frequency of other risk factors, eg cigarette smoking and hypertension. Within populations there is considerable variation in blood cholesterol level between individuals, reflecting in the main variability in both diet and genetic constitution. However, the marked international differences, as seen for South Japan and East Finland, are almost certainly nutritional in origin.

The British Regional Heart Study (BRHS)

This is a large prospective study of 7735 men aged 40–59 years at recruitment, drawn at random from the age-sex registers of representative general practices in 24 towns in England, Wales and Scotland. The study aims to determine the personal and environmental risk factors for CHD in Great Britain and to explain the reasons for the marked geographic variations in cardiovascular mortality (Shaper *et al.*, 1982). No attempt was made to exclude subjects with cardiovascular or other diseases, and 78% of those invited appeared for examination in 1978–80. The information on the prevalence of CHD, blood cholesterol, blood pressure and cigarette smoking presented in this paper is all drawn from the middle-aged men in this study.

Prevalence of CHD

Mortality statistics give us some idea of the likelihood of people in various age groups dying with a label of CHD, but they give us no feel for how commonly the 'man in the street' is affected by the disease. In the BRHS the men were administered a standardized WHO (Rose) questionnaire on chest pain (angina, possible myocardial infarction (MI)), and were asked 'Have you ever been told by a doctor that you have, or have had, angina, heart attack, coronary thrombosis, other heart trouble, high blood pressure, etc'. They also all had a resting electrocardiagram (ECG). Overall, about 25% of the men had some evidence of CHD at initial examination (Shaper *et al.*, 1984). This prevalence may seem very high, but on a town basis it correlated very strongly with the standardized mortality ratios (SMRs) for CHD in middle-aged men in the 24 towns, suggesting that the death certificates (on which the SMRs are based) are reflecting the true state of CHD in the population. Furthermore, men with angina on the WHO questionnaire had a 2.5-fold risk of heart attack on five-year follow-up compared with men who had no angina (Shaper *et al.*, 1985). For those with angina *and* possible myocardial infarction on the WHO questionnaire, the risk of a major CHD event was six times that of men with no chest pain. Only half of the men with definite MI on ECG at initial examination had any history of chest pain in the past or could recall a doctor diagnosis of CHD. This strongly supports the concept of 'silent MI', which may be more frequent than is usually realized. Only 6% of all the men could recall having been told by a doctor that they had angina or had suffered a heart attack. The vast majority of these men had evidence of angina or possible MI on their WHO chest-pain questionnaire. On follow-up, men who recalled a doctor diagnosis of CHD had six times the risk of a new major CHD event in the next five years compared with men who had no recall of such a diagnosis.

It is of considerable interest that all men who had chest pain on exertion on the WHO questionnaire had the same rates of major CHD events on follow-up, irrespective of whether they satisfied all the detailed criteria (site of pain, stopping when pain occurred, relief from stopping, relief within 10 minutes) or not. The strong suggestion is that all chest pain on exertion should be regarded as anginal in nature until proved otherwise (Cook *et al.*, 1989).

Blood cholesterol

There is considerable if not overwhelming evidence that a raised blood cholesterol level is the essential factor in determining the risk of CHD in individuals. The level of risk rises progressively with increasing concentrations

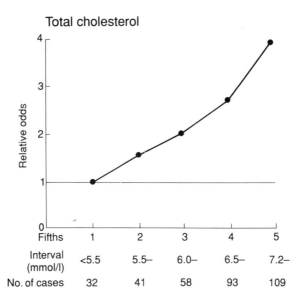

Figure 2.2: Relative odds of a major CHD event by fifths of the ranked distribution of serum total cholesterol. (Source: Shaper *et al.*, 1985.)

of blood cholesterol. This is seen in the BRHS men (Shaper *et al.*, 1985) (Figure 2.2) and in all the large studies such as the Multiple Risk Factor Intervention Trial (MRFIT) (Martin *et al.*, 1986) and the Seven Countries Study (Keys, 1980). In the BRHS some 20% of the major CHD events (fatal and non-fatal) in the first five years of follow-up occurred in the lower 40% of the blood cholesterol distribution (<6.0 mmol/l). However, it is unwise to regard these 'lower' levels of blood cholesterol in this British population as 'low-risk' levels: most of these 'lower' levels of blood cholesterol are well above the upper levels seen in populations at low risk of CHD.

Perhaps the most important observation to be made from Figure 2.2 is that the middle quintile, representing the 'man in the street' has a blood cholesterol level associated with a two-fold increase in risk of a major CHD event compared to men in the lowest quintile of the blood cholesterol distribution. This implies that 60% of middle-aged men in the UK have at least a two-fold risk of a major CHD event from their usual blood cholesterol level. Clearly, a problem of this magnitude can only be dealt with by a population-based strategy of dietary modification. This concept is further illustrated by looking at the relationship between the mean blood cholesterol concentrations in the middle-aged men in the 24 BRHS towns and the SMRs for all cardiovascular disease (CVD) in middle-aged men in those towns (Figure 2.3). It is evident that there is no relationship, and it would be easy to understand the concern of those who consider blood cholesterol fundamental to the CHD risk story and the pleasure

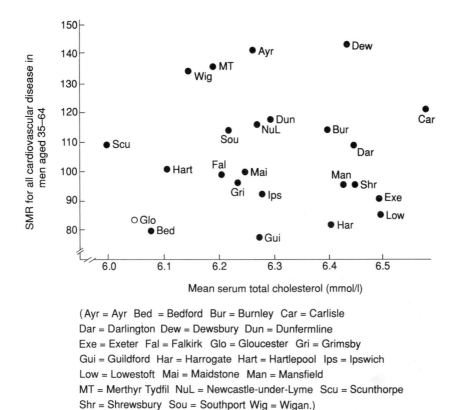

Figure 2.3: Mean total cholesterol concentrations and SMRs for CVD in 24 BRHS towns. (Source: Shaper *et al.*, 1982)

of those who regard the blood cholesterol story as untrue! However, it is important to keep the aetiological model in mind (Figure 2.1). The mean blood cholesterol level in all these British towns is above 6.0 mmol/l, well above the level of about 5.2 mmol/l regarded as optimal by the World Health Organization and other international bodies. Thus, in *every* town in the BRHS the men are highly susceptible to CHD and all that Figure 2.3 is showing is that mean blood cholesterol levels do not contribute to explaining the geographic variations in the incidence of and mortality from CHD in the UK. Indeed, in every UK town in which blood cholesterol has been measured in middle-age, the average blood cholesterol has been at or above 6.0 mmol/l both in men and women and in all social class groups. The data from the National Lipid Screening Project show that even in men and women aged 25–29 years of age blood cholesterol levels have already reached or passed the 'optimal' level recommended by WHO (Mann *et al.*, 1988).

Cigarette smoking

There is little doubt that in populations susceptible to CHD because they have diet-related hypercholesterolaemia, cigarette smoking is an important factor for increasing the risk of atherosclerosis and CHD. In the BRHS, cigarette smokers have almost three times the risk of major CHD events as those who have never smoked, and one of the early and disturbing findings from the study was that ex-smokers appeared to have a two-fold risk of major CHD events (Shaper *et al.*, 1985). Since those original observations, which included all men in the study irrespective of the presence or absence of pre-existing CHD and irrespective of the level of cigarette smoking, we have analysed the data in greater detail (Tang *et al.*, 1992).

A particularly revealing analysis used the simple measure of 'smoking years' and it was evident that there was a strong linear relationship between crude duration of exposure to cigarette smoking and risk of major CHD events. The lowest quintile of the 'smoking years' distribution consisted mainly of men who had never smoked and it was evident that for men in the next quintile of the distribution, risk had almost doubled (Shaper *et al.*, 1986). Thus almost 80% of these middle-aged men had increased risk of major CHD events from their current or past smoking experience (Figure 2.4). Obviously this is another situation which can only respond to a population-based strategy. Looked at on a town basis, there was a strong correlation between the percentage of middle-

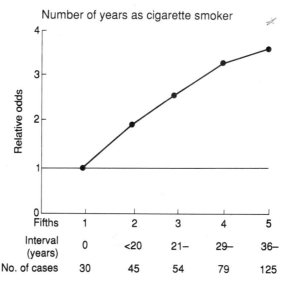

Figure 2.4: Relative odds of a major CHD event by fifths of the ranked distribution of 'smoking years'. (See Figure 2.3 for abbreviations.) (Source: Shaper *et al.*, 1986.)

aged men who were current smokers in a town and the SMRs for CVD. The implication of Figure 2.5 is that cigarette smoking is playing an important role in determining the geographic variations in CHD in Great Britain.

We have now examined the relative risk of a major CHD event after 2½ years' follow-up in the BRHS men who had no recall of a doctor-diagnosis of CHD, according to their smoking status, with those who had never smoked having a relative risk of 1.0 (Tang *et al.*, 1992). Current smokers at screening had a two-fold risk of a major CHD event during the follow-up period and those who had given up cigarettes and taken to a pipe or cigars, had a similar

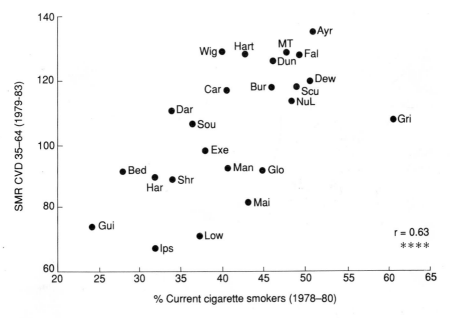

Figure 2.5: Current cigarette smoking (%) and SMRs for CVD in 24 BRHS towns. (Source: Shaper *et al.*, 1982.)

level of risk (Figure 2.6). In light smokers (<20/d) there was still an increased risk of CHD during the period 1–5 years after stopping smoking; thereafter, levels of risk were similar to men who had never smoked. In the heavier smokers (>20/d) relative risk remained increased for more than 20 years after stopping. The implications of these observations for both population and individual strategies are clear. We need to reduce the *incidence* of smoking in the young, to emphasize to cigarette smokers that switching to pipe or cigars is of little benefit from a cardiovascular standpoint, and to persuade persistent smokers that light smoking is more readily reversible than heavy smoking.

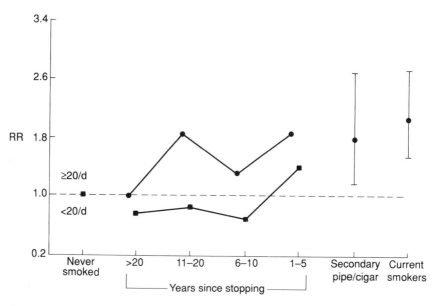

Figure 2.6: Relative risk (adjusted for age, systolic blood pressure and serum total cholesterol) of a major CHD even according to smoking status over 9.5 years follow-up in men without a doctor-diagnosis of CHD. (Source: Tang *et al.*, 1992.)

Blood pressure

Raised blood pressure levels are associated with a wide range of organic complications, including CHD and cerebrovascular disease (stroke). In countries where atherosclerosis and CHD are common, raised blood pressure is one of the most important established risk factors for CHD. Our aetiological model (*see* Figure 2.1) makes it clear that a population with high mean blood pressure, ie South Japan, can have a low incidence of CHD if the essential background, ie a raised mean blood cholesterol level, is not present. In the BRHS, a two-fold risk of CHD was apparent at systolic blood levels of ≥148 mmHg, even after taking other risk factors into account (Shaper *et al.*, 1985) (Figure 2.7). For diastolic blood pressure, the major risk was for those in the top quintile of the distribution (≥93 mmHg), but even those between 72 and 92 mmHg appeared to have some increased risk of CHD. The BRHS and many other studies have shown that systolic blood pressure is the major determinant of the risk associated with CHD, although diastolic pressure also contributes to the overall risk of CHD. The BRHS findings suggest that increased risk of CHD is present in middle-aged men at levels of systolic blood pressure that most clinicians would regard as completely acceptable (148–159 mmHg), and that at least 40% of middle-aged British men have systolic blood pressure levels associated with a twofold risk of CHD or higher. Obesity and alcohol intake are two factors with a well established relationship with blood pressure, and it is

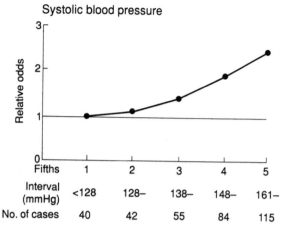

Figure 2.7: Relative odds of a major CHD event by quintiles of the ranked distribution of systolic blood pressure. (Source: Shaper *et al.*, 1985).

highly probable that the sodium/potassium ratio in the diet is also an important contributory factor (Bruce *et al.*, In press).

The relationship between the mean systolic blood pressure in the 24 BRHS towns and the SMRs for CVD is fairly strong, emphasizing the role that systolic blood pressure plays in determining the geographic variations in CHD in the UK (Figure 2.8). It is also important to note the very wide range of mean blood pressure levels in these towns, from 136–153 mmHg.

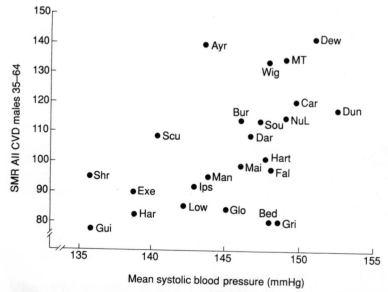

Figure 2.8: Mean systolic blood pressure and SMRs for CVD in 24 BRHS towns (see Figure 2.3 for abbreviations.) (Source: Shaper *et al.*, 1982).

The high-risk model

In trying to determine how important one risk factor is relative to another, we are often driven to think in rather simplistic terms. Table 2.1 shows the relative risk and the yield of CHD cases in the top quintile of the distribution of several risk factors (Shaper *et al.*, 1986). The relative risk is the incidence in the top quintile over the incidence in the lowest fifth of the ranked distribution of the risk factor. The 'yield' is the percentage of all major CHD events in the BRHS men falling into the top (high) quintile of the ranked distribution of the risk factor. The data are based on a five-year follow-up for all men in the study. It is seen that the relative risk ranges from 1.8 for body mass index (weight/height^2; kg/m^2) to 5.1 for 'smoking years'. The 'yield' ranges from 28% for body mass index to 38% for 'smoking years'. Clearly, no single risk factor has a particularly high relative risk and no factor has a particularly high 'yield'. Indeed, it might be said that knowing a middle-aged man's age is somewhat better than knowing his blood cholesterol concentration! Age, however, is presumably acting as a proxy for a lifetime exposure to all the other risk factors present. There is no doubt that this type of univariate comparison of the importance of risk factors is arbitrary and misleading, as it fails to take into account the complex interrelationships of the aetiological model, and in particular fails to recognize the essential role of the raised blood cholesterol concentration, without which there is unlikely to be a measurable rate of CHD in a population (Shaper 1988).

Ever since the Framingham study produced tables of risk for CHD based on a multivariate risk factor approach (Dawbar, 1980) we have been aware that a combination of factors provides a far better measure of risk of major CHD events than any single risk factor. The BRHS data have been used to produce a composite scoring system (Shaper *et al.*, 1986), in which the 'yield' increases to 59%, almost double that observed for any single risk factor, and with a relative risk of 30. A modified form of the scoring system (the GP score), without evidence from the ECG and without a blood cholesterol measurement, still yields 54% of the cases of major CHD events in the top quintile of the risk score distribution with a relative risk of 20. It is suggested that a score of this kind can be of use in a high-risk strategy, as those in the top quintile of the GP score have a 1:10 chance of a major CHD event in the next five years compared to a 1:250 chance experienced by those in the lowest quintile of the GP score distribution. It must be emphasized that the purpose of the score is *prediction*, as it clearly contains items that cannot be modified. On the other hand, it helps to identify a group of people who are at particularly high risk of a major CHD event within a relatively short time and in whom further investigations (such as ECG and measurement of blood lipids) may be indicated. For *action*, one must go beyond the items used to predict risk and consider issues such as diet, body weight, physical activity and stress (factors not used in the scoring system) as well as blood pressure and cigarette smoking, which are taken into account. All these issues both in relation to the population as a whole and those individuals at high risk demand more immediate intervention.

Factor	Relative risk	Yield in top fifth (%)
Age	4.7	34
Total cholesterol	3.1	31
Systolic BP	3.0	36
Diastolic BP	3.1	34
Body mass index	1.8	28
'Smoking years'	5.1	38

Table 2.1 Relative risk and yield of cases in the top fifth of the ranked distribution of risk factors in BRHS men after five years of follow-up. (Source: Shaper *et al.*, 1986.)

Acknowledgements

The British Regional Study is a British Heart Foundation Research Group and also receives support from the Department of Health and The Stroke Association.

References

Bruce NG *et al.* Lifestyle factors associated with geographic blood pressure variations among men and women in Great Britain. *Journal of Human Hypertension.* (In press.)

Cook DG *et al.* (1989) Using the WHO (Rose) angina questionnaire in cardiovascular epidemiological studies. *International Journal of Epidemiology.* 18:607–13.

Dawbar TR (1980) *The Framingham Study: the epidemiology of atherosclerotic disease.* Harvard University Press, Cambridge MA.

Keys A (1980) *Seven Countries: a multivariate analysis of death and coronary heart disease.* Harvard University Press, Cambridge MA.

Mann JI *et al.* (1988) Blood lipid concentrations and other cardiovascular risk factors: distribution, prevalence, and detection in Britain. *British Medical Journal* 296:1702–6.

Martin MJ *et al.* (1986) Serum cholesterol, blood pressure and mortality: implications from a cohort of 361,662 men. *The Lancet.* ii:933–6.

Rose G (1992) *The strategy of preventive medicine.* Oxford Medical Publications, Oxford.

Shaper AG *et al.* (1982) British Regional Heart Study: cardiovascular risk factors in middle-aged men in 24 towns. *British Medical Journal* 283:179–86.

Shaper AG *et al.* (1984) Prevalence of ischaemic heart disease in middle-aged British men. *British Heart Journal.* **51**:595–605.

Shaper AG *et al.* (1985) Risk factors for ischaemic heart disease: the prospective phase of the British Regional Heart Study. *Journal of Epidemiology and Community Health.* **39**:197–209.

Shaper AG *et al.* (1986) Identifying men at high risk of heart attacks: a strategy for use in general practice. *British Medical Journal.* **293**:474–9.

Shaper AG *et al.* (1987) A scoring system to identify men at high risk of a heart attack. *Health Trends.* **19**:37–9.

Shaper AG (1988) *Coronary heart disease: risks and reasons.* Current Medical Literature, London.

Tang J-L *et al.* (1992) Giving up smoking: how rapidly does the excess risk of ischaemic heart disease disappear? *Journal of Smoking Related Diseases.* **3**:203–15.

3

The Fetal Origins of Cardiovascular Disease

DJP BARKER

This chapter presents evidence that coronary heart disease (CHD), and its associated disorders hypertension and diabetes, originate during fetal life.

Programming

The phenomenon underlying this, 'programming', is the process whereby permanent alterations in structure, physiology and metabolism result from stimuli or damage during critical periods of early development. The phenomenon of programming is well known in animals (Dubos *et al.*, 1966; Winick and Noble, 1966; Blackwell *et al.*, 1968; Coates *et al.*, 1983; Hahn, 1984; Swenne *et al.*, 1987). For example, if a newborn rat is put on a low-protein diet for only three weeks its ability to produce insulin is permanently impaired (Swenne *et al.*, 1987). Underlying this must be permanent impairment of function of the beta cells of the pancreas, which produce insulin. Programming occurs because different systems and organs of the body develop in fetal life and infancy during critical and sometimes brief periods. There are windows of time during which maturation has to be achieved, and failure of maturation is to some extent irrecoverable. The kidney, for example, matures in the last few weeks of intra-uterine life. After birth there seems to be little ability to produce more nephrons (Hinchcliffe *et al.*, 1992). The same applies to other organs, although the precise time at which maturation has to be achieved is different for each.

Geographical studies

Suspicion that programming might be associated with cardiovascular disease (CVD) arose from geographical studies (Barker and Osmond, 1986; Barker *et al.*, 1989a). There are twofold variations in death rates from CHD between different areas of England and Wales. Rates are highest in northern industrial towns and some of the poorer rural areas such as North Wales. They are lowest in the south. These differences cannot be explained by differences in adult lifestyle. There are regional differences in smoking behaviour and in body build, but these go only a small way to explaining the large differences in death rates.

Being unable to explain the pattern of CHD through adult lifestyle, it is a logical step to think about earlier stages of life. The suggestion that events in childhood influence the pathogenesis of CVD is not new. Figure 3.1 shows the whole of England and Wales sub-divided into the 212 groupings which are usually used to divide the country: London boroughs, county boroughs (large towns) and within each county, rural districts and urban districts aggregated together. On the vertical axis is cardiovascular mortality (ie death rates from CHD and stroke) at ages 55–74 years in a recent 11-year period. On the horizontal axis are death rates in the first month of life between 1911 and 1915,

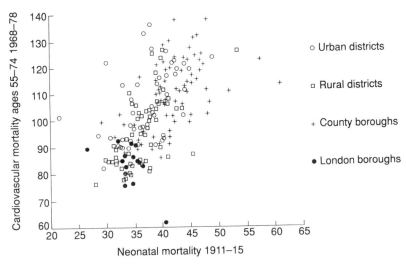

Figure 3.1: Standardized mortality ratios for CVD in 1968–78 and neonatal mortality per 1000 births in 1911–15 in the 212 areas of England and Wales.

around the time when the people dying of CVD were born. There is a strong correlation between current cardiovascular mortality and past neonatal mortality.

We know that areas which in the past had high neonatal mortality were characterized, at that time, by larger numbers of babies of low birthweight and mothers with worse physique, nutritional state and health (Barker *et al.*, 1989*a*). It is an important feature of these results that if post-neonatal mortality, that is the death of babies from one month to one year, were to be substituted for neonatal mortality in Figure 3.1, the correlation with cardiovascular mortality would not be so strong.

Death from CVD

The message from these geographical studies is that the search for environmental causes of CVD should not focus on the environment of children, their diets, homes, and illnesses, but rather should focus on babies and infants, whose mothers are the dominant environmental influence. This is a new point of departure for cardiovascular research. Accordingly the MRC Environmental Epidemiology Unit at Southampton sought out groups of men and women, now in middle to late life, whose early growth was recorded at the time, either by measurements made at birth or by measurements made during infancy. As a result of a systematic search, a number of collections of such records have come to light. The most important derives from Hertfordshire where, since 1911, every baby born in the county has been weighed at birth, followed up to one year by health visitors, and weighed again (Barker *et al.*, 1989*b*). The records for almost the entire county have been preserved. We have now traced 15 000 men and women, born in the county before 1931, whose early growth was recorded.

One of the early studies was of 6500 men born before 1931 in eight registration districts in East and West Hertfordshire. 469 of these 6500 men have died of CHD. The figures in Table 3.1 are the death rates expressed in relation to the national average of 100. The overall figure of 78 reflects the fact that Hertfordshire has below-average CHD rates. Table 3.1 shows that there is a sharp fall in the death rates between men with low weights at one year and those with high weights at one year. Such a fall in death rates is not shown by deaths from non-circulatory causes. A similar trend has now been shown in women (unpublished data) although change of name at marriage makes women more difficult to trace over long periods and studies on them

Weight at one year (lb)	Coronary heart disease	All non-circulatory disease
≤18	100 (36)	74 (39)
−20	84 (90)	99 (157)
−22	92 (180)	74 (215)
−24	70 (109)	67 (155)
−26	55 (44)	84 (99)
≥27	34 (10)	72 (31)
All	78 (469)	78 (696)

Table 3.1: Standardized mortality ratios for coronary heart disease according to weight at one year in 6500 men born during 1911–30. (Numbers of deaths in parentheses.)

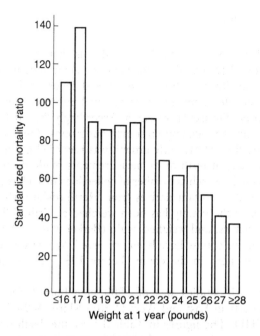

Figure 3.2: Mortality from CHD in 8175 men born during 1911–30 according to weight at one year.

take longer to complete. The Hertfordshire cohort has recently been extended to include 8175 men. Figure 3.2 shows death rates from CHD among men at each pound of weight at one year from 16 to 28. These findings suggest that powerful influences associated with early growth are determining CHD.

Birthweight is related to CHD in the same way as weight at one year, but less strongly (Barker *et al.*, 1989*b*). Birthweight, however is a summary description of fetal growth which includes weight, length and head size. In a study of 1585 men born in Sheffield before 1925, standardized mortality ratios from CVD were more strongly related to small head circumference and low ponderal index (weight/length^3) at birth than to birthweight (Barker *et al.*, 1993*a*). The relations with birth measurements were independent of duration of gestation. CVD is therefore associated with reduced fetal growth rather than preterm birth.

Hypertension

In Hertfordshire we have been able to examine samples of men and women still living in the county. We have made a series of measurements on them and have found that the trend of falling death rates from CHD with increasing early weight is matched by similar trends for each of the known risk factors for CHD

Birthweight (lb)	Number of men	Systolic pressure (mmHg)
≤5.5	10	173
>5.5–6.5	37	169
>6.5–7.5	106	168
>7.5–8.5	76	167
>8.5–9.5	39	163
>9.5	19	161
Total	287	167

Table 3.2: Mean systolic pressure in Hertfordshire men aged 66 and over.

and stroke (Barker 1992). The following are associated with reduced growth *in utero* or during infancy: high blood pressure (Table 3.2), impaired glucose tolerance, raised plasma concentrations of fibrinogen and factor VII, and lipid disorders. However, different risk factors are predicted by different patterns of early growth. High adult blood pressure is associated with low birthweight (Table 3.2) but not independently with weight at one year (Wadworth *et al.*, 1985; Barker *et al.*, 1990; Law *et al.*, 1991, 1993). Raised plasma fibrinogen concentrations are associated with low weight at one year but not independently with low birthweight (Barker *et al.*, 1992a). Serum concentrations of cholesterol are related to methods of infant feeding, which do not influence either blood pressure or plasma fibrinogen concentrations (Fall *et al.*, 1992).

Figure 3.3 brings together results from the three studies of adults of different ages and from a study in Farnborough where the blood pressure of children

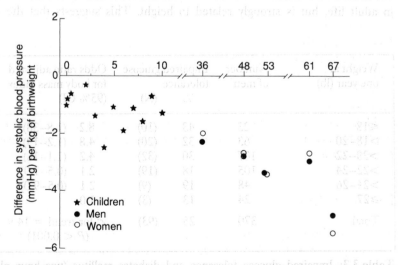

Figure 3.3: Relation between systolic blood pressure and birthweight in men and women at different ages.

was measured at intervals from birth up to 10 years (de Swiet *et al.*, 1992). The vertical axis gives, for each age, the strength of the association between birthweight and systolic blood pressure, expressed as the fall in pressure associated with a 1 kg increase in birthweight (Law *et al.*, 1993). The size of the fall increases with age. This may be interpreted as evidence that an effect initiated *in utero* is slowly amplified over the lifetime of an individual. Folkow (1978) first proposed the existence of these two components, initiation and amplification, in the aetiology of essential hypertension. The mechanisms underlying them are a matter of speculation. Initiation could depend on changes in feto-placental blood flow or increasing activity of trophins leading to changes in blood vessel structure (Lever and Harrap, 1992), associated with fetal growth retardation. Changes in blood-vessel compliance could underlie amplification. Reduced compliance increases blood pressure: increases in pulse pressure make vessel walls less compliant. Such a feedback could amplify an initially raised blood pressure from infancy to old age.

Non-insulin dependent diabetes

370 men, all born in Hertfordshire before 1931, had glucose tolerance tests (Hales *et al.*, 1991). The percentage with impaired glucose tolerance or non-insulin-dependent diabetes (NIDDM), defined as a two-hour plasma glucose concentration of 7.8 mmol/l and over, fell with increasing birthweight and weight at one year (Table 3.3). The risk of having impaired glucose tolerance or NIDDM at age 64 was eight times greater in those who weighed 18 lb or less at one year than in those who weighed more than 27 lb. This is a strong and graded relationship. Weight at one year is not necessarily related to fatness in adult life, but is strongly related to height. This suggests that the main

Weight at one year (lb)	Number of men	Impaired glucose tolerance %	(N)	Odds ratio adjusted for body mass index (95% CI)	
≤18	23	43	(10)	8.2	(1.8–38)
>18–20	63	32	(20)	4.8	(1.2–19)
>20–22	107	30	(32)	4.2	(1.1–16)
>22–24	105	18	(19)	2.1	(0.5–7.9)
>24–26	48	19	(9)	2.1	(0.5–9.0)
≥27	24	13	(3)	1.0	
Total	370	25	(93)	χ^2 for trend = 14.9 ($P < 0.001$)	

Table 3.3: Impaired glucose tolerance and diabetes mellitus (two-hour plasma glucose concentration $\geq$ 7.8 mmol/l) in men aged 59–70 years.

characteristic of those babies with large weight at one year was not greater fatness but greater length. Associations between reduced fetal growth and impaired glucose tolerance in adult life have been confirmed in a survey of 50-year-old men and women in Preston (Phipps *et al.*, 1993), among 50-year-old men and women in Sheffield (unpublished data) and in 21-year-old men (Robinson *et al.*, 1992).

We can make some progress in understanding the link between reduced early somatic growth and impaired glucose/insulin metabolism in adult life, because it is possible to measure 32–33 split pro-insulin concentrations in plasma (Hales *et al.*, 1991). 32–33 split pro-insulin is a precursor of insulin but is not thought to be biologically active in the concentration in which it is found in plasma. Higher plasma concentrations are thought to indicate impaired pancreatic beta-cell activity. The beta-cell complement of the pancreas is established largely before the age of one year. We found the highest 32–33 split pro-insulin concentrations among men who had the lowest infant weight, especially if they subsequently became obese. An interpretation of this is that men with low rates of early growth failed to develop an optimal functioning endocrine pancreas. This led to diabetes in adult life, especially if glucose/insulin metabolism was stressed by obesity. It is a matter for speculation whether suboptimal pancreatic function resulted from reduced numbers of β cells in the pancreas, impaired blood supply, modification of genes controlling metabolism, or some other mechanism.

Hypertension and diabetes—syndrome X

There is a group of adults who have both hypertension and NIDDM. They also have abnormal lipid metabolism, with high triglycerides and low high-density lipoprotein cholesterols, and are insulin resistant. This syndrome has been called 'syndrome X' (Reaven, 1988). In our Hertfordshire sample there were 56 men who had syndrome X. Table 3.4 shows that the prevalence of syndrome X falls from 30% in those who weighed 5½ lbs or less, to 6% in those who weighed 9 lb or more (Barker *et al.*, 1993*b*). After adjusting for current body mass, the risk falls from 18 to 1 from the lowest to the highest birthweight groups. This is a large spread of risk of an important and common disorder. Analysis of cases of syndrome X among 50-year-old men and women whose birth measurements were recorded in detail shows that it is associated with thinness at birth (Barker *et al.*, 1993*b*). A recent study in which 103 men and women were given insulin tolerance tests confirmed that thinness at birth is associated with insulin resistance in adult life (Phillips DIW, unpublished data). Thus reduced fetal growth may be associated with both insulin deficiency and resistance to insulin in later life.

The association of syndrome X and low birthweight is independent of possible confounding variables including cigarette smoking and alcohol consumption. It is found within each social class, defined currently or at birth. The

Birthweight (lb)	Total number of men	Syndrome X %	Syndrome X (N)	Odds ratio adjusted for body mass index (95% CI)
≤5.5	20	30	(6)	18 (2.6–118)
>5.5–6.5	54	19	(10)	8.4 (1.5–49)
>6.5–7.5	114	17	(19)	8.5 (1.5–46)
>7.5–8.5	123	12	(15)	4.9 (0.9–27)
>8.5–9.5	64	6	(4)	2.2 (0.3–14)
>9.5	32	6	(2)	1.0
Total	407	14	(56)	χ^2 for trend = 16.0 ($P < 0.001$)

Table 3.4: Percentages of men in Hertfordshire with syndrome X (hypertension, NIDDM and hypertriglyceridaemia) according to birthweight.

separate associations of blood pressure with birthweight (Table 3.2) and of impaired glucose tolerance and NIDDM with birthweight and weight at one year (Table 3.3) are similarly independent of known confounding variables. It is unlikely that unknown confounding variables related to adult lifestyle would produce large and graded relations such as that between birthweight and risk of syndrome X (Table 3.4). Such a confounding variable would have a stronger effect on the risk of syndrome X than any variable hitherto identified and its existence is likely to have been already known, or at least suspected.

Maternal nutrition

The conclusion that CHD, hypertension and NIDDM are programmed in fetal life raises two question. What are the influences which, acting through the mother, programme the fetus? What structural or physiological changes are set in place in fetal life and lead to abnormal function in adult life? We cannot answer either question, but there are interesting clues.

A set of obstetric records in Sharoe Green Hospital, Preston, gave us the opportunity to identify groups of men and women, now aged around 50, whose measurements at birth had been recorded in detail (Barker et al., 1990). Table 3.5 shows the mean systolic pressure of 327 men and women aged 50 living in Preston today (Barker et al., 1992b). They were all born after 38 completed weeks of gestation. The men and women are arranged by three birthweight groups, and in four groups of placental weight. There was, as expected, a fall in blood pressure associated with increasing birthweight. There was also an unsuspected increase in blood pressure with increasing placental weight. So, in Table 3.5, those with mean systolic pressures of 150 mmHg or more

Birthweight (lb)	Placental weight (lb)				
	≤ 1.0	−1.25	−1.5	>1.5	All
−6.5	149 (24)	152 (46)	151 (18)	167 (6)	152 (94)
−7.5	139 (16)	148 (63)	146 (35)	159 (23)	148 (137)
>7.5	131 (3)	143 (23)	148 (30)	153 (40)	149 (96)
All	144 (43)	148 (132)	148 (83)	156 (69)	149* (327)

*Standard deviation = 20.4

Table 3.5: Mean systolic blood pressure (mmHg) of men and women aged 46–54, born after 38 completed weeks of gestation, according to placental weight and birthweight (numbers of subjects in parentheses.)

comprise a group of babies who were relatively small in relation to the size of their placentas.

In man and animals, disproportionately large placental size may be a consequence of maternal undernutrition. It occurs in babies whose mothers were anaemic during pregnancy (Beischer et al., 1970; Godfrey et al., 1991). It can be produced in sheep by depriving the ewe of food in early pregnancy (Farchney and White, 1987; McCrabb et al., 1991). We therefore suspect that maternal undernutrition may be an important influence in determining high blood pressure in the next generation. Recent studies of four-year-old children in Salisbury have shown similar associations between birthweight, placental weight and blood pressure as were found in older people (Law et al., 1991). We therefore know that these associations depend on influences which still affect fetal growth today.

Examination of birth measurements additional to weight identifies two groups of babies who develop high blood pressure as adults (Barker et al., 1992b). One group, who also develop impaired glucose tolerance, have below-average birthweight, head circumference and a low ponderal index (weight/length^3) taking account of gestational age. Babies in this group are recognized as the result of suboptimal growth beginning in early pregnancy. A second group of babies who develop high blood pressure have above-average birthweight and head circumference but below-average length. These babies, who are not usually recognized clinically, have 'asymmetrical' growth retardation, thought to result from slowing of growth near full term. The mechanisms by which these two groups of babies subsequently develop high blood pressure may differ because of the different times when they were subject to adverse influences. 'Thin' and 'short' babies have different physiology and metabolism in adult life. For example, thin babies tend to develop syndrome X (Barker et al., 1993b), whereas short babies develop raised plasma concentrations of fibrinogen (Barker et al., 1992a).

Conclusions

The results described in this paper show that retarded growth in fetal life and infancy is strongly related both to mortality from CVD and to high blood pressure and NIDDM. Review of the associations between retarded early growth and other cardiovascular risk factors—lipid metabolism (Fall *et al.*, 1992), haemostatic factors (Barker *et al.*, 1992*a*) and body fat distribution (Law *et al.*, 1992)—is beyond the compass of this paper. One possible explanation for these relations is that genetic influences that first show themselves in early life as growth failure are revealed later in adult life through the occurrence of CVD. The implication is that the genes that determine low birthweight are the same as or are closely linked to the genes that determine CVD. This explanation is not likely to be correct because birthweight does not seem to be strongly genetically determined (Morton, 1955; Robson, 1955; Nance *et al.*, 1983; Carr-Hill *et al.*, 1987); nor is there much evidence that CVD has, in most people, a major genetic component.

We think that the relation between retarded growth in early life and risk of adult disease is due to long-term effects on physiology and metabolism imposed by an adverse environment during critical periods of development. This conclusion does not imply that the environment in adult life is unimportant, although it may explain why the known adult risk factors predict CVD in individuals so poorly. Further work is focusing on the nature and timing of environmental factors that influence the growth of the fetus and infant and programme its metabolism. Maternal nutrition is suspected to be important.

References

Barker DJP and Osmond C (1986) Infant mortality, childhood nutrition, and ischaemic heart disease in England and Wales. *The Lancet*; 1:1077–81.

Barker DJP *et al.* (1989*a*) The intrauterine and early postnatal origins of cardiovascular disease and chronic bronchitis. *Jounal of Epidemiology and Community Health*. 43:237–40.

Barker DJP *et al.* (1989*b*) Weight in infancy and death from ischaemic heart disease. *The Lancet*. ii:577–80.

Barker DJP *et al.* (1990) Fetal and placental size and risk of hypertension in adult life. *British Medical Journal*. 301:259–62.

Baker DJP (ed.) (1992) *Fetal and infant origins of adult disease*. British Medical Journal, London.

Barker DJP *et al.* (1992*a*). The relation of fetal and infant growth to plasma fibrinogen and factor VII in adult life. *British Medical Journal*. 304:148–52.

Barker DJP *et al.* (1992*b*): Relation of fetal length, ponderal index, and head circumference to blood pressure and risk of hypertension in adult life. *Paediatric and Perinatal Epidemiology.* **6**:35–44.

Barker DJP *et al.* (1993*a*). The relation of head size and thinness at birth to death from cardiovascular disease in adult life. *British Medical Journal.* **306**:422–6.

Barker DJP *et al.* (1993*b*) Type 2 (non-insulin dependent) diabetes mellitus, hypertension and hyperlipidaemia (syndrome X): relation to reduce fetal growth. *Diabetologia.* **36**:62–7.

Beischer NA *et al.* (1970) Placental hypertrophy in severe pregnancy anaemia. *Journal of Obsterics and Gynaecology, British Commonwealth.* **77**:398–409.

Blackwell NM *et al.* (1968) Further studies on growth and feed utilization in progeny of underfed mother rats. *Journal of Nutrition.* **97**:79–84.

Carr-Hill R *et al.* (1987) Is birthweight determined genetically? *British Medical Journal.* **295**:687–9.

Coates PM *et al.* (1983) Effect of early nutrition on serum cholesterol levels in adult rats challenged with a high fat diet. *Journal of Nurtrition.* **113**:1046–50.

de Swiet M *et al.* (1992) Blood pressure in first 10 years of life: the Brompton study. *British Medical Journal* **304**:23–6.

Dubos R *et al.* (1966) Biological Freudianism: lasting effects of early environmental influences. *Pediatrics* **38**:798–800.

Fall CHD *et al.* (1992) Relation of infant feeding to adult serum cholesterol concentration and death from ischaemic heart disease. *British Medical Journal.* **304**: 801–5.

Farchney GJ and White GA (1987) Effects of maternal nutritional status on fetal and placental growth and on fetal urea synthesis. *Australian Journal of Biological Science.* **40**:365–77.

Folkow B (1978) Cardiovascular structural adaptation: its role in the initiation and maintenance of primary hypertension. *Clinical Science.* **55**:3–22s.

Godfrey KM *et al.* (1991) The effect of maternal anaemia and iron deficiency on the ratio of fetal weight to placental weight. *British Jounal of Obstetrics and Gynaecology.* **98**:886–91.

Hahn P (1984) Effect of litter size on plasma cholesterol and insulin and some liver and adipose tissue enzymes in adult rodents. *Journal of Nutrition.* **114**:1231.

Hales CN *et al.* (1991) Fetal and infant growth and impaired glucose tolerance at age 64 years. *British Medical Journal.* **303**:1019–22.

Hinchcliffe SA *et al.* (1992) The effect of intra-uterine growth retardation in the development of renal nephrons. *British Journal of Obstetrics and Gynaecology.* **99**: 296–301.

Law CM *et al.* (1991) Maternal and fetal influences on blood pressure. *Archives of Disease in Childhood.* **66**:1291–5.

Law CM *et al.* (1992) Early growth and abdominal fatness in adult life. *Journal of Epidemiology and Community Health.* **46**:184–6.

Law CM *et al.* (1993) The initiation of hypertension *in utero* and its amplification throughout life. *British Medical Journal.* **306**:24–7.

Lever A and Harrap S (1992) Essential hypertension—a disorder of growth with origins in childhood. *Journal of Hypertension.* **10**:101–20.

McCrabb GJ *et al.* (1991) Maternal undernutrition during mid-pregnancy in sheep. Placental size and its relationship to calcium transfer during late pregnancy. *British Journal of Nutrition.* **65**:157–68.

Morton NE (1955) The inheritance of human birth weight. *Annals of Human Genetics.* **19**:125–34.

Nance WE *et al.* (1983) A causal analysis of birth weight in the offspring of monozygotic twins. *American Journal of Human Genetics.* **35**:143–51.

Phipps K *et al.* (1993) Fetal growth and impaired glucose tolerance in men and women. *Diabetologia.* **36**:225–8.

Reaven GM (1988) Role of insulin resistance in human disease. *Diabetes.* **37**: 1595–607.

Robinson SM *et al.* (1992) Relation of fetal growth to plasma glucose concentrations in young men. *Diabetologia.* **35**:444–6.

Robson EB (1955) Birthweight in cousins. *Annals of Human Genetics.* **19**:732.

Swenne I *et al.* (1987) Persistent impairment of insulin secretory response to glucose in adult rats after limited period of protein-calorie malnutrition early in life. *Diabetes.* **36**:454–8.

Wadsworth M *et al.* (1985) Blood pressure in a national birth cohort at the age of 36 years, related to social and familial factors, smoking and body mass. *British Medical Journal.* **291**:1534–8.

Winick M and Noble A (1966) Cellular response in rats during malnutrition at various ages. *Journal of Nutrition.* **89**:300–6.

4

Heart Disease Risk Factors in Women

ELIZABETH BARRETT-CONNOR

One of the most interesting questions in clinical medicine is why women live longer than men. This difference is apparent from birth, and increases with age wherever women no longer die frequently in childbirth. In most industrialized countries, the largest sex differential for mortality is due to coronary heart disease (CHD). Yet the sex ratio is remarkably consistent, ranging from 2.5 to 4.5, in countries with very different diets, habits and heart disease rates (Figure 4.1). This suggests that there is an intrinsic gender-mediated difference that could be most simply explained by differences in sex hormones. The simplest hypothesis is that oestrogen is protective.

Although women have higher endogenous oestrogen levels than men, they do not have more favourable levels of most heart disease risk factors. In general, women have higher blood pressure, higher plasma cholesterol levels, higher fibrinogen levels, are more obese and have more diabetes than men.

The few known exceptions, ie more favourable factors characteristic of women, are: less central or upper body obesity, higher high density lipoprotein (HDL) cholesterol, and lower triglyceride levels. These characteristics are all interrelated. In 1275 Rancho Bernardo women aged 50–89 years, the fasting plasma triglyceride level was positively correlated with waist-hip ratio (r = 0.30; p = 0.001) and inversely correlated with HDL cholesterol (r = 0.54; p = 0.001). Although this dyslipidaemia and body fat pattern occur in women with normal glucose tolerance, they are most characteristic of adult-onset diabetes. Diabetes is the only common condition which increases the female risk of heart disease to a level approaching that seen in men.

Central obesity

Central or upper body obesity was called android obesity by Vague in 1947 to reflect its male pattern; Vague also recognized the more recently rediscovered metabolic abnormalities that characterize this fat distribution, particularly when it is seen in women (Kissebah *et al.*, 1982). Central obesity has been shown to predict an increased risk of cardiovascular disease (CVD) in women.

Could the more favourable lower body fat distribution in women explain the sex difference in heart disease risk? It is difficult to answer this question in most

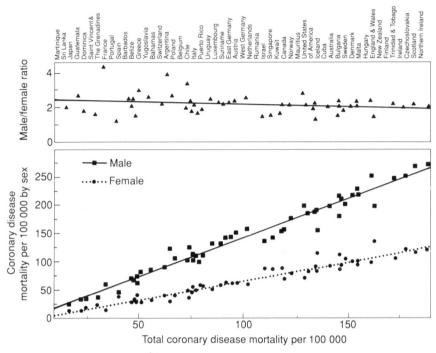

Figure 4.1: Age-standardized coronary disease death rates in 1987 for men and women from 52 countries. Both male and female coronary disease mortality correlate with total coronary disease mortality (for males, r = 0.98; for females, r = 0.97). The ratio of male to female mortality is constant at a mean value of 2.24 ± 0.08 (SEM). (Reproduced from Kalin and Zumoff, 1990, by permission.)

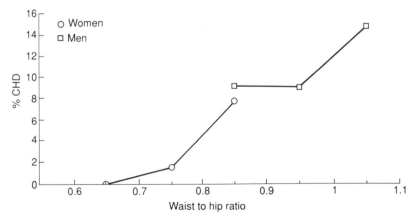

Figure 4.2: 12-year incidence of CHD by waist:hip ratio and sex (women aged 50, 54, and 60 years at base-line and men aged 54 years at base-line), Gothenburg, Sweden. (Men, 1967 to 1979; women, 1968/9–1980/1). (Reproduced from Larsson *et al.*, 1992, by permission.)

populations, where there is so little overlap between male and female waist-hip ratios (Figure 4.2) that adjusting for fat distribution is essentially adjusting for sex. Studies of ethnic groups (such as Near Eastern Indians), where male and female waist-hip ratios do overlap, may prove useful.

HDL cholesterol

In the prospective Donolo-Tel Aviv Study (Brunner *et al.*, 1987), women with hypercholesterolaemia appeared to tolerate relatively low levels of HDL choles- terol better than men (Table 4.1). In both Framingham and the Lipid Research Clinics, CVD mortality rates (Gordon *et al.*, 1989) were at least four times higher in low HDL than high HDL women. When female CVD mortality rates were compared with those of their male counterparts, the female survival advantage was limited to the middle and high HDL categories. After adjusting for other risk factors including blood pressure, cigarette smoking, and low- density lipoprotein (LDL) cholesterol, a theoretical increment in HDL of 1 mg/dl (0.026 mM) was associated with a slightly greater reduction in heart disease risk in women (3.2%) than in men (1.9–2.3%).

Total cholesterol	Men	Women
<200	140	87
200–224	194	76
225–249	234	94
250–264	252	81
>264	256	128

Table 4.1: Sex-specific 20-year incidence of definite coronary events/1000 in 1454 men and 1481 women aged 30–64 years with low HDL (<23% of total cholesterol) by cholesterol level (mg/dl): the Donolo-Tel Aviv Study. (Source: Brunner *et al.*, 1987.)

Triglycerides

Prospective population-based studies have found plasma triglyceride levels to be significantly associated with the risk of heart disease in women *before* adjusting for total or HDL cholesterol. For example, in the Lipid Research Clinics (Bush *et al.*, 1987*a*) cohort of 2270 women aged 40–69 years who were followed for 8.5 years, the age-specific quartile of triglyceride value was more consistently associated with the risk of subsequent CVD than the age-specific quartile of total LDL or HDL cholesterol. Compared with women who had the lowest quartile of triglyceride, women in the highest quartile had a relative risk of CVD death of 6.6, in the third quartile of 2.9 and in the second quartile of 1.9. However, triglyceride levels were not independently related to the risk of fatal CVD (R.R. = 1.00) in a multivariate Cox proportional hazards model, after adjusting for age, blood pressure, cholesterol, cigarette smoking, and use of exogenous oestrogen. In a separate model that included HDL and LDL instead of total cholesterol and triglyceride, HDL was independently and significantly inversely associated with subsequent CVD death.

The well documented, inverse association between HDL cholesterol and triglyceride (−0.2 to −0.7) and the relatively large intra-individual variation in triglyceride levels may explain why triglyceride does not emerge as an independent risk factor in multivariate models. In addition, as pointed out by Pyörälä and Laakso (1983) and by Austin (1989), interpretation of these multiply adjusted analyses is difficult because plasma triglyceride is biologically correlated positively with total plasma cholesterol and inversely with HDL cholesterol. The statistical models may 'overadjust' for complex metabolic processes.

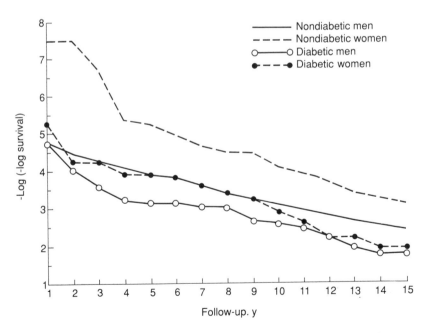

Figure 4.3: Age-adjusted ischaemic heart disease -log (-log survival) by sex and diabetes; Rancho Bernardo, California, 1972–88. Curves were estimated by a Cox model blocked on both sex and diabetes status and adjusted for age. (Reproduced from Barrett-Connor and Bush, 1991, by permission.)

Diabetes

Women with diabetes assume a risk of heart disease that closely approaches that of men (Figure 4.3) and is not entirely explained by the other classic heart disease risk factors. It is not clear whether the risk is independent of the upper body obesity, lower HDL cholesterol levels, and higher triglyceride levels seen in women with diabetes. These lipoprotein differences in women with and without diabetes are larger than the differences in men with and without diabetes, and cannot explain their reduced risk of heart disease. Triglyceride is said to contribute to the risk of heart disease particularly among diabetic women. Neither of these theses has been adequately tested (Janka, 1985; Fontbonne *et al.*, 1989).

Insulin is a current favourite among the cardiovascular risk factors. Hyperinsulinaemia or insulin resistance covaries with central obesity and the diabetic dyslipidaemia. Three prospective studies in men have found that higher levels of endogenous insulin predicted an increased risk of heart disease. The only prospective study that included women found no association of plasma insulin level with future heart disease. Since the glucose tolerance test and insulin levels in that study were obtained in non-fasting subjects who were examined throughout the day, a role for hyperinsulinaemia cannot be excluded as a heart-disease risk factor in women. However, a cross-sectional study also found a significant relation of insulin to heart disease in men but not women (Modan *et al.*, 1991), raising the possibility that women ordinarily possess inherent protection against insulin resistance or its covariates.

Menopause

If the more favourable female risk factors are explained by oestrogen, then patterns should become less favourable after the menopause. Cross-sectional studies such as Framingham (Figure 4.4) have shown that around age 50 the female LDL level increases and still remains higher than the level seen in men. Prospective studies suggest that HDL begins to fall several years before the last menstrual period, whereas the LDL rise is much more coincident with the end of menses (Jensen *et al.*, 1990). Mathews *et al.* (1989) found that menopause-related changes were greater in HDL and LDL than the lipid changes associated with ageing in the absence of menopause. Additional data from that same cohort also suggest an unfavourable shift in the haemostatic factors fibrinogen and factor VII at the time of menopause (Meilahn *et al.*, 1990). Some, but not all, studies have found serum oestradiol levels to be significantly associated with HDL levels in post-menopausal women (Kuller *et al.*, 1990).

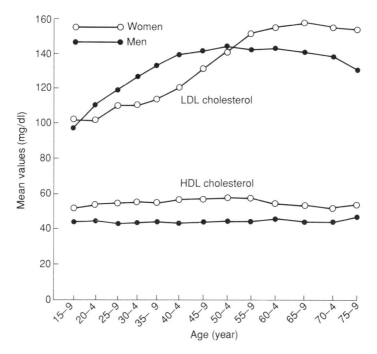

Figure 4.4: Trends of lipoprotein levels in men and women according to age. (Source: Kannel, 1988.)

Oestrogen replacement

Studies dating back to the early 1950s showed that oestrogen prevented atherosclerosis in animal models, that oestrogen raised HDL and lowered LDL levels in humans, and that prematurely oophorectomized women had an increased risk of heart disease. In 1959, Oliver and Boyd proposed 'the prescription of a little oestrogen for life' to prevent heart disease in all post-menopausal women. In 1978, Tikkanen proposed the use of oestrogen as a lipid-lowering agent for women with hypercholesterolaemia.

The Coronary Drug Project, however, an ambitious clinical trial of four lipid-lowering medications including two oestrogen regimens, was conducted in men. Very high doses of oestrogen (either 5 or 2.5 mg Premarin) were given daily. Regimens were chosen deliberately to cause gynaecomastia as a marker of successful feminization. Not surprisingly, in retrospect, these unphysiologic doses also caused impotence and thrombosis, leading to dropouts and discontinuation of these treatment arms (Coronary Drug Project Research Group, 1973).

Sadly, only one clinical trial has been reported in women. Nachtigall *et al.* (1979) reported a randomized trial of oestrogen plus a cyclic progestin in 168 institutionalized women who were followed for 10 years. Cardiovascular events were few, and the relative risk of 0.33 was not statistically significant. In the same year, Hammond *et al.* (1979) reported a large observational study showing significantly less heart disease and diabetes in women treated with oestrogen than in untreated women.

In the last 10 years, over 20 case-control and cohort studies have been published. Nearly all of them were based on unopposed conjugated equine oestrogen given without a progestin. A meta-analysis of these studies by Stampfer and Colditz (1991) found an overall risk reduction of about 50%. Three studies of women who underwent coronary angiography also found less atherosclerosis in oestrogen-treated women (Table 4.2).

These results are biologically plausible. The Lipid Research Clinics Study (Bush *et al.*, 1987*b*), and Gruchow *et al.*'s (1988) report on women with angiographic evidence of coronary artery disease, both suggest that the higher HDL levels found in hormone users are important, because adding HDL to the analytical model reduced the independent inverse association of oestrogen to heart-disease risk. Some data indicate that a portion of the apparent protection from heart-disease risk associated with oestrogen is reduced after hormone-replacement therapy is stopped (Criqui *et al.*, 1988), suggesting that oestrogen has a dynamic effect on blood flow, in addition to reducing atherosclerosis. All other known effects of oestrogen on heart-disease risk factors (with the possible exception of the coagulation and thrombolysis cascade) and on the endothelium are favourable (Barrett-Connor and Bush, 1991). Some think the results are sufficiently consistent to recommend oestrogen to nearly all post-menopausal women.

The data suggesting that hormone replacement prevents CHD are consistent and quite compelling. Nevertheless, the real risks and benefits of oestrogen can only be assessed by randomized placebo-controlled clinical trials. Much of the apparent benefit could reflect the various biases in characteristics of women before and after the prescription of hormones. Women who are prescribed oestrogen tend to be at lower risk at the outset, being on average of higher social class, more educated, leaner and with lower levels of heart-disease risk factors than untreated women. Women who take oestrogen for an extended period of time represent less than half of all women prescribed oestrogen; in clinical trials, compliance with placebo can reduce the risk of heart disease by 50%. There is also evidence for prevention bias; women taking oestrogen have regular medical care which often includes measurement (and management) of blood pressure and cholesterol, and other health advice.

Other practical questions remain. Is the effect of exogenous oestrogen the same as the effect of endogenous oestrogen? Will non-oral oestrogens or oestrogen plus progestin regimens have the same effect on heart disease? What is the optimal regimen in terms of benefit, safety and acceptability? Studies designed to answer these questions in post-menopausal women may help to answer the original question: is oestrogen the main reason why women have so much less heart disease then men?

Authors (year)	Study design	Study size	End point	Risk estimate
Sullivan (1988)	Case-control	Cases = 1444 Controls = 744	≥70% stenosis	0.44*
Gruchow et al. (1988)	Cross-sectional	Users = 154 Non-users = 779	Severe occlusion Moderate occlusion	0.37* 0.59*
McFarland (1989)	Case-control	Cases = 137 Controls = 208	≥70% stenosis	0.50*

*$P < 0.05$.

Table 4.2: Studies of oestrogen use in women and angiographically defined CHD. (Source: Barrett-Connor and Bush, 1991.)

References

Austin MA (1989) Plasma triglyceride as a risk factor for coronary heart disease: the epidemiologic evidence and beyond. *American Journal of Epidemiology*. **129**:249–59.

Barrett-Connor E and Bush TL (1991) Estrogen and coronary heart disease in women. *Journal of the American Medical Association*. **265**:1861–7.

Brunner D *et al.* (1987) Relation of serum total cholesterol and high-density lipoprotein cholesterol percentage to the incidence of definite coronary events: twenty-year followup of the Donolo-Tel Aviv Prospective Coronary Artery Disease Study. *American Journal of Cardiology*. **59**:1271–6.

Bush TL *et al.* (1987) Cardiovascular mortality and noncontraceptive use of estrogen in women: results from the Lipid Research Clinics Program follow-up study. *Circulation*. **75**:1102–9.

Bush TL *et al.* (1987) Cardiovascular disease mortality in women: results from the Lipid Research Clinics follow-up study. In: Baker ED *et al.* (eds) *Coronary heart disease in women*. Haymarket Doyma, New York. pp. 106–11.

Coronary Drug Project Research Group (1973) The Coronary Drug Project: findings leading to discontinuation of the 2.5 mg/day estrogen group. *Journal of the American Medical Association*. **226**:652–7.

Criqui MH *et al.* (1988) Postmenopausal estrogen use and mortality. Results from a prospective study in a defined, homogeneous community. *American Journal of Epidemiology*. **128**:606–14.

Fontbonne A *et al.* (1989) Hypertriglyceridemia as a risk factor of coronary heart disease mortality in subjects with impaired glucose tolerance or diabetes. *Diabetologia*. **32**:300–4.

Gordon DJ *et al.* (1989) High-density lipoprotein cholesterol and cardiovascular disease. Four prospective American studies. *Circulation*. **79**:8–15.

Gruchow HW *et al.* (1988) Postmenopausal use of estrogen and occlusion of coronary arteries. *American Heart Journal*. **115**:954–63.

Hammond CV *et al.* (1979) Effects of long-term estrogen replacement therapy, I: metabolic effects. *American Journal of Obstetrics and Gynecology*. **133**:525–36.

Janka HU (1985) Five-year incidence of major macrovascular complications in diabetes mellitus. *Hormone and Metabolic Resarch Supplement*. **15**:15–19.

Jensen J *et al.* (1990) Influence of menopause on serum lipids and lipoproteins. *Maturitas*. **12**:321–31.

Kalin MF and Zumoff B (1990) Sex hormones and coronary disease: a review of the clinical studies. *Steroids.* **55**:330–52.

Kannel WB (1988) Nutrition and the occurrence and prevention of cardiovascular disease in the elderly. *Nutrition Review.* **46**:66–78.

Kissebah AH *et al.* (1982) Relation of body fat distribution to metabolic complications of obesity. *Journal of Clinical Endocrinology and Metabolism.* **54**:254–60.

Kuller LH *et al.* (1990) Relationship of endogenous sex steroid hormones to lipids and apoproteins in postmenopausal women. *Atherosclerosis.* **10**:1058–66.

Larsson B *et al.* (1992) Is abdominal body fat distribution a major explanation for the sex difference in the incidence of myocardial infarction? *American Journal of Epidemiology.* **135**:266–73.

Mathews KA *et al.* (1989) Menopause and risk factors for coronary heart disease. *New England Journal of Medicine.* **321**:641–6.

McFarland LF *et al.* (1989) Risk factors and noncontraceptive estrogen use in women with and without coronary heart disease. *American Heart Journal.* **117**:1209–14.

Meilahn EN *et al.* (1990) Change in coagulation parameters over one year in postmenopausal women. *Circulation.* **81**:718.

Modan M *et al.* (1991) Hyperinsulinemia, sex, and risk of atherosclerotic cardiovascular disease. *Circulation.* **84**:1165–75.

Oliver MF and Boyd GS (1959) Effect of bilateral ovariectomy on coronary artery disease and serum-lipid levels. *The Lancet.* **ii**:690–4.

Pyörälä K and Laakso M (1983) Macrovascular disease in diabetes mellitus. In: Mann JI *et al.* (eds) *Diabetes in epidemiological perspective.* Churchill Livingstone, Edinburgh. pp. 183–264.

Stampfer MJ and Colditz GA (1991) Estrogen replacement therapy and coronary disease: a quantitative assessment of the epidemiological evidence. *Preventive Medicine.* **20**:47–63.

Sullivan JM *et al.* (1988) Postmenopausal estrogen use and coronary atherosclerosis. *Annals of Internal Medicine.* **108**:358–63.

Tikkanen MJ (1978) Natural oestrogen as an effective treatment for type-II hyperlipoproteinaemia in postmenopausal women. *The Lancet.* **ii**:490–1.

5

Insulin Resistance: A Unifying Hypothesis

ROBERT W STOUT

Atherosclerosis is a disease of the arterial wall which is characterized by cellular proliferation, lipid accumulation and connective tissue formation. The clinical manifestations of atherosclerosis, ischaemic heart disease (IHD), cerebrovascular disease, peripheral arterial disease and aortic aneurysm have been associated with a number of risk factors which have been identified in prospective epidemiological studies. For some of these risk factors there is evidence that treatment may reduce the frequency of clinical ischaemic vascular disease. Although an intervention which is shown by properly designed studies to reduce the frequency of the disease is clearly a significant advance our understanding of the relationship of risk factors to atherosclerosis is enhanced if there are credible mechanisms linking the epidemiological and biological aspects of the disease.

There is a cluster of cardiovascular risk factors which can be linked to abnormal insulin secretion which in turn may be related to the phenomenon of insulin resistance. Insulin resistance can be defined as a condition in which a normal amount of insulin produces a subnormal biological response. Although originally used in relation to insulin-treated diabetic patients requiring large doses of insulin for blood glucose control, it is now used more widely in a range of common physiological and pathological conditions in which high insulin levels occur in the presence of normal or increased blood glucose. Although the term 'insulin resistance' is used in a global sense, it is likely that insulin resistance does not apply uniformly to all tissues but may apply to one or other of the main sites of insulin action, e.g. muscle or liver.

This short review discusses the association of hyperinsulinaemia and insulin resistance with a number of cardiovascular risk factors. The risk factors considered are disorders of lipid metabolism, hypertension, obesity, diabetes and other multiple factors, together with evidence that high levels of insulin are themselves associated with cardiovascular risk.

Lipid metabolism

For many years there has been interest in disorders of lipid metabolism as risk factors for atherosclerosis. Particular attention has been paid to the role of raised blood cholesterol and low-density lipoprotein (LDL) levels and there is a linear association between cholesterol levels and cardiovascular risk. There is also some evidence that reduction of cholesterol levels in those with hypercholesterolaemia reduces cardiovascular risk. Rather less attention has been paid to other lipoproteins and to other lipid measurements. For many years there has been controversy on the relationship between raised triglyceride levels and cardiovascular disease (CVD), with studies that suggest a relationship being refuted by others which suggest the relationship is not independent. It is now clear, however, that there is a relationship between raised triglyceride levels and CVD. The major endogenous triglyceride carrying lipoprotein is the very low-density lipoprotein (VLDL). The other major lipoprotein class in the circulation is high-density lipoproteins (HDL), and the relationship between HDL and cardiovascular risk is inverse, high levels of HDL being protective against CVD. Triglyceride and HDL metabolism are closely linked and hence epidemiological relationships are complex. There is often an inverse relationship between triglyceride and HDL levels and both are frequently related to obesity.

In many populations the combination of high triglyceride and low HDL levels has been found in those at high cardiovascular risk. This has been a particular characteristic of the results of studies looking at ethnic factors in atherosclerosis. For example, there is a high prevalence of IHD in people from the Indian subcontinent, including those who have migrated to the UK. In comparison with European people, South Asian immigrants in London have a higher prevalence of diabetes, higher blood pressure, higher fasting and post-glucose serum insulin concentrations, higher plasma triglyceride and low HDL cholesterol concentrations, and higher waist–hip ratios. Other risk factors, including smoking, serum cholesterol, dietary fat and clotting factors were lower or similar in Asians and non-Asians. Similar findings have come from other population groups. The combination of high blood glucose and high insulin levels in these populations suggest the presence of insulin resistance, perhaps associated with central obesity.

Insulin has an important role in the regulation of lipid metabolism. Among the actions of insulin is inhibition of hormone-sensitive lipase, thereby reducing free fatty acid release into the circulation from adipose tissue sites and hence reducing substrate availability for triglyceride synthesis. Insulin is also necessary for the proper functioning of lipoprotein lipase and hence in states of insulin deficiency triglyceride catabolism is impaired, resulting in the accumulation of chylomicrons and VLDL in the circulation. Insulin probably also stimulates triglyceride synthesis in the liver. Insulin is involved, therefore, in both triglyceride synthesis and removal and triglyceride levels reflect the balance between the two. In many populations linear correlations between insulin and triglyceride levels have been described and it has been suggested that in states of insulin resistance, often associated with obesity, high insulin levels result in high triglyceride levels. Insulin resistance may also result in decreased insulin activity on lipoprotein lipase and as a result, there is decreased triglyceride breakdown and hence HDL levels are lowered. The trio of hyperinsulinaemia, raised triglyceride and VLDL levels and decreased HDL cholesterol levels is a common finding in patients with CVD. Studies using a hyperinsulinaemic clamp have shown a direct relationship between insulin resistance and triglyceride levels and an inverse relationship to HDL levels. A further study showed that insulin resistance, rather than high insulin levels, was associated with low HDL cholesterol and high total and VLDL triglyceride levels. These studies, associating impaired insulin-mediated glucose uptake to lipid and lipoprotein abnormalities, suggest that the association of high insulin levels with adverse lipid and lipoprotein changes may indirectly reflect the association of insulin resistance with lipid and lipoprotein changes.

Hypertension

Hypertension is an important risk factor for CVD and there is abundant evidence that reduction in high blood pressure reduces the incidence of stroke, although the evidence of a beneficial effect on myocardial infarction is less convincing. There have been a number of studies which have suggested a relationship between high insulin levels and hypertension. Although the first such study, published in 1966, showed that a small group of subjects with untreated hypertension had higher insulin levels than normotensive controls, it is only in the last decade that a considerable amount of interest has been taken in this association. A number of studies have reported high insulin levels in subjects with hypertension, with or without obesity and with or without diabetes. In the recently described syndrome of familial dyslipidaemic hypertension patients with familial hypertension have one or more of the following: high plasma triglycerides, high LDL cholesterol and low HDL cholesterol. In some of these increased fasting plasma insulin levels have been found. A study of young men with untreated essential hypertension found markedly impaired insulin-induced glucose uptake, ie insulin resistance, and several other studies have reported similar findings. Some of the drugs which are used to treat hypertension, including thiazide diuretics and some beta-blocking drugs, themselves cause insulin resistance and hyperglycaemia. However, studies relating insulin and insulin resistance to hypertension have used subjects who have been untreated. There are a number of possible mechanisms by which insulin might be causally related to hypertension. These include an effect of insulin on the renin–angiotension–aldosterone system, on renal sodium reabsorption or on sympathetic nervous system activity.

Body weight

For many years the role of obesity in CVD was controversial. While it was clear that obesity was associated with an increased mortality, epidemiological studies using multivariate analysis suggested that the relationship was not independent of other cardiovascular risk factors. Obesity is associated with a wide variety of metabolic abnormalities, including abnormal glucose, insulin and lipid levels. Blood pressure also tends to be higher in those who are overweight. Thus, the fact that any relationship between obesity and atherosclerosis may not be directly related to the excess body weight, but to some of its metabolic accompaniments, may simply be because independent statistical relationships have been sought between measurements which are not metabolically independent. Thus obesity may be the common factor behind a number of other cardiovascular risk factors, and reduction of weight in those who are overweight may prove to be an effective means of preventing CVD but one which has not been subject to rigorous investigation. Although much of the investigative work has looked at total body weight, attention has recently been paid to the distribution of adipose tissue between the upper and lower parts of the body. This may be measured as the waist-to-hip circumference ratio or subscapular skinfold thickness, higher values of each being indicators of abdominal, upper body or masculine body-fat distribution. CVD is most closely related to upper body adiposity and upper body adiposity is in turn related to diabetes, hypertension and to high triglyceride and low HDL cholesterol levels. Upper body adiposity is also associated with hyperinsulinaemia. In women upper body obesity was associated with increased glucose responses to an oral glucose test and an increase in insulin output. Upper body obesity is also associated with large fat cells which in turn tend to be resistant to the effects of insulin. Thus sites of body fat localization influence the degree of insulin sensitivity which in turn influences insulin levels and in turn plasma glucose and lipid levels. Sex hormone levels may also be involved in this relationship. Obesity is one of the best known insulin-resistant states, many different techniques demonstrating that insulin-mediated glucose uptake is reduced in states of obesity. Weight loss reduces the hyperinsulinaemia associated with obesity and is generally assumed to reduce insulin resistance.

Diabetes mellitus

Hyperinsulinaemia is common in diabetes. In non-insulin-dependent diabetes mellitus (NIDDM) this is probably related to the commonly associated obesity, although hyperinsulinaemia has also been found in subjects with NIDDM who are non-obese. It appears that the hyperinsulinaemia is due to insulin resistance and that insulin resistance and hyperinsulinaemia precede the development of hyperglycaemia in those who are developing diabetes. Hyperinsulinaemia has also been found in offspring of diabetic subjects and in non-diabetic populations in whom a high frequency of diabetes occurs. As glucose tolerance declines from normal, insulin responses to oral glucose become elevated but with severe glucose intolerance and fasting hyperglycaemia, insulin levels become normal or subnormal. It remains unclear whether impaired insulin action or impaired insulin secretion is the primary defect in NIDDM. As the two are closely related, it is difficult to solve this problem. Insulin resistance is, however, a prominent feature of NIDDM. In insulin-dependent diabetes (IDDM), insulin therapy is delivered in non-physiological ways with respect to both the route and regulation of delivery. Because of this, the insulin levels which are attained in those who are administered insulin by the subcutaneous route are higher than normal. Diabetes, both IDDM and NIDDM, is an important cardiovascular risk factor, since CVD is two to four times more frequent in those with diabetes than in those without. The risk is particularly high in women. The mechanism for the increased risk of CVD in diabetes remains unclear. Although diabetes is associated with other cardiovascular risk factors, such as impaired lipid metabolism and hypertension, these do not fully account for the increased risk in diabetes. Although there are few prospective studies, there is some evidence that high insulin levels are associated with CVD in those with diabetes.

Multiple risk factors

Although cardiovascular risk factors are often considered singly, subjects with CVD often have multiple risk factors. Abnormalities in lipids, in blood pressure and perhaps in body weight are particularly common, and in these circumstances high insulin levels are often found. In a number of small studies, high insulin levels have also been associated with some other cardiovascular risk factors including plasminogen activator inhibitor 1 (PAI-1), microalbuminuria, and type A behaviour.

Insulin and CVD

There are a considerable number of studies linking insulin to CVD. Most important of these are three prospective studies coming from Helsinki, Paris and Busselton (in Western Australia). These studies, which were all carried out in healthy non-diabetic people, showed that insulin is a risk factor for CVD. In all of the studies other cardiovascular risk factors were also studied and the effect of insulin was independent of the effects of cholesterol, blood pressure, body weight or cigarette smoking. HDL cholesterol was not measured in any of the studies. The Helsinki and Paris studies only looked at men. The Busselton Study looked at men and women, and the effect of insulin on cardiovascular risk was only found in men in the older age groups. In all cases the elevated insulin levels were associated with normal or slightly elevated blood glucose levels, a pattern which is usually associated with insulin resistance. High insulin levels have also been reported in more than 20 cross-sectional studies of subjects with CVD, as well as a small number of studies of patients with cerebrovascular disease and peripheral vascular disease. The high insulin levels were usually independent of other cardiovascular risk factors and were found in those who were not obese or diabetic and in those whose vascular disease was diagnosed by arteriography in the absence of tissue damage.

Conclusion

There is now compelling evidence that many cardiovascular risk factors, either singly or in combination, are associated with high circulating insulin levels. High insulin levels in the presence of normal or slightly elevated blood glucose levels signify a state of insulin resistance, and in some cases direct measurements of insulin resistance have confirmed this relationship. It seems reasonable to hypothesize, therefore, that a primary defect of insulin resistance occurs and that the associated high insulin levels may be causally related to some of the cardiovascular risk factors and—either independently or together with these risk factors—may also be associated with the development of atherosclerosis. An alternative suggestion is that the insulin resistance indicates a cellular defect which in some way is related to both cardiovascular risk factors and atherosclerosis. The latter, however, has not been demonstrated. Insulin has actions on arterial tissue which are potentially atherogenic. These include stimulation of proliferation and migration of arterial smooth muscle cells, stimulation of LDL receptor activity and stimulation of connective tissue synthesis. A hypothesis linking hyperinsulinaemia with atherosclerosis supports prominent advice on prevention of CVD, as avoidance of obesity and regular physical exercise are both known to reduce insulin resistance and reduce high insulin levels.

Bibliography

Detailed references to statements in the above review can be found in:
Stout RW (1990) Insulin and atheroma. 20-year perspective. *Diabetes Care*, **13**: 631–54.

Stout RW (ed.) (1992) *Diabetes and atherosclerosis*. Kluwer, Amsterdam.

6

Insulin Resistance and Risk Factors in Different Ethnic Groups

PAUL M McKEIGUE

Mortality from coronary heart disease (CHD) and prevalence of non-insulin-dependent diabetes mellitus (NIDDM) are higher in migrants from South Asia (India, Pakistan and Bangladesh) than in the general population of the United Kingdom. Similar findings have been reported for other overseas South Asian populations. The high coronary mortality is unexplained by smoking, blood pressure, serum cholesterol or haemostatic activity. Surveys of South Asian populations in the UK have identified a pattern of metabolic disturbances associated with insulin resistance—hyperinsulinaemia, high plasma triglyceride and low high-density lipoprotein (HDL) cholesterol—of which high diabetes prevalence is only one manifestation. These disturbances are associated with a pronounced tendency to central obesity in South Asians, even though average body-mass index is no higher in South Asian than in European men. Comparisons between different South Asian communities point to metabolic disturbances associated with central obesity and insulin resistance as the most plausible explanation of the increased coronary risk. This increased risk may be mediated through disturbances of triglyceride metabolism, rather than through hypertension or low HDL cholesterol. The occurrence in South Asians of central obesity without generalized obesity contrasts with other populations at high risk for NIDDM and emphasizes the close relationship of the insulin resistance syndrome to body-fat distribution. Insulin resistance may underlie the high rates of CHD and diabetes emerging in some other non-European populations.

Epidemiology of CHD and NIDDM in South Asians

From the 1950s onwards reports began to appear of unusually high rates of CHD in South Asian people settled overseas in comparison with other ethnic groups in the same countries (Danaraj et al., 1959; Adelstein, 1963; Sorokin, 1975). Recent mortality data for South Asians overseas are summarized in Table 6.1. In comparison with high-risk populations such as Europeans in South Africa or the UK, the relative risk for CHD mortality associated with South Asian origin is about 1.4 (Steinberg et al., 1988; OPCS, 1990), and in comparison with relatively low-risk groups such as Chinese in Singapore

Country	Years	Groups contrasted	Age	CHD mortality ratio	Reference
Singapore	1980–86	S.Asian/Chinese	30–69	3.8	Hughes et al., 1990a
Fiji	1980	S.Asian/Melanesian	40–59	3.0	Tuomilehto et al., 1984
Trinidad	1977–86	S.Asian/African	35–69	2.4	Miller et al., 1989
South Africa	1985	S.Asian/European	35–74	1.4	Steinberg et al., 1988
England	1979–83	S.Asian/European	20–69	1.4	OPCS, 1990

Table 6.1: Mortality from CHD in South Asians overseas.

(Hughes *et al.*, 1990*a*) or Africans in Trinidad (Miller *et al.*, 1989) the relative risk is about 3. Reliable population-based coronary mortality data from South Asia are not available but in two northern Indian cities the prevalence of Minnesota-coded major Q waves on electrocardiograms has been reported to be at least as high as in European populations (Sarvotham and Berry, 1968; Chadha *et al.*, 1990). In contrast, very low prevalence rates have been recorded in rural India (Dewan *et al.*, 1974; Jajoo *et al.*, 1988).

In England and Wales high coronary mortality is common to Hindus originating from Gujarat in western India, to Sikhs originating from Punjab in northern India, and to Muslims from Pakistan and Bangladesh (Balarajan *et al.*, 1984; McKeigue and Marmot, 1988). The consistency of the high CHD risk in urban South Asian populations around the world, affecting both sexes and with early onset in men, suggests a common underlying cause.

Where average plasma cholesterol levels differ between South Asians and Europeans in the UK, the differences are in the opposite direction to that which would explain the high CHD risk in people of South Asian origin (McKeigue *et al.*, 1988, 1991; Miller *et al.*, 1988). Average cholesterol levels are lowest in Gujarati Hindus, who are generally vegetarian, but even in Sikhs and Muslims, who are not vegetarian, average cholesterol levels are no higher than the national average (McKeigue *et al.*, 1991). Smoking rates in Hindu and Muslim men are similar to the national average, and very low in Sikh men and in all groups of South Asian women (McKeigue *et al.*, 1991). In comparison with Europeans, average blood pressures are higher in Punjabis, similar in Gujaratis and lower in Bangladeshis even though all these groups share the excess coronary risk (McKeigue *et al.*, 1988, 1991). Thus the three classic major risk factors for CHD—smoking, hypertension and elevated plasma cholesterol— fail to explain the high coronary disease rates in South Asians, and so do some of the newer risk factors such as fibrinogen and factor VII clotting activity (McKeigue *et al.*, 1988; Miller *et al.*, 1988).

One clue to the high CHD risk is that prevalence of NIDDM is high in all overseas South Asian populations for which data are available (Table 6.2). In South Asian men and women aged 40–69 years in the UK, the prevalence is 19% (McKeigue *et al.*, 1991), which is remarkably consistent with surveys in other overseas South Asian populations and with a study of an urban population in southern India (Ramachandran *et al.*, 1988). For comparison, in this age group the prevalence of diabetes in men and women of European descent in the UK is about 4% (McKeigue *et al.*, 1991). Most South Asian patients with coronary disease are not diabetic (Hughes *et al.*, 1989), and glucose intolerance cannot alone explain more than a small proportion of the excess coronary risk in South Asian people (Miller *et al.*, 1989).

Country	Year	Age	Prevalence	Reference
Trinidad	1977	35–69	21%	Miller et al., 1989
Fiji	1983	35–64	25%	Zimmet et al., 1983
South Africa	1985	30 and over*	22%	Omar et al., 1985
Singapore	1990	40–69	25%	Hughes et al., 1990b
Mauritius	1990	35–64	20%	Dowse et al., 1990
England	1991	40–69	19%	McKeigue et al., 1991
Prevalence in Europeans, for comparison				
London	1991	40–69	4%	McKeigue et al., 1991

*No upper age limit

Table 6.2: Prevalence of NIDDM in South Asians overseas.

Evidence for metabolic disturbances associated with insulin resistance in South Asians

In an early study comparing Bangladeshi migrants to east London with native Europeans, a pattern of intercorrelated metabolic disturbances was identified in Bangladeshi men and women: high prevalence of NIDDM, high levels of insulin and triglyceride after a glucose load, and low HDL cholesterol (McKeigue et al., 1988). This pattern corresponds to the insulin resistance syndrome described by others (Reaven, 1988; DeFronzo and Ferrannini, 1991). The high prevalence of this syndrome in South Asians was confirmed in a larger study of Indian and Pakistani subjects in west London—the Southall Study (Table 6.3) (McKeigue et al., 1991). At two hours, after a glucose load, mean insulin levels are about twice as high in South Asians as in Europeans. South Asian men and women have a more central distribution of body fat than Europeans, with thicker trunk skinfolds and markedly higher mean waist-hip girth ratios for a given level of body-mass index. Glucose intolerance and two-hour insulin are more strongly associated with waist-hip ratio than with body-mass index, especially in South Asian women (McKeigue et al., 1992). Although base-line data from the Southall Study (unpublished) show strong cross-sectional associations of electrocardiographic Q waves in South Asian men with glucose intolerance, elevated insulin and triglyceride levels, confirmation that this accounts for the high CHD risk will depend on prospective studies.

	Men		Women	
	European	South Asian	European	South Asian
Body-mass index (kg m^{-2})	25.9	25.7	25.2	27.0
Waist-hip girth ratio	0.94	0.98	0.76	0.85
Median systolic blood pressure (mmHg)	121	126	120	126
Diabetes prevalence	5%	20%	2%	16%
2-hour insulin (mU/l)	19	41	21	44
Total cholesterol (mmol/l)	6.1	6.0	6.3	6.0
HDL cholesterol (mmol/l)	1.25	1.16	1.58	1.38
2-hour triglyceride (mmol/l)	1.39	1.72	1.01	1.27

Table 6.3: Mean levels of coronary risk factors in South Asians and Europeans in the Southall Study (adapted from McKeigue et al., 1991).

Implications for understanding the insulin resistance syndrome and its relation to CHD risk

Central obesity appears to be a characteristic feature of the insulin resistance syndrome in South Asian populations. In both Europeans and South Asians, glucose intolerance, insulin, triglyceride and HDL cholesterol are related to waist-hip ratio. The strongest associations are the inverse correlations between HDL and plasma triglyceride, and the positive correlations of plasma triglyceride with insulin and waist-hip ratio. The mechanisms underlying these assocations are poorly understood. Failure of insulin to suppress release of non-esterified fatty acids from adipose tissue may lead to increased production of very-low-density lipoprotein (VLDL) triglyceride (Yki-Jarvinen and Taskinen, 1988). Raised triglyceride levels in turn may lower plasma HDL cholesterol and cause changes in the composition and size of particles in the LDL fraction (Austin *et al.*, 1990). Although raised blood pressure is associated with glucose intolerance and hyperinsulinaemia, the associations between elevated blood pressure and disturbances of lipid metabolism are weak, suggesting that the association of insulin resistance with dyslipidaemia and the association with hypertension are mediated through different mechanisms.

If the hypothesis that the insulin resistance syndrome is the explanation for high CHD risk in South Asians is correct, then the disturbances which cause CHD must be consistently present in all the groups originating from South Asia who share the high CHD risk. Table 6.4 summarizes the results of comparisons between these groups. Although systolic and diastolic blood pressures are correlated with insulin levels in South Asians as in other populations, it is only in Sikhs and Hindus of Punjabi origin that average blood pressures are higher than in Europeans (McKeigue *et al.*, 1991). Average HDL cholesterol is lower in Hindu and Muslim South Asian men than in the native British population, but in Sikh men average HDL cholesterol is no lower than in native British men (McKeigue *et al.*, 1991). It follows that if the high coronary risk common to all groups originating from South Asia results from insulin resistance, this effect cannot be mediated mainly through blood pressure or HDL cholesterol. Common to all South Asian populations at high risk

Common to all South Asian populations at risk	Not common to all South Asian populations at risk
Central obesity Hyperinsulinaemia High diabetes prevalence High post-glucose triglyceride	High blood pressure (not Muslims) Low HDL cholesterol (not Sikhs) High fasting triglyceride (not Gujarati Hindus)

Table 6.4: Which features of the insulin resistance syndrome are common to all the South Asian groups who share high CHD risk?

of CHD are central obesity, hyperinsulinaemia and high diabetes prevalence. In all South Asian groups studied, triglyceride levels after a glucose load are higher than in Europeans (McKeigue *et al.*, 1988; McKeigue *et al.*, 1991); this may be a marker for other disturbances of lipoprotein metabolism which are associated with insulin resistance (Austin *et al.*, 1990).

Comparison with other populations at high risk for NIDDM

The tendency for South Asians to accumulate intra-abdominal fat without necessarily developing generalized obesity contrasts with other populations at high risk of diabetes, such as Pima Americans (Knowler *et al.*, 1981) and Nauruans (Zimmet *et al.*, 1977), in whom average body mass indices are considerably higher than in populations of European origin. Although Mexican-American women have a more central pattern of subcutaneous fat distribution than non-Hispanic European women, waist-hip ratios in Mexican-American men and women are no higher than in non-Hispanic Europeans when allowance is made for differences in body mass index (Stern and Haffner, 1988). There are few studies of other populations at high risk of NIDDM which permit similar comparisons.

NIDDM is commoner in Afro-Caribbeans and African-Americans than in Europeans: the ratio of diabetes prevalence in people of African descent to that in Europeans was 1.8 in the United States (Harris *et al.*, 1987) and 2.4 in Trinidad (Beckles *et al.*, 1986). In contrast to the high CHD mortality of South Asian people settled overseas, national data for England and Wales in 1979–83 showed that the relative risk of CHD mortality was 0.45 for Afro-Caribbeans compared with Europeans (OPCS, 1990). In the Southall Study prevalence of NIDDM in Afro-Caribbean men was almost as high as in South Asian men but, in contrast to South Asians, fasting and serum insulin levels were similar in Afro-Caribbean and European men (McKeigue *et al.*, 1991). Plasma triglyceride levels are consistently lower and HDL cholesterol levels consistently higher in Afro-Caribbean and African-American men than in men of European descent (Slack *et al.*, 1977; Morrison *et al.*, 1981; McKeigue *et al.*, 1991); in these respects Afro-Caribbean men resemble European women. Mean waist-hip ratios are no higher in Afro-Caribbean than in European men (McKeigue *et al.*, 1991). Other studies have found insulin levels to be higher in Afro-Caribbeans than in Europeans but confirm that Afro-Caribbean men are not more centrally obese or more dyslipidaemic than European men (Cruickshank *et al.*, 1991). These findings suggest that the aetiology of NIDDM in Afro-Caribbeans differs from that in South Asians and that the insulin resistance syndrome is not the cause of the high rates in Afro-Caribbeans. Despite the high prevalence of diabetes and hypertension in Afro-Caribbean and African-American men, the low triglyceride and high HDL cholesterol in these groups compared with European men is the opposite of what would be predicted from the insulin resistance syndrome hypothesis. This favourable lipoprotein pattern may be one reason for the low CHD mortality of Afro-Caribbean men.

Conclusion

Epidemiological studies of CHD and diabetes in South Asians provide compelling evidence for the existence of a syndrome of metabolic disturbances associated with insulin resistance and with increased risk of CHD. Some disturbance of lipoprotein metabolism, related to increased synthesis of VLDL triglyceride, is the most likely mediator of the increased CHD risk associated with insulin resistance. High prevalence of NIDDM and other metabolic disturbances associated with insulin resistance occur in people of South Asian descent in widely different environments and persist several generations after migration. It is therefore likely that some genetic predisposition to develop insulin resistance exists in this group. The ability to store fat in intra-abdominal depots and to rely on non-esterified fatty acids rather than glucose as fuel for muscle may have been an advantage in times of unreliable food supply. Control of obesity and increased physical activity are likely to be the most effective means of reducing the risk of coronary disease in South Asians if the insulin resistance hypothesis is correct. It is possible that metabolic disturbances associated with insulin resistance underlie some of the recent increases in CHD mortality in urban populations in developing countries where susceptibility to NIDDM is high.

References

Adelstein AM (1963) Some aspects of cardiovascular mortality in South Africa. *British Journal of Preventive and Social Medicine.* 17:29–40.

Austin MA *et al.,* (1990) Atherogenic lipoprotein phenotype: a proposed genetic marker for coronary heart disease risk. *Circulation.* 82:495–506.

Balarajan R *et al.,* (1984) Patterns of mortality among migrants to England and Wales from the Indian subcontinent. *British Medical Journal.* 289:1185–7.

Beckles GLA *et al.,* (1986) High total and cardiovascular disease mortality in adults of Indian descent in Trinidad, unexplained by major coronary risk factors. *The Lancet.* i:1298–301.

Chadha SL *et al.,* (1990) Epidemiological study of coronary heart disease in urban population of Delhi. *Indian Journal of Medical Research.* 92:424–30.

Cruickshank JK *et al.,* (1991) Ethnic differences in fasting C-peptide and insulin in relation to glucose tolerance and blood pressure. *The Lancet.* 338:842–7.

Danaraj TJ *et al.*, (1959) Ethnic group differences in coronary heart disease in Singapore: an analysis of necropsy records. *American Heart Journal*. **58**:516–26.

DeFronzo RA and Ferrannini E (1991) Insulin resistance: a multifaceted syndrome responsible for NIDDM, obesity, hypertension, dyslipidemia, and atherosclerotic cardiovascular disease. *Diabetes Care*. **14**:173–94.

Dewan BD *et al.*, (1974) Epidemiological study of coronary heart disease in a rural community in Haryana. *Indian Heart Journal*. **26**:68–78.

Dowse GK *et al.*, (1990) High prevalence of NIDDM and impaired glucose tolerance in Indian, Creole and Chinese Mauritians. *Diabetes*. **39**:390–6.

Harris MI *et al.*, (1987) Prevalence of diabetes and impaired glucose tolerance and plasma glucose levels in US population aged 20–74 yr. *Diabetes*. **36**:523–34.

Hughes K *et al.*, (1990*a*) Cardiovascular diseases in Chinese, Malays and Indians in Singapore. I. Differences in mortality. *Journal of Epidemiology and Community Health*. **44**:24–8.

Hughes K *et al.*, (1990*b*) Cardiovascular diseases in Chinese, Malays and Indians in Singapore. II. Differences in risk factor levels. *Journal of Epidemiology and Community Health*. **44**:29–35.

Hughes LO *et al.*, (1989) Disturbances of insulin in British Asian and white men surviving myocardial infarction. *British Medical Journal*. **299**:537–41.

Jajoo UN *et al.*, (1988) The prevalence of coronary heart disease in rural population from central India. *Journal of the Association of Physicians of India*. **36**:689–93.

Knowler WC *et al.*, (1981) Diabetes incidence in Pima Indians: contributions of obesity and parental diabetes. *American Journal of Epidemiology*. **113**:144–56.

McKeigue PM and Marmot MG (1988) Mortality from coronary heart disease in Asian communities in London. *British Medical Journal*. **297**:903.

McKeigue PM *et al.*, (1988) Diabetes, hyperinsulinaemia and coronary risk factors in Bangladeshis in east London. *British Heart Journal*. **60**:390–6.

McKeigue PM *et al.*, (1991) Relation of central obesity and insulin resistance with high diabetes prevalence and cardiovascular risk in South Asians. *The Lancet*. **337**:382–6.

McKeigue PM *et al.*, (1992) Relationship of glucose intolerance and hyperinsulinaemia to body fat pattern in South Asians and Europeans. *Diabetologia*. **35**:785–91.

Miller GJ *et al.*, (1988) Dietary and other characteristics relevant for coronary heart disease in men of Indian, West Indian and European descent in London. *Atherosclerosis*. **70**:63–72.

Miller GJ *et al.*, (1989) Ethnicity and other characteristics predictive of coronary heart disease in a developing country—principal results of the St James survey, Trinidad. *International Journal of Epidemiology.* **18**:808–17.

Morrison JA *et al.*, (1981) Lipid and lipoprotein distributions in black adults. The Cincinnati Lipid Research Clinic's Princeton School Study. *Journal of the American Medical Association.* **245**:939–42.

Omar MAK *et al.*, (1985) The prevalence of diabetes mellitus in a large group of South African Indians. *South African Medical Journal.* **67**:924–6.

OPCS (1990) *Mortality and geography: a review in the mid-1980s. The Registrar-General's decennial supplement for England and Wales, series DS no. 9.* HMSO, London.

Ramachandran A *et al.*, (1988) High prevalence of diabetes in an urban population in south India. *British Medical Journal.* **297**:587–90.

Reaven GM (1988) Role of insulin resistance in human disease. *Diabetes.* **37**: 1595–607.

Sarvotham SG and Berry JN (1968) Prevalence of coronary heart disease in an urban population in northern India. *Circulation.* **37**:939–53.

Slack J *et al.*, (1977) Lipid and lipoprotein concentrations in 1604 men and women in working populations in north-west London. *British Medical Journal.* **2**:353–6.

Sorokin M (1975) Hospital morbidity in the Fiji islands with special reference to the saccharine disease. *South African Medical Journal.* **49**:1481–5.

Steinberg WJ *et al.*, (1988) Decline in the ischaemic heart disease mortality rates of South Africans, 1968–1985. *South African Medical Journal.* **74**:547–50.

Stern MP and Haffner SM (1988) Do anthropometric differences between Mexican-Americans and Non-Hispanic Whites explain ethnic differences in metabolic variables? *Acta Medica Scandinavica.* **723** (Suppl):37–44.

Tuomilehto J *et al.*, (1984) Cardiovascular diseases in Fiji: analysis of mortality, morbidity and risk factors. *Bulletin of the World Health Organization.* **62**:133–43.

Yki-Jarvinen H and Taskinen M-R (1988) Interrelationships among insulin's antilipolytic and glucoregulatory effects and plasma triglycerides in nondiabetic and diabetic patients with endogenous hypertriglyceridemia. *Diabetes.* **37**:1271–8.

Zimmet P *et al.*, (1977) The high prevalence of diabetes on a Central Pacific island. *Diabetologia.* **13**:111–15.

Zimmet P *et al.*, (1983) Prevalence of diabetes and impaired glucose tolerance in the biracial (Melanesian and Indian) population of Fiji: a rural-urban comparison. *American Journal of Epidemiology.* **118**:673–88.

7

Cardiovascular Disease in Blacks, Whites and Asians in Birmingham

JOHN WEIL AND DG BEEVERS

International comparative data have demonstrated wide differences in the prevalence and incidence of cardiovascular diseases (CVD) in different countries. Coronary heart disease (CHD) is rare in Africa and the West Indies but relatively common in urban India and Pakistan. Many of these comparisons are, however, subject to inaccuracies because of differences in clinical practice, diagnostic fashions and the accuracy of International Classification of Diseases (ICD) coding. Within individual countries, however, there is abundant evidence that there are major differences in CHD and stroke rates in different ethnic groups. In black Americans, hypertension and stroke disease are more common than in whites whereas CHD appears to be less common. (Hypertension Detection and Follow-up Program Cooperative Group, 1977). In Trinidad, CHD is also rare in blacks but very common in the substantial Asian minority (Miller *et al.*, 1988).

The United Kingdom (UK) is in a nearly unique position to investigate inter-ethnic cardiovascular epidemiology because, in addition to the majority white population, there are significant Afro-Caribbean communities as well as 'Asian' populations who have migrated from Pakistan, India and East Africa. Both of these groups came to the UK in the 1960s and early 1970s and it soon became apparent that there were wide differences in the heart disease and stroke rates (Tunstall-Pedoe *et al.*, 1975).

Data available from death certificates from the Office of Population Census and Surveys have demonstrated an excess incidence of hypertensive-related deaths amongst people born in the West Indies and in Africa, and by comparison a high incidence of CHD deaths amongst people born in India, Pakistan and Bangladesh (Marmot, 1984).

Information based on proportional hospital admission rates in patients from these three ethnic groups to Dudley Road Hospital in West Birmingham between 1974 and 1978 largely confirmed the trends described above (Cruickshank *et al.*, 1980), and have the advantage of including both fatal and non-fatal cases. The updated information presented here suggests that the differences in CHD between the Asians and the other ethnic groups are increasing. The Asian community in West Birmingham is mainly Sikh or Muslim from the Punjab with a smaller number from the Sylhet area of Bangladesh. Between 1976 and 1986, a total of 121 834 men and women aged 40–69 were admitted to Dudley Road Hospital. The figures are based on hospital activity analysis coding for diagnosis and for place of birth. The numbers of admissions where place of birth was coded as 'unknown' were 16 613 (13.6%); for the purposes of this analysis it is assumed that there is no ethnic bias for inclusion of patients into this category. The numerator for calculating hospital admission rates was the number of admissions for heart attack or stroke for each age-band and each ethnic group; the denominator was the total number of admissions for all causes in the same age-bands and ethnic groups.

These data confirm the higher frequency of CHD admissions in people born in the Indian subcontinent as well as the considerably lower rate in Afro-Caribbean-born people (Figure 7.1). By sharp contrast, stroke disease was commonest in Afro-Caribbeans, particularly amongst females. Stroke admissions were, also common in Asian patients when compared with white, however, although the rate was still lower than in black people (Figure 7.2). Comparisons of the two time intervals, 1976–1980 and 1981–1986, demonstrate that these trends remain; although the absolute numbers of people

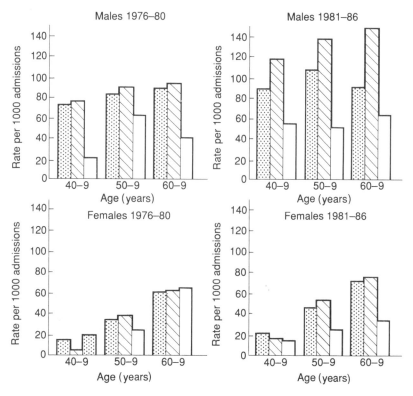

Figure 7.1: Proportional admission rates to Dudley Road Hospital for CHD in men and women born in England and Wales ▨, the Indian subcontinent ▧ and the Caribbean □. Data from 1976–80 and 1981–86 are presented separately.

admitted with CHD rose in both UK born and Asian born patients. This is surprising, given falling CHD mortality rates in England and Wales through this period. There was a trend, however, for the proportion of Asians to be greater during the second time period. For example, the ratio of observed to expected Asian admissions in the 50–59 year band increased from 1.11 to 1.45 between 1976–1980 and 1981–1986. Numbers for female admissions are too small to draw any definite conclusions.

Given these data, any ethnic differences in the cardiovascular risk factors would have clear importance in any strategy for prevention. The three main environmental risk factors for CHD are high blood pressure, raised levels of serum cholesterol and the frequency of cigarette smoking. The Birmingham Factory Screening Project was established specifically to investigate ethnic differences in these risk factors (Cruickshank *et al.*, 1985). The project was conducted in censussed populations based on the workforce in several large light industrial factories in Central and West Birmingham.

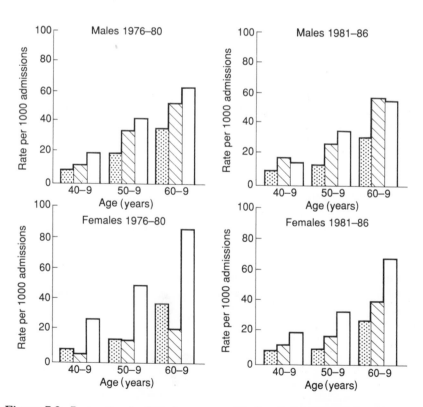

Figure 7.2: Proportional admission rates to Dudley Road Hospital for strokes in men and women born in England and Wales ▨, the Indian subcontinent ◺ and the Caribbean ☐. Data for 1976–80 and 1981–86 are presented separately.

The prevalence of hypertension

The Birmingham Factory Screening Project was able to demonstrate only a modest excess prevalence of hypertension amongst the black examinees when compared with whites. In the Asian examinees, hypertension was also very common. One curious finding of the Birmingham Factory Screening Project was that the average blood pressure of the three ethnic groups did not differ substantially even though high blood pressure was particularly common in black people. These findings, which were independent of body mass index and alcohol intake, are at odds with those obtained from the Northwick Park Heart Study (Meade *et al.*, 1978) but are similar to those obtained from a general practitioner-based screening survey in north London (Haines *et al.*, 1987). Most studies conducted in North America have suggested hypertension is considerably more common in blacks than in whites even after adjustment for body mass index, social class, age, sex and occupational group (Stamler *et al.*, 1975). However, the Birmingham findings are not substantially different from those obtained in a survey conducted in Jamaica in the 1960s, where hypertension did not appear to be particularly common (Miall *et al.*, 1961). It remains possible, therefore, that blacks of West Indian origin living in Britain differ from blacks living in the USA and possibly from first-generation black migrants from Africa.

Taking an overview of the data on hypertension in blacks, it seems that it is genuinely more common than in the white population, which may in part explain why stroke disease is also more common. However, the amount of data available on hypertension in the Asian community in Britain is not sufficient to draw any firm conclusions.

Cigarette smoking

In the Birmingham Factory Screening Project, detailed smoking histories were obtained from all examinees. These demonstrated that smoking was relatively uncommon in people of Asian origin, was more frequent in black populations but was most common in whites (Jackson *et al.*, 1981). These data, therefore, do not in any way provide an explanation as to why CHD is so prevalent in the Asian community.

Lipoproteins

Serum total cholesterol levels show a consistent correlation with coronary artery disease (CAD) both at an international and national (Martin *et al.*, 1986) level. However, ethnic differences in total cholesterol have not been found to be sufficiently marked to explain the high rates of Asians in Trinidad (Beckles *et al.*, 1986), Singapore (Saha, 1987) or the UK (McKeigue *et al.*, 1988). Low CHD rates in black males have been related to low levels of serum cholesterol in the Evans County Study from the USA (Tyroler *et al.*, 1975), although the small number in that study limits this interpretation. Fewer data on black/white differences are available from the UK but a pilot study conducted in West Birmingham (Zezulka *et al.*, 1988) was able to demonstrate no significant difference in non-fasting plasma total cholesterol levels in healthy black, white and Asian people visiting hospital, although there was a trend for black people to have lower serum cholesterol levels.

Lipoprotein abnormalities with raised serum triglyceride and low high-density lipoprotein (HDL) levels as well as high prevalence of diabetes have been consistently reported in South Asian communities overseas. McKeigue *et al.* (1991) found a high insulin response to a glucose load in a sample of 121 Bangladeshis and have suggested that hyperinsulinaemia may be the link between the metabolic disturbances and CAD in South Asians.

Vasculotoxic lipids

Serum cholesterol levels measured in the non-fasting state are not particularly good as predictors for CHD. There has been a recent interest in free radical activity, diene conjugated lipids and also anti-oxidants in the aetiology of CHD. The study of diene conjugated lipids amongst blacks, whites and Asians in West Birmingham did show a trend which might explain the ethnic differences of CHD. Circulating diene conjugated lipids, which are incorporated into atheromatous plaques, were highest in people of Asian origin and least common in people of Afro-Caribbean origin. These data were more significantly different than those obtained on serum total non-fasting cholesterol levels alone. There were no significant differences in free radical scavenging activity as assessed by measurement of non-fasting vitamin E levels (Zezulka *et al.*, 1988).

At an individual level, the relationship between serum cholesterol and dietary fats is not close. However, preliminary results from a survey of the shopping habits of housewives from the three ethnic groups in Birmingham suggest that differences in animal fat intake may go some way to explain the high incidence of CHD amongst Asians. The average dietary consumption of fat in Asian households was 1007.7 (SEM 58.6)g/person/week. By comparison the intake amongst white households was 890.2 (42.7) and in black households was 757.8 (37.5). It has been suggested that ghee made from clarified butter used in Asian-style cooking, may be a potent factor in CHD in Asians. Ghee contains a high proportion of oxidized lipids which may act synergistically with diene conjugates to cause atheroma deposition in coronary arteries as described above (Jacobson, 1987).

Prevention

It must be stressed that, while there are important differences in CHD and stroke rates in the three main ethnic groups in England, these diseases remain unacceptably common in all groups. Heart attacks are seen in Afro-Caribbean people and strokes are common in Asians. Any strategies for the prevention of diseases must be applied to the whole community within the context of good primary care. The ethnic differences in arterial diseases described here do, however, have some practical implications. First, stroke disease is particularly common in blacks and this is in part related to a higher prevalence and mortality from both malignant and non-malignant hypertension (Clough *et al.*, 1990). There is some evidence that black people are more salt-sensitive than whites and this difference may in part explain why plasma renin levels are much lower in blacks. There is a trend for circulating renin levels partly to explain the marked differences in response of blacks to antihypertensive drugs. There is good evidence that the beta-adrenergic blocking drugs and the angiotensin converting enzyme inhibitors are relatively ineffective in black hypertensive patients, while the thiazide diuretics and the calcium slow-channel blockers are effective (Hall, 1990). Thus, an awareness of the increased salt-sensitivity of black people can lead to specific counselling on the value of dietary salt restriction and an awareness of ethnic differences in drug response can lead to a more appropriate choice of anti-hypertensive agent.

Turning to the Asian community, there are no striking pathophysiological differences when compared with whites although non-insulin-dependent diabetes mellitus, insulin insensitivity as well as central obesity are commoner and there is a higher prevalence of atheromatous disease which may, in part, be related to a higher intake of saturated fats. Specific targeted counselling on the avoidance of obesity and a restriction in saturated (largely animal) fat intake seems worthwhile. Drugs like the thiazide diuretics and beta-blockers which adversely affect serum lipid profiles, blood glucose and insulin sensitivity are best avoided and regular measurement of serum lipid levels should be undertaken.

Whilst the practical points outlined above can be helpful, it must be stressed that it is the duty of the primary health-care clinician to ensure that the optimum preventative care should be given to *all* people. The rules of primary cardiovascular prevention are the same, regardless of ethnic origin.

Acknowledgements

We are grateful to Mrs E Thomas, Medical Records Department at Dudley Road Hospital for ensuring accuracy of data on place of birth in our hospital admission data, and we are indebted to Ms Fay Cox for secretarial assistance.

References

Beckles GLA *et al.* (1986) High total and cardiovascular disease mortality in adults of Indian descent in Trinidad, unexplained by major coronary risk factors. *The Lancet.* **i**:1298–301.

Clough CG *et al.* (1990) The survival of malignant hypertension in blacks, whites and asians in Britain. *Journal of Human Hypertension.* **4**:94–6.

Cruickshank JK *et al.* (1980) Heart attack, stroke, diabetes and hypertension in West Indians, Asians and Whites in Birmingham, England. *British Medical Journal.* **281**:1108.

Cruickshank JK *et al.* (1985) Similarity of blood pressure in blacks, whites and asians in England: the Birmingham Factory Study. *Journal of Hypertension.* **3**:365–71.

Haines AP *et al.* (1987) Blood pressure, smoking, obesity and alcohol consumption in blacks and whites in general practice. *Journal of Human Hypertension.* **1**:39–46.

Hall WD (1990) Pathophysiology of hypertension in blacks. *American Journal of Hypertension* **3**:366–71s.

Hypertension Detection and Follow-up Program Cooperative Group (1977) Race, education and prevalence of hypertension. *American Journal of Epidemiology.* **106**: 351-61.

Jackson SHD *et al.* (1981) Ethnic differences in respiratory disease. *Postgraduate Medical Journal.* **57**:777–8.

Jacobson M (1987) Cholesterol oxides in Indian ghee: a possible cause of unexplained high risk of atherosclerosis in Indian immigrant populations. *The Lancet.* **ii**:656–8.

Marmot MG (1984) Lessons from the study of immigrant mortality. *The Lancet.* **i**:1455–8.

Martin MJ *et al.* (1986) Serum cholesterol, blood pressure and mortality: implications from a cohort of 361,622 men. *The Lancet.* **ii**:933–6.

McKeigue PM *et al.* (1988) Diabetes, hyperinsulinaemia and coronary risk factors in Bangladeshis in East London. *British Heart Journal.* **60**:390–6.

McKeigue PM *et al.* (1991) Relation of central obesity and insulin resistance with high diabetes prevalence and cardiovascular risk in South Asians. *The Lancet.* **337**:382–6.

Meade TW *et al.* (1978) Ethnic group comparisons of variables associated with ischaemic heart disease. *British Heart Journal.* **40**:789–95.

Miall WE *et al.* (1961) Factors influencing the arterial pressure in the general population in Jamaica. *British Medical Journal.* **2**:497–506.

Miller GJ *et al.* (1988) Adult male all cause cardiovascular and cerebrovascular mortality in relation to ethnic group, systolic blood pressure and blood glucose concentration in Trinidad, West Indies. *International Journal of Epidemiology.* **17**: 62–9.

Saha N (1987) Serum high density lipoprotein cholesterol, apoliprotein A-I, A-II and B levels in Singapore ethnic groups. *Atherosclerosis.* **68**:117–21.

Stamler J *et al.* (1975) Multivariate analysis of the relationship of seven variables to blood pressure. *Journal of Chronic Diseases.* **28**:527–48.

Tunstall-Pedoe H *et al.* (1975) Coronary heart attacks in East London. *The Lancet.* **ii**: 833–8.

Tyroler HA *et al.* (1975) Black-white differences in serum lipids and lipoproteins in Evans County. *Preventive Medicine.* **4**:541–9.

Zezulka AV *et al.* (1988) Racial differences in coronary disease and diene conjugated lipids. *Journal of Human Hypertension.* **2**:297.

8

Coronary Heart Disease Screening: Logistics and Risk Scores

LEWIS D RITCHIE

In the United Kingdom (UK) there is a growing desire for action to prevent coronary heart disease (CHD). The Government recently targeted a 40% reduction for CHD mortality in the under-65 age-group by the year 2000 (Secretary of State for Health, 1992). There has been considerable debate on how to address the prevention of CHD, and in particular on the merits and demerits of a 'population' versus 'high-risk' strategy. In reality, there is no dichotomy and both approaches should be regarded as complementary.

Much of the responsibility for the 'high-risk' approach has been devolved to primary care, with the expectation that effective screening activities will be implemented by general practitioners (GPs) and their staff. Faced with this responsibility there are several major issues to be resolved:

- should patients be screened?
- which patients should be screened?
- how should screening be performed?
- what constitute adequate measures of success?

The first of these questions is outside the scope of this chapter. Definitive evidence of the worth of CHD risk-factor screening is still awaited. Two large UK general practice-based trials, the OXCHECK Study (Imperial Cancer Research Fund OXCHECK Study Group, 1991) and the Family Heart Association Study (D.Wood, personal communication) are under way to address whether health checks by nurses are effective in helping to reduce the risk of heart disease, cancer and stroke.

Which patients should be screened?

Should the target group of patients be determined by age/sex considerations alone, or should priorities be dictated by other factors such as pre-existing risk (previous diagnosis of CHD, hypertension, diabetes or lipid disorder), smoking, obesity or positive family history of premature CHD? Taken together, these would account for well over half of all adult patients in an average general practice list. There is a balance between extended target groups (what may seem desirable) and available resources (what is feasible). The issue of resource requirements is particularly important, not only in relation to initial screening and rescreening, but also in the considerable and perhaps underestimated workload (Imperial Cancer Research Fund OXCHECK Study Group, 1991) generated by follow-up assessment and treatment of those individuals with newly discovered abnormalities.

The targeting dilemma has been addressed by the Coronary Prevention Group and British Heart Foundation, who recently published guidelines based on formal risk assessment using the Dundee coronary risk-disk (Tunstall-Pedoe, 1991; Working Group of the Coronary Prevention Group and the British Heart Foundation, 1991). They proposed a division of risk based on two groups: first, a 'clinical risk' group—those individuals with pre-existing CHD or diabetes or who are already receiving drug treatment for hypertension or hyperlipidaemia—and secondly a 'multiple risk' group. This latter group would consist of individuals at increased risk for CHD, as determined by the Dundee coronary risk-disk (Working Group of the Coronary Prevention Group and the British Heart Foundation, 1991). All assessed patients would receive general advice and those at 'clinical risk' or 'multiple risk' would be allocated to 'special care' follow-up. This selective approach seems sensible, and the extent of screening and follow-up may be determined by the availability of local resources.

Risk scores: development and attributes

The development of risk scores recognizes that risk factors interact synergistically, and that a unifactorial approach for CHD risk assessment and management is inadequate. However, this does not gainsay the requirement for clear guidelines on how individual factors need to be tackled, set in the context of a multifactorial assessment of risk. There are a number of risk scores currently in use in the UK, and these are now described.

Lifestyle management score

This score is loosely based on US data from the Pooling Project (Anggard *et al.*, 1986). It operates on an additive rather than a multiplicative basis, and therefore does not predict risk. It should be regarded rather as a tool for motivating change and for monitoring progress in the individual following lifestyle interventions. It assumes measurement of cholesterol in all assessed patients using a desktop dry chemistry analyser (Reflotron, Boehringer Mannheim) allowing immediate patient feedback. The score also takes into account sex, family history, smoking habits, obesity and both systolic and diastolic blood pressures. All parameters are entered directly to a microcomputer which then automatically calculates a score which the nurse interprets to the patient. There is no automatic range-checking of data entered to the computer. For patients who are asked to return, a patient-held record card ('health passport') is annotated with a score graphic and progress is charted at subsequent visits (Figure 8.1). The strengths are that it is computer-based, with simple guide-

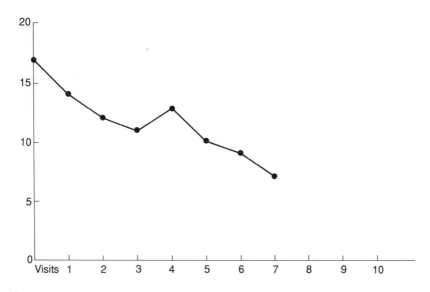

Figure 8.1: Score graphic from patient-held 'health passport'; score is registered on Y axis plotted against follow-up visits on X axis.

lines, and readily understood by patients and staff. Unfortunately scores are unvalidated and non-predictive, and arguably undue emphasis is given to cholesterol as one component of the risk score.

Shaper score

This score is based on the British Regional Heart Study dataset (Shaper *et al.*, 1986, 1987). It takes account of cigarette smoking, mean blood pressure, history of pre-existing CHD or diabetes mellitus and parental history of death from CHD; the presence of angina is assessed by questionnaire. This predictive score has been internally validated and does not necessarily require the measurement of cholesterol levels. It allows an individual at increased risk to be placed into a risk group permitting tailored advice/intervention to be given. It is validated and predictive, and has been well received by both staff and patients (Wilson and Morrell, 1991). Its weaknesses are that it is restricted to men and is paper-based in a standard format. As such, it involves multiple calculations and *may* be prone to computation error and problems of practicability. Arguably it underemphasizes cholesterol as a CHD risk component.

Dundee coronary risk-disk

This scoring and ranking method was devised by Tunstall-Pedoe based on data from the Scottish Heart Health Study and has been externally validated against the Whitehall Study dataset. (Tunstall-Pedoe, 1991; Working Group of the Coronary Prevention Group and the British Heart Foundation, 1991). It takes into account sex, systolic blood pressure, smoking habit and cholesterol concentration (which is estimated at first and can then be selectively measured in appropriate patients). Unlike the two previous scores, calculation is confined to modifiable risk, age is preset to 50 (with adjustments for female age), and previous personal or family history of CHD is not considered. The score also allows the calculation of a Dundee risk rank which places individuals in a percentile-based queue of 1 (front of queue, high risk, priority action) to 100 (back of queue, low risk, general advice). It is available in standard format, as a circular slide-rule risk-disk, and has also been published in the form of a computer software program. This score has recently been subject to a computerized simulation based on the OXCHECK dataset (Imperial Cancer Research Fund OXCHECK Study Group, 1991; Randall *et al.*, 1992). The authors concluded that the Coronary Prevention Group Guidelines (Working Group of the Coronary Prevention Group and the British Heart Foundation, 1991) and the Dundee coronary risk-disk (Tunstall-Pedoe, 1991) may help to make the best use of resources within specific age-sex groups but also concluded that: 'sound protocols for unifactorial assessment remain essential' (Randall *et al.*, 1992). In an accompanying article (Tunstall-Pedoe, 1992), the originator pointed out that calculation of a patient score was not just about categories of risk but also about motivation for change, and that unifactorial risk assessment was too naïve. Although it is validated and predictive, and has been well received by some professionals (Tunstall-Pedoe, 1992), in risk-disk form it *may* be prone to calculation error and problems of practicability.

Risk scores: an assessment

Risk score developments are at an early stage. No publications have as yet appeared describing rigorous evaluation studies of their implementation within general practice and their impact on motivating risk-factor change. There are many questions to be answered: should they take the form of a simple guideline or complex predictive score? Should they be manual or computerized? Computerization may transform a complex calculation into a readily understood score; however, computer-based risk scores are not necessarily better than manual alternatives. Although calculation errors should be eliminated and speed enhanced by using computers, correct scoring relies on accurate entry of data. In the future, all computer-based scores should include range-checking software to vet all data entries, although even this precaution can only reject the impossible and query the implausible (Ritchie, 1992*a*).

How useful are risk scores? In principle, they seem worthwhile as tools for risk measurement and for influencing beneficial changes in risk factors, but appropriate randomized study designs are necessary for a more robust assessment of their worth. There are certainly traps for unwary users of risk scores: the need for adequate staff training and quality control is paramount, and there must be careful translation of the significance of the score by health professional to patient. Availability of a score does not equate to actual usage—in the Lifestyle Management Programme, the score was not calculated in approximately 30% of follow-up visits (Änggard *et al.*, 1986). Finally, in relation to the utility of a score, it may be that practicability (which influences extent of use) outweighs scientific elegance, comprehensiveness or educational value.

How should screening be done?

Having identified which patients should be screened, and having considered their possible assessment by risk scores, how should screening be performed? Patients may be screened opportunistically; this pivots on the attendance of patients at surgeries and medical centres for some unrelated reason. 70% of patients can be expected to attend a GP at least once a year, and 95% attend at least once in five years. Opportunistic screening retains its reputation as being ineffective because of previous experience with the detection and recording of hypertension in the 1970s and early 1980s (Heller and Rose, 1977; Ritchie and Currie, 1983). This should be reappraised in the light of enhanced health promotional activity in general practice and a heightened awareness among both doctors and patients. The other major method in use is by formal invitation (by letter or by phone) to attend specifically for screening. This method is organization-intensive and prone to the risks of sending letters to wrong addresses and of receiving refusals. Which is the preferred option? Again there is no dichotomy. Screening by letters of invitation may be the preferred method when numbers are relatively small or when the timescale is more critical. An example might be the invitation of a selected group of patients with known risk factors—eg hypertensives, diabetics or individuals with previous CHD. Opportunistic screening may be the most sensible option when numbers are large or the timescale is less critical; for CHD risk assessment, this should be the usual method of recruiting individuals with unknown risk factors.

Opportunistic cholesterol screening has recently been subjected to a favourable cost-effectiveness analysis by the Standing Medical Advisory Committee on Blood Cholesterol Testing (Standing Medical Advisory Committee to the Secretary of State, 1990). If a screening clinic is established in a practice, then it is also likely that patients will attend without formal invitations or by opportunistic prompting by primary care staff. In the Lifestyle Management Programme, of 80 504 patients recruited, around 60% of attendances were prompted by primary care staff, around 25% by encouragement of friends and relatives, and the remainder by self-referral.

Ingredients for risk-factor screening

Protocols

A complete protocol must be developed which not only takes account of target groups as discussed earlier, but which also defines precise guidelines on what are trigger levels for action. This would include agreement on the interventions to be used—lifestyle advice and drugs, when necessary, and the adoption of a tailored, individual approach. Numerous guidelines are available to assist the management of individuals with detected abnormalities—for example hypertension (British Hypertension Society Working Party Report, 1989) and hyperlipidaemia, (Shepherd *et al.*, 1987; Royal College of General Practitioners, 1992).

Delegation

Coronary risk factor screening may be successfully delegated to nurses (Änggard *et al.*, 1986; Imperial Cancer Research Fund OXCHECK Study Group, 1991) who require appropriate training and professional support from GP colleagues. In the Lifestyle Management Programme, all of the initial screening and many of the follow-up activities were successfully delegated to nurses. This is also the mechanism being tested in the OXCHECK and Family Heart Association Studies.

Special equipment—microcomputers and desk-top analysers

Because of the continuous nature of screening and follow-up visits, serious consideration should be given to computer-based records to facilitate collection, retrieval and analysis of data, and (as discussed earlier) for use with risk scores (Ritchie, 1986, 1989).

Many practices are now using desk-top dry chemistry devices for rapid measurement of cholesterol on capillary non-fasted blood specimens, allowing immediate feedback to patients. Like risk scores, immediate cholesterol feedback may be regarded as a means of assessing this factor, for monitoring progress at subsequent visits, and for having a possible motivational effect on patients. Devices available include the Reflotron and Lipotrend C (Boehringer Mannheim), the Seralyser (Ames), Vision (Abbott), and Ektakem (Kodak). Major concerns have been expressed in relation to the accuracy and precision of these devices (eg Broughton *et al.*, 1989). In trained hands, these devices can approximate to standard wet chemistry techniques, with a coefficient of variation between 3 and 5%. Practices using these devices *must* enrol in external quality control programmes. For the moment, desk-top analysers should be regarded as screening tools only and diagnostic confirmation of a lipid abnormality should be made on fasting lipoprotein profile specimens sent to a biochemistry laboratory. Because of differences between local laboratories, GPs must first liaise with clinical biochemists on the nature and extent of services which might be needed and made available—otherwise requirements may not marry with actual provision.

Space and administrative requirements

Apparently mundane but essential logistic requirements for CHD screening are adequate space in which to conduct screening, and administrative back-up to arrange scheduling of appointments for screening clinics. Lack of 'screening space' may be a problem in premises which are already overcrowded. Similarly, there is an extra administrative overhead for office and receptionist staff as a result of screening. Although predominantly a nurse-centred activity with GP support, the administrative workload should not be overlooked.

Publicity and educational materials

Informing patients of the availability of screening may be done in several ways: by posters, by leaflets or by invitation cards which can be made available opportunistically during attendances. Alternatively, as discussed above, patients may be canvassed to attend by letters of invitation. This can be done most efficiently by using 'mail-merged' standard letters, a facility available on most general practice computer systems currently in use. There is also a requirement for a continuous supply of educational materials for general 'healthy heart' lifestyle advice and specifically for hypertension, hyperlipidaemia, diet (including weight reduction and lipid lowering materials), smoking, alcohol and physical exercise. These are available from a number of sources including the Health Education Authority, the Health Education Board for Scotland, local health promotion departments of District Health Authorities, from many commercial organizations involved in food marketing and from charities such as the British Heart Foundation and Family Heart Association. Consideration should also be given to providing a patient held record card, such as the 'health passport' (Figure 8.1) which documents the progress of patients at each followup visit, explains the aims of the screening programme, allows recording of treatments and records the time of future appointments (Änggard *et al.*, 1986).

Training

Staff training is a requirement in relation to the conduct of the screening process, for the use and maintenance of technology (risk scores, computers, analysers) and for the monitoring of patient attendance and default.

Relationships

A CHD screening programme should be seen as an opportunity to cement relationships with local specialists including laboratory staff, dietitians and hospital consultants. Although screening programmes take place within primary care, they clearly generate investigations and referrals for colleagues in secondary care, with an attendant increase in workload.

Resources

Staff time, new technology, laboratory investigations and hospital referrals have already been considered. The funding for these is not necessarily guaranteed and need to be carefully planned. Following the introduction of health promotion clinic payments in the 1990 Contract for GPs, screening costs can be defrayed against additional practice income from this source. It is likely that this form of contractual funding will be revised and more closely aligned to local health priorities set against the background of national targets (Secretary of State for Health, 1992). This may be co-ordinated by local directors of public health and consultants in public health medicine who will wish to ensure some equity in relation to CHD reduction initiatives in individual health districts and boards.

What constitute adequate measures of success?

This might best be considered as audit of process and outcome, and it, constitutes an essential ingredient of any screening programme. The definition of target groups, the elaboration of operational protocols and the implementation of screening are not complete without a mechanism for measuring success or otherwise. A number of questions can be posed and answers offered:

Q. What are we trying to achieve?
A. Reduced CHD mortality, reduced CHD morbidity, overall mortality reduction, and improved patient wellbeing—patients' perceptions of *quality* of life are usually more immediate than *quantity*.

Q. What do we measure?
A1. CHD mortality and morbidity reductions. Penalty: extended timescale, large numbers and need for controls; verdict: impracticable measurement for most general practitioners; *may* be within scope of public health medicine consultants.
A2. Observed changes in risk factors. Penalty: proxy and therefore *soft* measures of outcome; verdict: practicable measurements, acceptable timescale, but should also incorporate additional process measures of patient characteristics, including—rate of target recruitment, compliance/default, diagnoses, drugs prescribed (mainly antihypertensive and lipid lowering agents) and secondary referrals.

Q. What are the associated costs?
A. Medical, nursing, administrative, drug prescriptions, laboratory and referral costs; indirect patient costs, e.g. inconvenience, time off work, travel; opportunity costs—other activities sacrificed in order to screen patients; psychological costs—may incur patient anxieties with potential negative impact of labelling.

The measurement of success in relation to CHD screening is therefore a complex process and, as such, is multidimensional, multiprofessional and evolving.

References

Änggard EE *et al.* (1986) Prevention of cardiovascular disease in general practice: a proposed model. *British Medical Journal.* **293**:177–80.

British Hypertension Society Working Party Report (1989) Treating mild hypertension. *British Medical Journal.* **298**:694–8.

Broughton PMG *et al.* (1989) Quality of plasma cholesterol measurements in primary care. *British Medical Journal.* **298**:297–8.

Heller RF and Rose GA (1977) Current management of hypertension in general practice. *British Medical Journal.* i:1442–4.

Imperial Cancer Research Fund OXCHECK Study Group (1991) Prevalence of risk factors for heart disease in OXCHECK trial: implications for screening in primary care. *British Medical Journal.* **302**:1057–60.

Randall T *et al.* (1992) Choosing the preventive workload in general practice: practical application of the Coronary Prevention Group guidelines and Dundee coronary risk-disk. *British Medical Journal.* **305**:227–31.

Ritchie LD and Currie AM (1983) Blood pressure recording by general practitioners in northeast Scotland. *British Medical Journal.* **286**:107–9.

Ritchie LD (1986) *Computers in primary care.* 2nd ed. Heinemann Medical, London.

Ritchie LD (1989) Finding patients at risk of coronary heart disease: what can computers contribute? In: Shepherd *et al.* (eds) *Coronary risk factors revisited.* Excerpta Medica, Amsterdam. pp. 87–92.

Ritchie LD (1992*a*) Computers in screening and surveillance In: Hart CR and Burke P (eds) *Screening and surveillance in general practice.* Churchill Livingstone, Edinburgh. pp. 55–63.

Ritchie LD (1992) Cholesterol screening in general practice: halting between two opinions. *Update.* **44**:232–8.

Royal College of General Practitioners (1992) *Guidelines for the management of hyperlipidaemia in general practice—towards the primary prevention of coronary heart disease.* Occasional Paper 55. Royal College of General Practitioners, London.

Secretary of State for Health (1992) *Health of the nation.* HMSO, London.

Shaper AG *et al.* (1986) Identifying men at high risk of heart attacks: strategy for use in general practice. *British Medical Journal.* **293**:474–9.

Shaper AG *et al.* (1987) A scoring system to identify men at high risk of a heart attack. *Health Trends.* **19**:37–9.

Shepherd J *et al.* (1987) Strategies for reducing heart disease and desirable limits for blood lipid concentrations: guidelines from the British Hyperlipidaemia Association. *British Medical Journal.* **295**:1245–6.

Standing Medical Advisory Committee to the Secretary of State (1990) *Blood cholesterol testing: the cost effectiveness of opportunistic blood screening*. Department of Health, London.

Tunstall-Pedoe H (1991) The Dundee coronary risk-disk for management of change in risk factors. *British Medical Journal*. **303**:744–7.

Tunstall-Pedoe H (1992) Value of the Dundee coronary risk disk: a defence. *British Medical Journal*. **305**:231–2.

Wilson A and Morrell J (1991) Prevention of heart disease in general practice: the use of a risk score. *Health Trends*. **23**:69–73.

Working Group of the Coronary Prevention Group and the British Heart Foundation (1991) An action plan for preventing coronary heart disease in primary care. *British Medical Journal*. **303**:748–50.

9

Risk Factors: Are They Relevant in the Elderly?

KAY-TEE KHAW

The proportion of the population of England and Wales aged 65 years and over, now 16% of the total or approximately 8 million persons, is projected to increase to 20% of the population, or 9.5 million persons by 2020. Cardiovascular disease (CVD) mortality increases exponentially with increasing age and CVD is the leading cause of death in the elderly, accounting for about half the deaths. More importantly, it is also a leading cause of disability and morbidity, at least as measured by health-service utilization: diseases of the circulatory system are the leading causes of hospital bed occupancy and general practice consultations. CVD thus constitutes a major burden of potentially preventable disability in the elderly.

The role of classic risk factors: blood pressure, cholesterol and cigarette smoking

The plethora of reported risk factors for CVD (over 280 in one recent review) should not obscure the fact that just three classic risk factors—blood pressure, serum cholesterol and smoking—are enormously powerful predictors of cardiovascular events and have been so documented in virtually every prospective population study where they have been measured. The largest of these, those screened for the Multiple Risk Factor Intervention Trial (MRFIT) (Stamler et al., 1986) showed a 15-fold difference in coronary heart disease (CHD) between men who were non-smokers and had diastolic blood pressure less than 90 mmHg and serum cholesterol in the lowest quintile, compared to men who were current smokers, had diastolic blood pressure greater than or equal to 90 mmHg and serum cholesterol in the top quintile. Indeed, based on extrapolations of data from the Framingham Study, a 60-year-old man with no risk factors might be estimated to have a similar CHD mortality risk to that of a 45-year-old male cigarette smoker with hypertension and hypercholesteraemia (Grundy, 1986).

However, it has been suggested that at older ages (65 years and over), the classic risk factors are no longer predictive of CVD mortality in the elderly. Although some studies of the very old (over 75 or 80 years) have reported a paradoxical inverse relationship of blood pressure with mortality (Mattila et al.,

1988), the current commentary will focus on the elderly defined as those aged 60 years and over.

Do CVD risk factors predict CVD morbidity or mortality in the elderly?

Early reports from prospective studies had conflicting results about the predictive contribution of the classic risk factors in older adults. For example, in an early follow-up of the Framingham Study of men and women aged 49–82, total cholesterol was not predictive after age 60 (Gordon *et al.*, 1977). However, later analyses reported that serum cholesterol did indeed predict mortality in later life (Castelli *et al.*, 1989). The Busselton Study of 3390 adults reported that neither blood pressure nor cholesterol was predictive in subjects aged over 60 (Weldorn and Wearne, 1979). Later prospective studies, however, including the Rancho Bernardo Study (Barrett-Connor *et al.*, 1984), found that even in men and women aged 65–79 years at base-line, cholesterol predicted ischaemic heart disease (IHD) mortality. Benfante reported in the Honolulu heart study (Benfante *et al.*, 1989; Benfante and Reed, 1990) that in men aged 65–74 years followed up for 12 years, serum cholesterol levels were independently related to CHD risk, with a 1.64 upper to lower quartile relative risk for serum cholesterol level, a relative risk identical to that for men aged 52–59 years; the Puerto Rican Study (Kittner *et al.*, 1983) found similar relative risks for CHD associated with cholesterol level in middle-aged and older men. The Honolulu Heart Study (Benfante *et al.*, 1989; Benfante and Reed, 1990) also reported significantly increased CHD risks associated with raised systolic blood pressure and cigarette smoking. Tables 9.1 and 9.2 summarize findings from the Rancho Bernardo and Honolulu Heart Studies.

One possible explanation is that, in populations where coronary rates are lower, the impact of selective mortality from hypercholesterolaemia or other risk factors may be delayed so that cholesterol level, blood pressure or cigarette smoking still has expression at older ages; early studies showing no association may reflect earlier selective mortality in high-risk cohorts. In an era of rapid secular decline in CHD, major risk factors remain significant at older ages. A recent overview of 25 populations examining the value of serum total cholesterol measurement in predicting CHD concluded that total cholesterol predicted fatal CHD in middle-aged (<65 years) and older (>=65 years) men and women, although the strength and consistency of these relationships in older women were diminished (Manolio *et al.*, 1992).

The relationship between cigarette smoking and CHD, while apparent in most studies at all ages, has (as with cholesterol) varied in magnitude with different ages. Doll and Peto (1976) reported that the relative risk for CHD death in male doctors smoking 25 or more cigarettes daily compared to non-smokers was 2.2 for those aged 45–54, 1.6 for those aged 55–64, and 1.5 for those aged 65–74 years.

Risk factor (SD)	50–64 years		65–79 years	
	All causes	IHD	All causes	IHD
Age (per 7.2 years)	1.8*	1.6	2.2**	2.8**
Cholesterol (per 0.95 mmol/l)	1.5**	1.8**	1.1	1.4**
Systolic blood pressure (per 22.7 mmHg)	1.4*	1.4	1.2**	1.2
Cigarette smoking (current/ never)	1.4	1.1	1.8**	1.1

$*P = < 0.05$
$**P = < 0.01$

Table 9.1: Relative risk of selected factors from all cause and ischaemic heart disease mortality among men aged 50–64 and 65–79 years in Rancho Bernardo. (Source: Barrett-Connor *et al.*, 1984.)

Risk factor	Relative risk (95% confidence interval)	
Serum cholesterol (per 80 mg/dl)*	1.65	(1.14–2.37)
Systolic blood pressure (per 47 mmHg)	1.87	(1.34–2.61)
Cigarettes smoking (per 30 cigarettes daily)	1.56	(1.01–2.40)
History of diabetes (yes/no)	1.74	(2.32–2.51)

*1 mg % = 0.02586 mmol/l

Table 9.2: Inter-quartile relative risks of CHD for selected risk factors measured in men aged 65 years and older, Honolulu Heart Program. (Source: Benfante *et al.*, 1989; Benfante and Reed 1990.)

To summarize, prospective studies in general consistently report that smoking, blood pressure and cholesterol still predict CHD in older persons, although the relative risk associated with these risk factors tends to decrease with increasing age. Nevertheless, because the absolute risk of CVD increases so sharply with increasing age, the absolute risk associated with these risk factors in fact increases with age.

Does reduction of CVD risk factors reduce mortality and morbidity in the elderly?

If risk factors do predict cardiovascular mortality in the elderly, the question remains whether intervention to reduce blood pressure and serum cholesterol or to stop cigarette smoking will reduce mortality and morbidity. Since the

		35–44 years	45–54 years	55–64 years
Number treated to prevent one	Men	862	234	104
event	Women	4649	1112	315
Number of events prevented	Men	1371	4695	11 568
	Women	144	1230	6057

Table 9.3: Estimated numbers of persons with cholesterol level > 6.5 mmol/l treated for five years to prevent one CHD death within five years in different age categories in England and Wales, and estimated numbers of events prevented. (Source: Khaw and Rose, 1989.)

absolute risk associated with risk factors increases with age, the potential individual absolute benefit, as well as the population absolute benefit, may be greater in older than in younger persons (Gordon and Rifkind, 1989; Khaw and Rose, 1989) Table 9.3 shows some estimates of the individual and population absolute risks.

Although several trials of cholesterol-lowering agents have reported an approximate 20% reduction CHD in middle-aged men, there have been no trials of the effect of cholesterol-lowering medication in older persons (Stamler, 1988; Tyroler, 1989).

There have also been no randomized trials of smoking cessation in older persons but the CASS study found that the relative risk of myocardial infarction or death in those who continued smoking compared those who stopped was in fact greatest in those aged 70–74 years (RR 2.9, whereas in those aged 55–59 it was 1.5) (Hermanson et al., 1988).

Results from several hypertension treatment trials in the elderly have consistently shown reductions in cardiovascular morbidity and mortality associated with treatment; these have been reviewed elsewhere (Wilhemsen, 1988; Dahlof et al., 1991; SHEP Cooperative Research Group, 1991; Medical Research Council Working Party, 1992). The absolute magnitude of the benefits has been greater than in trials conducted on younger populations; for example, the SHEP trial of treatment of isolated systolic hypertension in the persons aged 60 years and over found a 36% reduction in stroke (30 events prevented per 1000 treated over five years) and 13% reduction in all CVD events (55 events prevented per 1000 treated over five years) (SHEP Cooperative Research Group, 1991). The European trial of hypertension in persons aged 60 years and over reported 58 cardiovascular events prevented per 1000 persons treated (Amery et al., 1985).

Conclusions

The major burden of CVD is in the old, but the majority of the prospective studies and trials of cardiovascular risk factors and the effects of their reduction have been in middle-aged population groups. However, there now is little doubt that the classic risk factors (cigarette smoking, raised blood pressure and raised serum cholesterol) remain predictive of CVD well into older ages. While caution is needed in extrapolating from one age-group to another, and indeed from one study cohort to another, there is also evidence that reduction of risk factors such as cessation of cigarette smoking and treatment of hypertension is associated with substantial cardiovascular benefits. There are concerns that in older persons, other endpoints become increasingly important—in particular, quality of life and morbidity from any cause including stroke and cancer—so that prevention of CHD mortality cannot be considered in isolation. All interventions need to be evaluated with regard to potential risks and benefits. In the elderly, in particular, the impact on other health endpoints such as quality of life may not be weighted in the same way as in younger populations.

Nevertheless, the elderly should not, *a priori*, be precluded from considering risk factor reduction. Large secular trends already observed, with increasing numbers of surviving healthy older persons and changing distributions of risk factors, necessitate continuing research: in particular, trials that focus more on endpoints of importance in the elderly, such as all-cause morbidity and quality of life.

While this commentary has focused on the classic high risk-factor intervention approach to prevention of CVD in the elderly, it should not be forgotten that all older persons, irrespective of risk factor levels, are likely to benefit from general advice and support for modest changes in lifestyles which are recognized as being associated not just with improved cardiovascular but also with general health, eg increasing fresh fruit and vegetable and fish intake, and undertaking regular exercise such as walking.

Summary

The burden of morbidity as well as mortality from CVD is greatest in the elderly since incidence rises exponentially with increasing age. Data from numerous prospective studies indicate that classic CVD risk factors, including high blood pressure, raised serum cholesterol and cigarette smoking, still predict CVD in persons aged 60 years and over. Observational studies indicate that stopping smoking is associated with risk reduction even at older ages. Several trials have clearly demonstrated benefit from treatment of hypertension in the elderly, but the overall risk-benefit balance of pharmacological reduction of raised serum cholesterol levels in the elderly is yet to be determined in trials. Although the relative risks associated with the classic risk factors may be lower in elderly than in younger persons, the absolute risks—and hence the potential absolute benefits of risk-factor reduction—are greater in the elderly. Since older persons have a higher prevalence of hypertension and higher lipid levels than younger persons, the potential public health consequences of risk-factor intervention in the elderly are considerable. Although there are concerns about preventive measures compromising quality of life in older persons, these should not preclude older persons from considering treatment of hypertension and possibly hypercholesterolaemia. There is also abundant evidence that feasible lifestyle changes, such as physical activity and dietary sodium reduction, might in fact have greater cardiovascular as well as other health benefits in older persons.

References

Amery A *et al.* (1985) Mortality and morbidity results from the European working party on high blood pressure in the elderly trial. *The Lancet.* i:1349–54.

Barrett-Connor E *et al.* (1984) Ischemic heart disease risk factors over age 50. *Journal of Chronic Diseases.* 37:903–8.

Benfante RJ *et al.* (1989) Risk factors in middle age that predict early and late onset of coronary heart disease. *Journal of Clinical Epidemiology.* 42:95–104.

Benfante RJ and Reed D (1990) Is elevated serum cholesterol level a risk factor for coronary heart disease in the elderly? *Journal of the American Medical Association.* 263:393–6.

Castelli WP *et al.* (1989) Cardiovascular risk factors in the elderly. *American Journal of Cardiology.* 63:12–19H.

Dahlof B (1991) Morbidity and mortality in the Swedish trial in old patients with hypertension (STOP-Hypertension). *The Lancet.* 338:1281–5.

Doll R and Peto R (1975) Mortality in relation to smoking; 20 years' observations on male British doctors. *British Medical Journal.* ii:1525–36.

Gordon T *et al.* (1977) High density lipoprotein as a protective factors against coronary heart disease. The Framingham Study. *American Journal of Medicine.* 62:707–14.

Gordon DJ and Rifkind BM (1989) Treating high blood cholesterol in the older patient. *American Journal of Cardiology.* 63:48–52H.

Grundy SM (1986) Cholesterol and coronary heart disease. A new era. *Journal of the American Medical Association.* 256:2849–58.

Hermanson B *et al.* (1988) Beneficial six-year outcome of smoking cessation in older men and women with coronary artery disease: results from the CASS Registry. *New England Journal of Medicine.* 319:1365–9.

Khaw K-T and Rose G (1989) Cholesterol screening programmes: how much potential benefit? *British Medical Journal.* 299:606–7.

Kittner SJ *et al.* (1983) Alcohol and coronary heart disease in Puerto Rico. *American Journal of Epidemiology.* **117**:538–50.

Manolio TA *et al.* (1992) Cholesterol and heart disease in older persons and women. *Annals of Epidemiology.* **2**:161–76.

Mattila K *et al.* (1988) Blood pressure and 5 year survival in the very old. *British Medical Journal.* **296**:887–9.

Medical Research Council Working Party (1992) Medical Research Council trial of treatment of hypertension in older adults: principal results. *British Medical Journal.* **304**:405–12.

SHEP Cooperative Research Group (1991) Prevention of stroke by antihypertensive drug treatment in older persons with isolated systolic hypertension. *Journal of the American Medical Association.* **265**:3255–64.

Stamler J *et al.* (1986) Is the relationship between serum choelsterol and risk of premature death from coronary heart disease continuous and graded? *Journal of the American Medical Association.* **256**:2823–8.

Stamler J (1989) Risk factor modification trials: implications for the elderly. *European Heart Journal.* **9**:(Suppl. D): 9–53.

Tyroler HA (1989) Overview of clinical trials of cholesterol lowering in relationship to epidemiologic studies. *American Journal of Medicine.* **87** (Suppl. 4A):14–19S.

Welborn TA and Wearne K (1979) Coronary heart disease incidence and cardiovascular mortality in Busselton with reference to glucose and insulin concentrations. *Diabetes Care.* **2**:154–60.

Wilhelmsen L (1988) Trials in coronary heart disease and hypertension with special reference to the elderly. *European Heart Journal.* **9**:207–14.

10

Are we Living Longer or Dying Longer?

ELIZABETH BARRETT-CONNOR

The fastest growing segment of the population in most industrialized countries is the elderly, who consume a disproportionate amount of the health-care budget. The consequences of an ever-increasing number of older adults has focused attention on cardiovascular disease (CVD), the most common cause of death and one of the leading causes of morbidity in the elderly.

Only two broad topics are addressed in this brief review.

1   Are the major heart disease risk factors still important after age 65 and, if so, does reversing them after age 65 matter, or is it 'too late'?
2   What are the consequences to the individual and to society of preventing or postponing CHD?

The heart disease risk-factor review is based on selected international publications. US data are used to describe the societal costs of a decline in heart disease death rates. Data from the Rancho Bernardo Heart and Chronic Disease Study are used to illustrate individual consequences of heart disease prevention and increased longevity in a California cohort of older adults whose standardized mortality ratio (SMR) for ischaemic heart disease is already less than half the national rate.

Possible heart disease risk factors after age 65

Hypertension

Hypertension, the best studied of the three classic risk factors for CHD in the elderly, has been shown to predict an increased risk of fatal CVD in almost every cohort studied—at least to age 75 or 80. Systolic and diastolic blood pressure seem to be equally important, but since systolic hypertension is more common than combined or diastolic hypertension in older adults, the percentage of disease attributable to systolic hypertension is larger. Several clinical trials have shown a significant reduction in stroke (although not necessarily CHD) when older adults with diastolic hypertension were treated (Dahlof et al., 1991). Recently the Systolic Hypertension in the Elderly Program (SHEP) study showed the benefit of treating isolated *systolic* hypertension in otherwise healthy older adults (SHEP Cooperative Research Group, 1991).

The disappointing effect of blood pressure control on the prevention of fatal CHD in many clinical trials, in contrast to the striking reduction in stroke risk, is well known and still puzzling. In most trials in elderly hypertensives, there

Trial (age range, years)	Sample size	Stroke	Cardiac	Total mortality
HDFP* 60–69	2376	47*	23*	16
EWPHE 60–97	840	32	38	9
Cooper and Warrender 60–79	884	30	22	3
SHEP ⩾60	4736	36	27	13
STOP 70–84	1627	47	28	43
MRC 65–74	4396	25	19	4

*Age-specific data not available

Table 10.1: Percentage reduction in mortality in older adults: controls vs antihypertensive drugs

were more strokes than heart attacks in both the placebo and treated groups. In the European Working Party on Hypertension in the Elderly (EWPHE) trial there was a 26% reduction in CVD mortality but only a 7% reduction in total mortality in treated hypertensive adults aged 60–97. Table 10.1 shows a wide range of all-cause mortality rates in large antihypertensive trials in the elderly, but no evidence that antihypertensives increase overall mortality rates.

Despite this, studies from Finland (Mattila *et al.*, 1988) and Rancho Bernardo (Langer *et al.* 1989) found the very old who had low blood pressure were less likely to survive. A similar pattern was observed in the EWPHE randomized controlled trial. In that study of persons aged 65 and older with diastolic hypertension, the treated group had better survival and less CVD up to about age 80, when a crossover phenomenon appeared. This paradoxical survival pattern could be merely a marker for a premortal condition, but requires further investigation. It is biologically plausible that either spontaneous low blood pressure or therapeutically induced low blood pressure could dangerously impair cerebral or coronary blood flow in older adults with a stiff or atherosclerotic arterial system. For example, low blood pressure might lead to inadequate coronary perfusion because coronary arteries normally fill during diastole.

Do antihypertensives disturb the quality of life? The SHEP trial paid special attention to possible adverse effects in the elderly and reported no serious sequelae: specifically, no depression or impairment of cognitive function associated with lowering systolic blood pressure. Clinical trials tend to include healthier people than the general population, in whom many factors contribute to a possible increased risk of pharmacologic intervention.

Cholesterol

Until recently there were only scattered reports on the relation of plasma cholesterol measured after age 65 to outcome (Barrett-Connor *et al.*, 1984). In 1990 the National Heart Lung and Blood Institute convened an international workshop where many investigators reported the relation of serum cholesterol to CHD among cohorts aged 65 and older (Manolio *et al.*, 1992). After follow-up intervals ranging from three to 23 years, the relative risk associated with a cholesterol of 1.6 mmol/l or higher exceeded one in 10 of 16 studies in women and 21 of 24 studies in men (Figure 10.1, 10.2). Nevertheless, in both sexes the average relative risk was less than two, and only one study of older women and eight of the studies of older men found a statistically significant excess risk. Thus total plasma cholesterol remains a coronary risk factor in older men, but the association is less convincing in women.

Although the average age of the cohorts varied widely, the workshop did not address risks among the very old. Recent reports from Framingham and elsewhere suggest that low cholesterol levels may not be healthy in the very old. The Glostrup study followed 70-year-old Danes to age 80 and found that serum cholesterol levels were unassociated with the risk of dying in either sex, although there was a positive graded relation between serum cholesterol and CHD, and an inverse graded relation of serum cholesterol with cancer death (Agner, 1985). Because the elderly are more apt to have other diseases and to die (half of the Glostrup cohort died between ages 70 and 80), it is difficult to determine whether low cholesterol is a risk factor or marker for existing disease in the elderly.

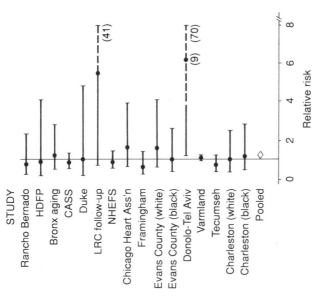

Figure 10.2: Relative risk and 95% confidence interval of fatal CHD associated with cholesterol levels of 6.20 mmol/l or higher compared to cholesterol levels less than 5.17 mmol/l in older women. (Reproduced from Manolio *et al.*, 1992, by permission.)

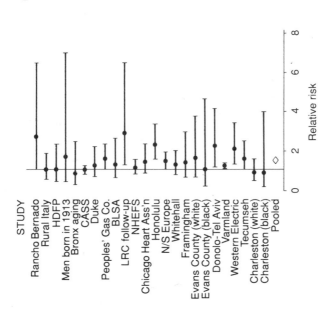

Figure 10.1: Relative risk and 95% confidence interval of fatal CHD associated with cholesterol levels of 6.20 mmol/l or higher compared to cholesterol levels less than 5.17 mmol/l in older men. (Reproduced from Manolio *et al.*, 1992, by permission.)

The major clinical trials of lipid lowering for primary prevention of CHD have excluded older adults. One exception is the Veterans' Administration Domiciliary Study, where institutionalized men were randomly assigned to a low saturated, high polyunsaturated fat diet or to a typical (high saturated fat) US diet (Dayton *et al.*, 1970). At the close of the trial, there were significantly fewer cardiovascular events in treated than in untreated men less than 65 years of age, but no significant differences in those aged 66–89. Somewhat more promising results were reported from the unblinded Stockholm trial, where men aged 60–69 who were randomly assigned to clofibrate and niacin had 36% lower total mortality rates than those assigned to placebo (Carlson *et al.*, 1988). For the present, the benefit of cholesterol lowering to prevent heart disease after age 65 remains unproven.

It should be noted that the value of general recommendations for cholesterol lowering in middle-aged men is also under scrutiny, because several trials of lipid-lowering medications have found no reduction or even an increase in total mortality (Oliver, 1992). This issue has not been addressed in the elderly. It is possible that lipid-lowering diets or drugs might cause more untoward effects in the aged, in whom dietary restriction or polypharmacy could increase the risk of other illness.

Cigarette smoking

Several studies of older adult men with and without heart disease show a greater probability of survival in those who quit compared to those who continue to smoke (La Croix *et al.*, 1991). Data from the American Cancer Society (Surgeon General's Report, 1990) showed a reduced risk of CVD in both sexes, even when smoking stopped after age 70. Hermanson *et al.* (1988) found that giving up cigarettes significantly reduced the risk of death and of new coronary events in elderly patients with known heart disease, to the same or greater degree than in younger patients (Table 10.2).

Overall, the evidence suggests that the three classic CHD risk factors continue to increase risk in the elderly, at least up to the age of 75 or 80. However, clinical trial data supporting active intervention are available only for treatment of hypertension. In the high-risk patient, decisions not to intervene are difficult to support and are rarely influenced by the absence of data. Prevention for the 'usual risk patient' implies a different risk-benefit ratio, even though most cases come from the population in the middle of the risk-factor distribution. According to Rose (1985), interventions that mimic the evolutionary norm (such as not smoking, eating less fat and salt, and getting more exercise) can be recommended to the general public without a trial, with little fear of harm. Survival of more than half of any population to age 50 is a very recent phenomenon, however. At the turn of this century, 75% of people in the western world died before age 65; now 75% die after age 65 (Brody and Miles, 1990). The elderly do not represent the evolutionary norm!

| | Death | Myocardial infarction or death |
Age group	Relative risk (95% CL)	Relative risk (95% CL)
55–9	1.5 (1.1,2.0)	1.5 (1.2,1.9)
60–4	2.0 (1.5,2.6)	1.4 (1.1,1.9)
65–9	1.4 (0.9,2.0)	1.5 (1.0,2.3)
70+	3.3 (1.5,7.1)	2.9 (1.4,5.9)

Table 10.2: Effects of smoking vs cessation in elderly patients with heart disease. Source: Hermanson *et al.* (1988)

Individual and societal implications

What are the consequences of CHD prevention? In most developed countries, life expectancy at age 65 is now increasing more rapidly than life expectancy at birth, largely because of the reduction in CVD before age 65 (Kinsella, 1992). In the United States, CHD death rates have fallen since 1970, and over half of the fall in total mortality rates has been attributed to a decrease in heart disease deaths. With the postponement of premature mortality, 80% of CHD deaths occur after age 65. The absolute number of heart disease deaths continues to rise, even in countries such as the United States, where CHD death rates have fallen, because the number of elderly at risk is increasing.

The prevention of death from CHD results in more prevalent cases, and raises the spectre of more disabled sick individuals and a greater cost to society. According to the National Heart Lung and Blood Institute, between 1977 and 1987 the decline in the CHD death rate in the USA was parallelled by an 80% increase in the prevalence of CHD and a 150% increase in morbidity costs (Rosen *et al.*, 1990). Because incidence appears to have decreased in all age groups, the increased prevalence presumably represents improved survival with heart disease. Costs rose less than expected because the average duration of hospitalization was reduced by nearly 50% during this same period. Nevertheless, Webster *et al.* (1990) found that heart disease and heart attack account for the largest number of Medicare dollars spent in the last year of life (although heart disease ranks after nephritis, cancer, diabetes and emphysema for cost per patient).

In addition to cost, important questions are being asked about quality of life and active life years. Patients, physicians, and health policy planners question whether we are living longer or dying longer. Brody *et al.* (1990) are concerned that active life expectancy has increased little in proportion to the number of years being lived with disabilities. In contrast, Fries (1980) has proposed a finite life expectancy with a 'compression of morbidity'. The latter more optimistic view is plausible with regard to heart disease prevention. A delay in CHD death should be a delay in morbidity, because many changes in cardiovascular function now attributed to ageing may in fact reflect occult heart disease or the consequences of lifestyle (Geokas *et al.*, 1990). Current recommendations to prevent or postpone heart disease, such as not smoking, exercise, a low-fat high-fibre diet, match advice intended to promote general health and to prevent cancer.

What are the negative consequences of preventing heart disease? There is a widespread belief that behaviour change and improved risk-factor status will replace a sudden cardiovascular death with a slow deterioration or a painful death from cancer. Elderly patients sometimes explain that they will not change a noxious habit because they would prefer to die quickly of a heart attack. There are, however, no guarantees that the heart attack will be fatal. The public does not recognize that heart disease is a major disabler. The Health Interview Survey in the USA found that more than one in four men and women aged 65 and older had known heart disease, of whom one in 10 were disabled (Verbrugge, 1984). Others have reported disability rates as high as 70% in patients with heart disease (Frishman *et al.*, 1987). In a follow-up study of ambulatory men and women aged 80 and older, cardiovascular problems were the main reason reported to cause a change in the ability to walk a quarter of a mile or climb 10 steps (Harris *et al.*, 1989).

There is a price to pay for increasing longevity. Women spend a greater fraction of their lives in a disabled or dependent state, negating some of the benefit of greater female longevity (Kinsella, 1992). One estimate indicated that each year of increased active life expectancy incurs almost four years of compromised healthy living (Guralnik *et al.*, 1986). The number of persons who are blind or deaf, or incapacitated with arthritis, hip fracture or dementia, increases concordantly with the increasing number of persons who do not die before the ages when these conditions become common (Brody *et al.*, 1987). Unless improved survival delays the onset of these diseases, surviving an additional 15 years of quality life beyond age 65 also increases the risk of the conditions that lead to dependency before death.

Among the healthy elderly, dependency is more dreaded than death. Perhaps the largest single concern is the fear of dementia. Some evidence suggests that blood pressure control will reduce multi-infarct dementia (Meyer *et al.*, 1986). Aronson *et al.* (1990) found that women who had known CHD were more likely to become demented than those without heart disease. Nevertheless, Alzheimer's disease is a more common cause of dementia than multi-infarct dementia, and it is likely that measures intended to prevent heart disease will increase longevity and thereby the risk of dementia.

What of hospitalization, institutionalization and community services during these years of extended life? In a study of six health districts in England, Henderson *et al.* (1990) found that the percentage of people aged 65 and older who had had at least one hospital admission in the year before death increased significantly in the decade between 1976 and 1985—but the oldest were less likely to be hospitalized before death than those less than 75 years of age. This somewhat surprising result could be because they are already in a nursing home, because doctors believe interventions to be inappropriate in the elderly, or because the very old represent those who are unusually healthy, as evidence by their having outlived their peers, and who remain quite healthy until just shortly before death.

In a British study (Hall *et al.*, 1990), the proportion of the elderly population who were fit and active was much smaller than the proportion of survivors who were institutionalized or housebound. In the long-lived Rancho Bernardo cohort, where the SMR for CHD was less than half the national average, dependency requiring institutional or community-based service use increased with age, and only 29% of men and 14% of women died without some period of dependency (Barrett-Connor *et al.*, 1991). However, less than 20% were dependent for two or more years before death.

A study in the UK, the USA, Japan and Hungary found that the average duration of illness is inversely proportional to the mortality rate (Riley, 1990). Women seem to use more services than men, and not because they have less or later heart disease. A study of the elderly in Massachusetts found that the percentage of independent remaining years was smaller in women than men at every age (Katz *et al.*, 1983). In Rancho Bernardo, women were more likely to be in a nursing home than men at all ages. In women, the probability of being in a nursing home increased with the number of living children, while the reverse was true for men, suggesting that men are more likely than women to be cared for by a spouse or child in the last year(s) of their life (Barrett-Connor *et al.*, 1991).

What are we to make of all this? Measures to improve the health of the patient and the public appear to have reduced CVD morbidity and mortality and to have played a role in increasing longevity. As Rose and Shipley (1990) noted, '*To the extent that preventive measures succeed in reducing the lifetime probability of death from cardiovascular disease, then there will be a compensatory increase in the probability of death from other causes.*' But just as we would not want to return to the period before 1950—ie before vaccines and antibiotics and sanitation extended the active life years beyond age 50—so we cannot reverse the period from 1950 to the present, when prevention, treatment and lifestyle changes appear to have reduced the risk of CVD and extended the median life expectancy beyond 75 years. We now need to pay more attention to the serious public health and policy questions raised by the fact that we are living long and dying longer.

References

Agner E (1985) Epidemiology of coronary heart disease in the elderly patient. In: Coodley EL (ed.) *Geriatric heart disease*. PSG Publishing, Littleton, Mass. pp. 111–26.

Aronson MK *et al.* (1990) Women, myocardial infarction, and dementia in the very old. *Neurology.* **40**:1102–6.

Barrett-Connor E *et al.* (1984) Ischemic heart disease risk factors after age 50. *Journal of Chronic Disease.* **37**:903–8.

Barrett-Connor E *et al.* (1991) Heart disease risk factors as determinants of dependency and death in an older cohort: the Rancho Bernardo Study. *Journal of Ageing and Health.* **3**:247–61.

Brody JA *et al.* (1987) Trends in the health of the elderly population. *Annual Review of Public Health.* **8**:211–34.

Brody JA and Miles TP (1990) Mortality postponed and the unmasking of age-dependent non-fatal condition. *Ageing.* **2**:283–9.

Carlson LA *et al.* (1988) Reduction of mortality in the Stockholm Ischaemic Heart Disease Secondary Prevention Study by combined treatment with clofibrate and nicotinic acid. *Acta Medica Scandinavica.* **223**:405–18.

Coope J and Warrender TS (1986) Randomised trial of treatment of hypertension in the elderly patients in primary care. *British Medical Journal.* **293**:1145.

Dahlof B *et al.* (1991) Morbidity and mortality in the Swedish Trial in Old Patients with Hypertension (STOP-Hypertension). *The Lancet.* **338**:1281–5.

Dayton S *et al.* (1970) The VA Domicillary Study. Cholesterol, atherosclerosis, ischemic heart disease and stroke. *Annals of Internal Medicine.* **72**:97–109.

Fries JF (1980) Aging, natural death and compression of morbidity. *New England Journal of Medicine.* **303**:130–5.

Frishman WH *et al.* (1987) CV disease in the elderly: clinical assessment. *Journal of the American College of Cardiology.* **10**:48–51A.

Geokas MC *et al.* (1990) The aging process. *Annals of Internal Medicine.* **113**: 455–66.

Guralnik JM *et al.* (1986) Aging in America. A demographic perspective. *Geriatric Cardiology.* **4**:175–86.

Hall RCP *et al.* (1990) Age, pattern of consultation, and functional disability in elderly patients in one general practice. *British Medical Journal.* **301**:42–8.

Harris T *et al.* (1989) Longitudinal study of physical ability in the oldest old. *American Journal of Public Health.* **79**:698–702.

HDFP (1979) Five-years' findings of the Hypertension Detection and Follow-up Program (HDFP). *Journal of the American Medical Association.* **242**: 252–7.

Henderson J *et al.* (1990) Hospital care for the elderly in the final year of life; a population based study. *British Medical Journal.* **301**:17–19.

Hermanson B *et al.* (1988) Beneficial six-year outcome of smoking cessation in older men and women with coronary artery disease: results from the CASS registry. *New England Journal of Medicine.* **319**:1365–9.

Katz S *et al.* (1983) Active life expectancy. *New England Journal of Medicine.* **309**: 1218–24.

Kinsella KG (1992) Changes in life expectancy. *American Journal of Clinical Nutrition.* **55**:1196–202S.

LaCroix AZ *et al.* (1991) Smoking and mortality among older men and women in three communities. *New England Journal of Medicine.* **32**:1619–25.

Langer RD *et al.* (1989) Paradoxical survival of elderly men with high blood pressure. *British Medical Journal.* **298**:1356–8.

Manolio TA *et al.* (1992) Cholesterol and heart disease in older persons and women. Review of the NHLBI Workshop. *Annals of Epidemiology.* **2**:161–76.

Mattila K *et al.* (1988) Blood pressure and five-year survival in the very old. *British Journal of Clinical Research.* **296**:887–9.

Meyer JS *et al.* (1986) Improved cognition after control of risk factors for multi-infarct dementia. *Journal of the American Medical Association.* **26**:2203–9.

MRC Working Party (1992) Medical Research Council trial of treatment of hypertension in older adults: principal results. *British Medical Journal.* **304**:405–12.

Oliver MF (1992) Doubts about preventing coronary heart disease. *British Medical Journal.* **30**:393–4.

Riley JC (1990) Long term morbidity and mortality trends: inverse transition. In: Caldwell JC *et al.* (eds) *What we know about health transition: the cultural, social and behavioral determinants of health. Vol. 1.* Canberra, Australia: Australian National University, Canberra. pp. 165–88.

Rose G (1985) Sick individuals and sick populations. *International Journal of Epidemiology.* **14**:32–8.

Rose G and Shipley M (1990) Effects of coronary risk reduction on the pattern of mortality. *The Lancet.* **335**:275–7.

Rosen RM *et al.* (1990) The report of the American Heart Association Task Force on strategies to increase federal research funding. *Circulation.* **82**:1551–9.

SHEP Cooperative Research Group (1991) Prevention of stroke by antihypertensive drug treatment in older persons with isolated systolic hypertension. *Journal of the American Medical Association.* **265**:3255–64.

Surgeon General's Report (1990) *The health benefits of smoking cessation: a report of the Surgeon General,* 1990 Rockland Md: US Dept of Health and Human Services, Public Health Service, Centers for Disease Control, Center for Chronic Disease Prevention and Health Promotion, Office on Smoking and Health, Washington DC.

Webster JR *et al.* (1990) Ethics and economic realities. *Archives of Internal Medicine.* **150**:1795–7.

Verbrugge LM (1984) Health Interview Survey. A health profile of older women with comparisons to older men. *Research on Aging.* **6**:291–322.

11

Cost-Effective Purchasing of Health Care

RON AKEHURST

The separation of purchasers from providers of health care, which was introduced by the April 1992 reforms to the National Health Service, has produced significant changes in the way health-service managers think about their role. It therefore has great potential for affecting the way in which health care is provided. Traditionally, health-service managers have concentrated on the demands of maintaining a service. The creation of a class of managers solely responsible for purchasing health care has produced a focus on a new range of issues. Initially, and perhaps inevitably, purchasers have had so much to do —writing and agreeing contracts which reflect current practice, and setting up their own organizations—that more fundamental issues have had relatively little attention. Nevertheless, there is an underlying desire and determination to pursue cost-effective purchasing of health care. This chapter explores some of the issues which face a purchasing authority when it sets out to purchase cost-effectively.

Competing desirable ends and scarce means

Economics is the study of choice between competing desirable ends, when the means are too scarce to achieve all of them. Many more services could be provided for a population than can be afforded, and the purchaser has to make hard choices. This is a classic problem of economics, although it may also relate to politics, epidemiology or management theory. Purchasers must maximize the health gain to the population for which they are responsible, and this requires cost-effective purchasing of health care.

Maximizing health gain

The logic of maximization requires that purchasing should be so organized that no net gain could be achieved by switching resources from one set of purchases to another. Being confident that this is the case requires purchasers to answer three very basic questions:

(a) What are the consequences for health of the increased purchases?
(b) What are the consequences for health of the decreased purchases?
(c) How are the consequences of (a) and (b) valued?

These questions are quite simple. However, providing answers will continue to tax a whole research industry. The issues of valuation raised in question (c) are not the subject of this paper. Judgements have to be made, and these are the responsibility of the purchaser. Much effort and debate has gone into generating indices of value, the best known of which is probably the QALY (Quality Adjusted Life Year). However, before such judgements can be applied, whether they employ explicit valuation instruments or not, it is necessary to have knowledge of the health status consequences (however measured) of health interventions, and to understand the resource implications of changes that may be made.

Questions (a) and (b) require further exploration. Every manager who is responsible for purchasing for a population, and who wishes to pursue cost-effectiveness, faces a set of concerns which apply nationally.

What interventions are available? There is a large but finite set of interventions that can be pursued by purchasers, and the first problem is to identify and classify them in some useful form.

What are the key choices on how those interventions are made? Given, for example, that an intervention identified is that of prevention of heart disease by changing dietary habits, there are choices to be made about how it is achieved.

What are the consequences for patients/populations of interventions? If one choice of intervention or style of particular intervention is made, what will the effect be, measured in whatever units are natural or appropriate to the area in question?

What are the resource consequences of making one choice rather than another? For example, what does it cost to pursue one form of prevention of coronary heart disease (CHD) rather than another?

How do the outcome and resource consequences vary with the characteristics of populations? For example, the effectiveness of particular interventions may vary with the sickness of the population. Particular social groups may be resistant to changing their behaviour unless very large sums are spent, whereas other groups may respond more cheaply.

How do the outcomes and resource implications of choice vary with the scale of provision? What happens to the relationship between costs and benefits at the margin as provision is increased? For example, as the rate of coronary artery bypass graft (CABG) in a population goes up, does the marginal benefit decline because all of the necessary quadruple and triple bypasses have been done first? Conversely, do the marginal costs of the operation decline because of economies of scale?

If answers to these questions could be found nationally then they could be applied locally, with local research needed only on the characteristics of the local population and on local cost structures.

Current information

There is little information currently available to an interested purchaser. A classification of available interventions which is both appropriate to contracting and which allows the research literature to be drawn upon has not yet been achieved, and likewise the key choices in each area of intervention have not been identified. Consequences for patients may be known, but many areas of medical practice have been subjected to little or no research on outcomes. Similarly, true resource consequences of choices are rarely known by either purchasers or providers. Sophistications, such as variations with population characteristics or scale effects, are doubly scarce.

There has been a slow realization that information appropriate to assisting purchasing decisions is not readily available, and there are the beginnings of efforts to remedy the situation. Health authorities, both at district and regional level, have tackled particular areas. There is concern at the lack of co-ordination of such efforts. Most authorities have independently looked at CHD and scores of searches have been made of the same literature. The Department of Health has recently announced funding for a clearing house for such efforts which may reduce some of the duplication. The Department has also funded research on outcome measurement at the Universities of Leeds and Aberdeen and on the effectiveness of particular interventions at the Universities of York and Leeds.

Research at the York Health Economics Consortium

Trent and Mersey Regional Health Authorities have funded research at the Health Economics Consortium at the University of York which, in an ambitious manner, tries to overcome several weaknesses of current information in one approach. The approach exploits the fact that most published research on health outcomes is disease-based (rather than specialty-based, which is what purchasing contracts tend to be), but tries to organize the information in such a way that it could be used in contracts led by specialty.

The method used in the Consortium work begins by describing, in the form of a network flow-chart, how patients may first come or be brought into contact with the health services, and then how they may flow through, around, out and back into it. In constructing the network, every effort is made to identify the full range of treatment choices available—partly through discussions with clinicians and partly by looking at practice across a number of health districts. Every branch in the pathway through the system identifies either a choice or the population characteristics that are relevant for determining the number of patients that we would expect to take one path rather than another. The choice nodes define the set of choices about which the purchaser could potentially make decisions and the chance nodes and the probabilities attached to them will reflect the influence of local population characteristics on the outcomes of choices.

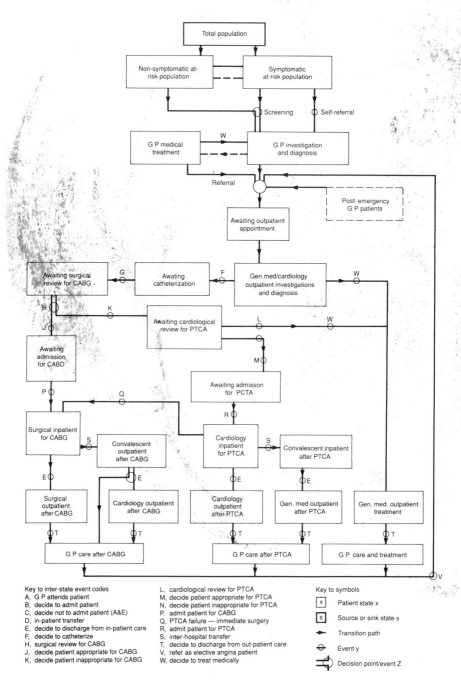

Key to inter-state event codes
A, G P attends patient
B, decide to admit patient
C, decide not to admit patient (A&E)
D, in-patient transfer
E, decide to discharge from in-patient care
F, decide to catheterize
H, surgical review for CABG
J, decide patient appropriate for CABG
K, decide patient inappropriate for CABG

L, cardiological review for PTCA
M, decide patient appropriate for PTCA
N, decide patient inappropriate for PTCA
P, admit patient for CABG
Q, PTCA failure — immediate surgery
R, admit patient for PTCA
S, inter-hospital transfer
T, decide to discharge from out-patient care
V, refer as elective angina patient
W, decide to treat medically

Key to symbols

| x | Patient state x |

| s | Source or sink state s |

➤ Transition path

⊖ Event y

⊟⇒ Decision point/event Z

Figure 11.1: CHD treatment paths: elective patients/angina. All states are self-repeating, and have transition paths to death (sink) and to emergency stream.

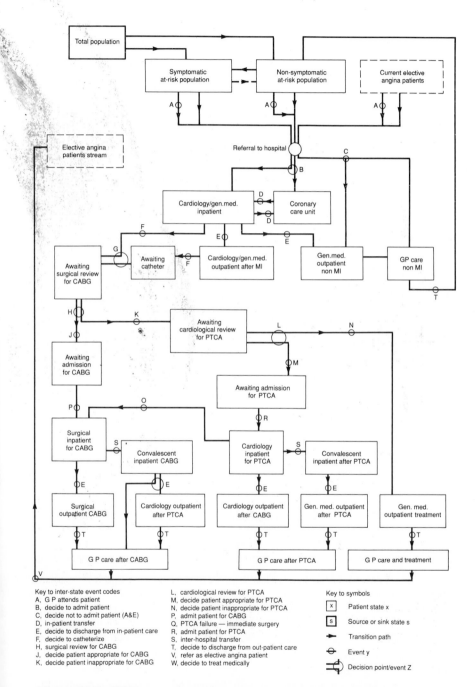

Key to inter-state event codes
A, G P attends patient
B, decide to admit patient
C, decide not to admit patient (A&E)
D, in-patient transfer
E, decide to discharge from in-patient care
F, decide to catheterize
H, surgical review for CABG
J, decide patient appropriate for CABG
K, decide patient inappropriate for CABG

L, cardiological review for PTCA
M, decide patient appropriate for PTCA
N, decide patient inappropriate for PTCA
P, admit patient for CABG
Q, PTCA failure — immediate surgery
R, admit patient for PTCA
S, inter-hospital transfer
T, decide to discharge from out-patient care
V, refer as elective angina patient
W, decide to treat medically

Key to symbols

| x | Patient state x

| s | Source or sink state s

→ Transition path

⊖ Event y

⇒ Decision point/event Z

Figure 11.2: CHD treatment paths: emergency patients – ? M.I./cres. angina. All states are self-repeating, and have transition paths to death (sink).

The network flow charts are used to organize the further gathering information. The steps are as follows:

1 Identify the key choices.
2 Add information on what the splits are likely to be at the chance nodes, and relate that to population characteristics and the scale of provision.
3 Identify likely outcomes down each leg. This might be done using evidence published from clinical trials or from reports of consensus conferences or, if all else fails, using the opinions of clinicians.
4 Identify the resources likely to be used down each leg.

Examples of flow-charts relating to CHD with particular emphasis on surgery, are shown in Figures 11.1 and 11.2.

Use of the information from the network flow-charts

So far, work has made substantial progress in the following areas:

- lung cancer
- CHD
- childhood deafness
- maternity services
- schizophrenia.

Work is at an early stage on:

- asthma
- stroke
- epilepsy
- visual impairment.

For each of the areas covered, a document shows how the flow-chart was created and records the literature review relating to the key choices identified. This is used to produce a smaller and more readable purchasers' guide which identifies the cost and effectiveness (and other) issues which are relevant at each key choice node. The guide may make strong statements about desirable or undesirable choices. It will distinguish between circumstances where there is good evidence of ineffectiveness and where there is no evidence one way or the other.

More ambitiously, software will be produced to allow the purchaser to answer hypothetical questions. For example, what would the cost and outcome consequences be of purchasing a further 100 CABGs per year? What would the consequences be of purchasing an extra 300 cardiology out-patient attendances? Are there bottlenecks in the system which prevent benefits being achieved? So far, such software has only been produced for lung cancer, but work is proceeding in other areas.

Once such software is available for many areas, the questions could move from how services should be provided to how much of each should be provided. If radical radiotherapy and chemotherapy for lung cancer sufferers is reduced, what resources could be saved and what consequences would there be for health? If the same sum could be made available for CHD treatment, what would be gained there? The purchaser would still have to make a hard judgement on whether funds should be transferred, but it would be based on firmer information than in the current situation where information is almost totally lacking.

The future

It is quite clear that organizing information needed to support purchasing will take a long time, and that information will always be imperfect. Nevertheless, the questions now being asked will mean that new information will be assembled. A focus on both broad and detailed cost-effectiveness issues will develop further and show itself in contract specifications and the mix of services to be bought. The most profound effects of the NHS reforms are yet to come.

12

Atherosclerosis—The Link Between Arterial Intimal Lesions and Myocardial Infarction

MJ DAVIES

The vast majority of human myocardial infarcts are due to coronary atherosclerosis. This chapter explores the link between the two conditions and considers how risk factors operate.

The basic process of atherosclerosis

Atherosclerosis is a focal rather than a diffuse intimal disease. It is a disease of large and medium-sized arteries but some, such as the internal mammary, are spared. Coronary, aortic and cerebral involvement is frequently disparate in the same individual. The focal plaques of atherosclerosis are best appreciated when arteries are slit open and the intimal surface is viewed *en face*. Each plaque contains two major components, lipid and collagen. These two components form the bulk of plaque and contribute to one facet of the clinical symptomatology in that the plaque may directly encroach on the lumen. In the coronary arteries a flow-limiting stenosis may be produced, leading to stable angina.

A second facet of atherosclerosis is that one or more plaques may enter an unstable phase and be complicated by thrombosis. The result is unstable angina or acute infarction. A third feature is that atherosclerotic vessels have diffuse abnormalities of vascular tonal responses which favour vasoconstriction (Ganz *et al.*, 1991) on exercise. The final feature of atherosclerosis is that, although it is an intimal disease, there is a secondary medial loss which may result in aneurysm formation.

Against this background there are some more detailed aspects of the plaque which are important in understanding how clinical symptoms develop, and the pathogenesis of the disease itself. The amount of lipid varies widely from plaque to plaque even in the same individual. The lipid may be either extracellular or intracellular; the intracellular lipid is contained predominantly in foam cells of monocyte origin. The connective tissue matrix proteins—collagen, elastin and proteoglycans—form the basic framework of the plaque, and without them the whole plaque would collapse. These matrix proteins are produced by smooth muscle cells acting in their synthetic phenotype.

Calcification is common in atherosclerotic plaques and forms in both lipid and collagen as nodular or lamellar masses. Since it is deposited on pre-existing plaque constituents it does not contribute to plaque growth or volume itself.

Atherosclerotic plaques are increasingly being regarded as the site of an inflammatory response to vessel wall injury. In addition to monocyte-macrophage foam cells, numerous T lymphocytes are present (Hansson *et al.*, 1989). Numerous cytokines and adhesion molecules are expressed by cells within the plaque. Lipid, particularly when it has undergone oxidation (Steinberg *et al.*, 1989), is one of the factors inducing inflammatory activation.

Progression of atherosclerotic lesions in man

Morphological studies of atherosclerosis have been dominated by descriptions of the lesions as seen *en face* in arteries opened at autopsy. Viewed in this manner the intimal surface of the human aorta affected by atherosclerosis can be seen to contain plaques which vary in size and appearance. The appearances at autopsy represent just one point in time in a disease evolving over years. It was probably safe only to assume that large plaques grow from smaller plaques. The work by Stary (1989) has been a major advance in understanding the disease. In his study the aortae and coronary arteries of subjects dying from accidents or other clear non-cardiac causes were examined in great detail. Cohorts of individuals were gathered in five-year steps from infancy onward. In this way the age at which lesions of a particular type appeared could be noted, and the evolutionary sequence of plaque types inferred.

The study has shown that all human infant hearts develop intimal thickening in the coronary arteries, and that this thickening is focally accentuated at points of branching. The intimal thickening contains smooth muscle cells which are presumed to have migrated in from the media. Stary has argued that this intimal thickening is adaptive, and should not be regarded as atherosclerosis. However, it may mean that human arteries are presensitized to the development of atherosclerosis if certain conditions prevail in later life. The coronary arteries of many small animals such as the rabbit do not have intimal smooth muscle cells, and for these species a necessary prerequisite of atherosclerosis is migration of smooth muscle cells from the media.

The development of atherosclerosis begins with flat yellow dots or streaks on the intimal surface. These consist of lipid-filled foam cells accumulating in the intima. There is evidence from comparative geographic studies that while fatty streaks are the earliest atherosclerotic lesion many must either remain static or even vanish. Fatty streaks appear in the parts of the coronary artery tree where in later life advanced plaques appear. If, on the other hand, hearts are examined from young subjects drawn from populations in which little or no advanced atherosclerosis occurs they also have an eqivalent number of fatty streaks (Freedman *et al.*, 1988). The question of the relationship of fatty streaks to advanced lesions is of more than academic interest. Short-term animal models of atherosclerosis induced by high dietary lipid reproduce essentially the fatty streak stage of human disease; yet it is in such models that drugs are often tested for their anti-atherogenic affect.

The Stary study suggests that fatty streaks are succeeded by a stage in which extracellular lipid appears within the intima. Smooth muscle proliferation occurs next and forms a layer separating the extracellular lipid from the lumen. Collagen and elastin are produced in increasingly greater amounts; the plaque grows and is now raised above the surface. Stary termed this 'advanced plaque formation': at this stage, elevated plaques are usually oval in shape with the long axis in the direction of blood flow, and often a centimetre or more in length in the aorta. Most individuals from the developed world will have some such advanced plaques by the age of 20 to 30 years.

The advanced plaque is more usually called the raised fibrolipid plaque. As seen in the aorta, it is a raised lesion ranging in colour from yellow (if there is a preponderance of lipid) to white (if collagen is preponderant).

There is abundant epidemiological and geographic information from large autopsy studies on the relevance of the raised plaque to symptoms (Robertson and Strong, 1968; Strong et al., 1968; Deupree et al., 1973). The amount of the intimal surface of the aorta and coronary arteries covered by raised plaques, in a particular population, closely mirrors the actual frequency of death from ischaemic heart disease in that population. The inference is that the greater the number of atherosclerotic plaques in an individual, the greater is the risk of clinically expressed disease. While this is so, it must be remembered that there will always be unlucky individuals who die from one strategically placed plaque, and who have little atherosclerosis elsewhere.

Comparative autopsy studies (PDAY Research Group, 1990) also show that groups such as diabetics, smokers, those with hypertension and those with elevated plasma lipids all have more raised plaques in the coronary arteries than subjects without these risk factors. The inference is that one way in which risk factors operate in atheroslcerosis is simply to increase the number of raised plaques rather than altering the nature of plaques.

The evolution of clinical symptoms in man

The substrate on which the clinical symptoms of atherosclerosis develop is the advanced raised fibrolipid plaque. Atherosclerosis can be considered as a two-stage process: first, raised plaques are formed, and then complications of these plaques lead to symptoms.

Advanced fibrolipid plaques cannot necessarily be seen on angiography. The angiogram is nothing more than a cast of the lumen, and provides few data on the arterial wall itself. The angiogram underestimates the amount of wall disease by a variable and unpredictable degree. There are two reasons for this insensitivity. The first is that the vessel wall has considerable capacity for remodelling (Glagov et al., 1987). As atherosclerosis develops, the media remodels to accommodate the intimal plaques, preserving lumen dimensions by increasing the external diameter of the vessel. Only when this remodelling potential is exhausted does narrowing of the lumen occur. Secondly the media behind atherosclerotic plaques undergo marked atrophy of the smooth muscle cells, and the internal elastic lamina fragments and ruptures. The result is that the plaque bulges outward rather than inward. In extreme cases a plaque is extruded almost completely from the original outline of the vessel wall. Thus a normal coronary angiogram can conceal large plaques. The Stary study suggests that 'new' lesions appearing in a coronary angiogram, far from being new, represent a change in a lesion which have been there for perhaps 10–15 years.

Microanatomy of raised fibrolipid plaques

In vessels which have been distended at physiological pressures the plaques are usually eccentric, ie involving only one segment of the vessel wall. The plaque bulges outward rather than inward and the lumen retains a circular shape. The plaque has a central core of extracellular lipid comprised of cholesterol, some of which is esterfied and some crystalline. The lipid cord of the plaque is often devoid of connective tissue: ie there is a potential space within the plaque. This space is filled with the lipid 'gruel' which is so typical of atherosclerosis. External pressure on the plaque in the autopsy room can extrude material with the consistency of toothpaste from the lipid core. The lipid core itself is a highly thrombogenic material containing Tissue Factor released from lipid-filled foam cells, collagen fibrils and lipid surfaces. In the stable intact plaque the lipid core is separated from the arterial lumen by the cap. Cap tissue has considerable tensile strength, being formed of a matrix of collagen and elastin. The lumenal surface of the plaque cap is covered by endothelial cells but they do not contribute to the mechanical strength of the cap. The lipid core is thought to be derived from the death of lipid-filled macrophage foam cells, but surrounding the core there is usually a layer of surviving foam cells.

The proportion of total plaque volume occupied by the lipid core varies widely even in the same individual. At one extreme the lipid core may occupy up to 80% of the plaque; at the other extreme it may be absent and the plaque consists almost entirely of collagen. The relation between these two components of plaque volume is uncertain. It is possible that plaques which consist almost entirely of collagen may once have had a lipid pool which has been replaced by fibrous tissue. In primate animal models, lipid lowering will lead to lipid-rich plaques becoming more solid. On the other hand, solid fibrous plaques in humans may have a different pathogenesis from the start.

Plaque progression

Advanced fibrolipid plaques advance by one of two mechanisms (Figure 12.1). The primary processes of atherosclerosis are lipid accumulation and collagen production. Either can increase the total plaque volume, but the two processes are not directly coupled. These primary processes of atherosclerosis may cause the volume of an individual plaque to reach the stage where remodelling within the arterial wall is overcome. The result is increasing stenosis at one point in the arterial tree. In general, very high-grade stenosis (>70% diameter stenosis) is

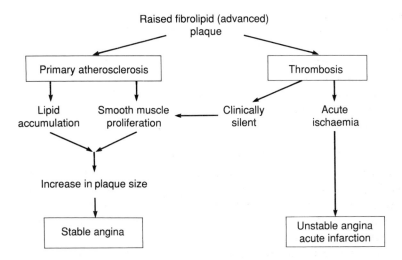

Figure 12.1: Diagrammatic representation of the possible pathways for progression of a coronary advanced plaque to clinical symptoms.

associated with plaques which are predominantly fibrous, while lipid-rich plaques are more common at lower grades of obstruction. The second way in which plaques progress is by becoming unstable and undergoing thrombosis. This thrombosis may be either clinically silent, or clinically expressed as type B unstable angina and acute myocardial infarction. There are good clinical, pathological and theoretical grounds for believing that silent thrombosis is a major factor in driving smooth muscle proliferation and increasing plaque size in many subjects with coronary atherosclerosis, irrespective of whether thrombosis has been recognized clinically. A major part of this evidence is the finding of small recent plaque fissures in up to 16% of individuals with coronary atherosclerosis but who died of non-cardiac causes (Davies *et al.*, 1989).

Mechanisms of thrombosis over plaques

Two distinct mechanisms exist for the induction of thrombosis over plaques (Fuster *et al.*, 1992*a,b*). In superficial intimal injury the endothelium alone is lost. Subendothelial connective tissue is exposed and there is platelet adhesion and activation. In deep intimal injury a plaque tears open, exposing its thrombogenic centre to the blood in the lumen. Blood initially enters the plaque from the lumen and the thrombosis is initially within the plaque itself.

Superficial intimal injury

Animal models of atherosclerosis show that the initiation of atherosclerosis involves the migration of monocytes into the intima through an intact endothelial surface (Faggiotto *et al.*, 1984). There is no exposure of the subendothelial collagen and no platelet adhesion to the vessel wall. Platelet-derived growth factors cannot be a factor initiating smooth muscle cell proliferation.

Animal models (Faggiotto and Ross, 1984) are in agreement that, once raised plaques are established, breaks do appear in the endothelial surface and platelets do adhere. Such endothelial denudation is almost ubiquitous over raised human plaques (Burrig, 1991; Davies *et al.*, 1988*a,b*). The platelets are deposited as a monolayer, restricted to areas to where endothelial cells have been lost, and are ultramicroscopic, being demonstrated by scanning electron microscopy. Nevertheless they are a potential source of growth factors for smooth muscle cell plaques.

Ultramicroscopic thrombi are very different in size from anything that would be visible angiographically. However, endothelial denudation may occur over a large area; it is then associated with larger thrombi which may become visible macroscopically at autopsy, or on angiography in life. Occlusive thrombi may develop, particularly in smaller coronary vessels such as the left marginal or posterior descending coronary arteries.

Deep intimal injury

Splits, fissures or tears into the plaque from the lumen allow the ingress of blood and lead initially to a platelet-rich thrombus developing within the plaque itself (Davies and Thomas, 1985). This may be followed by healing, with smooth muscle proliferation resealing the tear, or by the development of thrombosis within the arterial lumen. In the latter case, clinical symptoms may develop due to acute myocardial ischaemia. The process was described by pathologists as long ago as the last century, but only recently has it been accorded its rightful place as the major factor precipitating coronary thrombosis. This followed more detailed pathological studies using angiography, and studies of live subjects using angioscopy.

The magnitude of the tear in the plaque varies between 100 and 200 μm to several millimetres. The larger the tear the more likely is there to be a large intraplaque thrombosis distorting and expanding the plaque. The larger the plaque tear, the greater is the exposure of thrombogenic surfaces and the greater the likelihood of intraluminal thrombosis. Plaque fissuring should be seen first, as a relatively common process, and second as a stimulus to the formation of intraluminal thrombosis. Numerous factors probably govern whether such thrombosis does occur. Some are local within the plaque itself, and include the degree of plaque disruption; others are systemic, and include the thrombogenic and thrombolytic potential of the subject at the time. One way in which risk factors operate is to increase the risk of thrombosis when an episode of plaque fissuring and instability occurs (Meade and North, 1980).

Intraluminal thrombosis is first mural, develops over the site of plaque disruption and is largely platelet-derived. At this stage, distal embolization of platelet-rich fragments of thrombus into the myocardium occurs (Falk, 1985; Davies *et al.*, 1986). Such emboli are associated with focal myocardial necrosis and with episodes of resting angina. This stage of the evolution of coronary thrombosis is typical of that found in unstable angina and there is a highly characteristic angiographic appearance, with the culprit lesion showing a ragged eccentric stenosis with an overlying intraluminal filling defect. Some patients stay in this stage until healing of the plaque occurs, while others progress to the formation of an occlusive thrombus.

The final occluding stage of the thrombotic process is different in that fibrin and red cells predominate. It is therefore not surprising that this final element of the thrombus is very susceptible to fibrinolysis whether this is therapeutically administered or spontaneous. Restoration of antegrade flow will once again reveal an unstable plaque with overlying mural thrombus. The factors which govern the transition from mural to occlusive thrombus (Fuster *et al.*, 1992*a,b*) must include the degree of exposure of lipid and the residual antegrade flow. Marked reduction of flow over the lesion—whether this is due to rapid expansion of the plaque by intraplaque thrombosis, local spasm, or a rise in distal resistance—will all favour occluding thrombus formation.

Pathogenesis of plaque fissuring

A key consideration in plaque stability is the mechanical strength of the cap tissue. The larger the proportion of the total plaque volume occupied by extracellular lipid, the greater the risk of an episode of fissuring or tearing in the cap (Richardson *et al.*, 1989; Mizuno *et al.*, 1991). One factor is that the lipid core is not capable of carrying a mechanical load; circumferential wall stress during systole is therefore redistributed and concentrated on the cap tissue (Richardson *et al.*, 1989). Alongside this elevation of stress, the cap tissue may undergo changes in structure which weaken its ability to resist fracture. These changes include a reduction in collagen content, infiltration by lipid-filled macrophages and a loss of smooth muscle cells. The key factor may be increasing degrees of 'inflammatory' activity disturbing the normal balance between smooth muscle cell proliferation and monocyte infiltration. In this regard, smooth muscle proliferation may be the stabilizing factor in plaques, and any reduction increases the risk of thrombosis. Any factor which increases the inflammatory activity and lipid content of plaques will enhance instability; conversely anything which reverses these factors may stabilize plaques and reduce the subsequent risk of acute ischaemic events. It is the nature of the plaque itself which governs the risk of instability and not the degree of stenosis. Clinical studies suggest that the risk is greatest with plaques which are either not visible or cause minor stenosis on angiography. Intravascular ultrasound (Nissen *et al.*, 1991), with its ability to visualize the vessel wall, may be the method of detecting potentially dangerous plaques in the future.

Pathogenesis of acute myocardial infarction

Regional infarction is now clearly recognized to be due to thrombosis in the artery subtending that segment of myocardium (Davies *et al.*, 1990). Of these, around 70% are due to plaque fissuring, 30% due to more superficial intimal injury over a plaque. When angiographic studies are carried out in life, the shorter the interval between the onset of symptoms and the angiogram, the higher is the frequency of occlusive thrombosis without antegrade flow (DeWood et al., 1985; Stadius et al., 1985). The frequency of total occlusion falls with time, even without fibrinolytic therapy, emphasizing the labile nature of thrombosis and the natural repair responses of the arterial wall.

References

Burrig K (1991) The endothelium of advanced arteriosclerotic plaques in humans. *Arteriosclerosis and Thrombosis*. **11**:1678–89.

Davies M and Thomas A (1985) Plaque fissuring—the cause of acute myocardial infarction, sudden ischaemic death and crescendo angina. *British Heart Journal*. **53**:363–73.

Davies M et al. (1986) Intramyocardial platelet aggregation in patients with unstable angina suffering sudden ischaemic cardiac death. *Circulation*. **73**:418–27.

Davies et al. (1988a) Endothelial integrity in human coronary arteries. *British Heart Journal*. **59**:101.

Davies M et al. (1988b) Morphology of the endothelium over atherosclerotic plaques in human coronary arteries. *British Heart Journal*. **60**:459–64.

Davies M et al. (1989) Factors influencing the presence or absence of acute coronary artery thrombi in sudden ischaemic death. *European Heart Journal*. **10**:203–8.

Davies M (1990) A macroscopic and microscopic view of coronary thrombi. *Circulation*. **82**:1138–46.

Deupree R et al. (1973) Atherosclerotic lesions and coronary heart disease. Key relationships in necropsied cases. *Laboratory Investigation*. **28**:252–62.

DeWood M et al. (1985) Prevalence and significance of spontaneous thrombolysis in transmural myocardial infarction. *European Heart Journal*. **6**:33.

Faggiotto A et al. (1984) Studies of hypercholesterolaemia in the non-human primate. I Changes that lead to fatty streak formation. *Arteriosclerosis*. **4**:323–40.

Faggiotto A and Ross R (1984) Studies of hypercholesterolaemia in non-human primates. II Fatty streak conversion to fibrous plaque. *Arteriosclerosis*. **4**:341–56.

Falk E (1985) Unstable angina with fatal outcome: dynamic coronary thrombosis leading to infarction and/or sudden death. *Circulation*. **71**:699–708.

Freedman D et al. (1989) Black-white differences in aortic fatty streaks in adolescence and early adulthood: the Bogalusa Heart Study. *Circulation*. **77**:856.

Fuster V *et al*. (1992*a*) Mechanisms of disease: the pathogenesis of coronary artery disease and the acute coronary syndromes I. *New England Journal of Medicine*. **326**:242–50.

Fuster V *et al*. (1992*b*) The pathogenesis of coronary artery disease and the acute coronary syndrome II. *New England Journal of Medicine*. **326**:310–18.

Ganz P *et al*. (1991) Coronary vasospasm in humans: the role of atherosclerosis and of impaired endothelial vasodilator function. *Basic Research in Cardiology*. **86**:215–22.

Glagov S *et al*. (1987) Compensatory enlargement of human atherosclerotic coronary arteries. *New England Journal of Medicine*. **316**:1371–5.

Hansson G *et al*. (1989) Immune mechanisms in atherosclerosis. *Arteriosclerosis*. **9**:567–78.

Meade T *et al*. (1980) Haemostatic function and cardiovascular death: early results of a prospective study. *The Lancet*. **i**:1050–4.

Mizuno K *et al*. (1991) Angioscopic coronary macromorphology in patients with acute coronary disorders. *The Lancet*. **337**:809–12.

Nissen S *et al*. (1991) Differences in ultravascular plaque morphology in stable and unstable patients. *Circulation*. **84**:436A.

PDAY Research Group (1990) Relationship of atherosclerosis in young men to serum lipoprotein cholesterol concentrations and smoking. A preliminary report from the pathological determinant of atherosclerosis in youth study. *Journal of the American Medical Association*. **264**:3018–24.

Richardson P *et al*. (1989) Influence of plaque configuration and stress distribution on fissuring of coronary atherosclerotic plaques. *The Lancet*. **ii**:941–4.

Robertson W and Strong J (1968) Atherosclerosis in persons with hypertension and diabetes mellitus. *Laboratory Investigation*. **18**:538–51.

Stadius M *et al*. (1985) Coronary anatomy and left ventricular function in the first 12 hours of acute myocardial infarction: the Western Washington randomized intracoronary streptokinase trial. *Circulation*. **72**:292–301.

Stary H (1989) Evolution and progression of atherosclerotic lesions in coronary arteries of children and young adults. *Arteriosclerosis*. **9**:1–19.

Steinberg D *et al*. (1989) Beyond cholesterol. Modifications of low-density lipoprotein that increases its atherogenicity. *New England Journal of Medicine*. **320**:915–24.

Strong J *et al*. (1968) Atherosclerosis in persons with coronary heart disease. *Laboratory Investigation*. **18**:527–37.

13

Dietary Fat and Coronary Heart Disease

PN DURRINGTON

The two major nutritional influences on coronary heart disease (CHD) risk are obesity and the type of dietary fat. Obesity is discussed in Chapter 17. However, in a society such as ours in which fat averages 40% of dietary energy, fat intake and obesity are intimately associated. In 1984 the Committee on the Medical Aspects of Food Policy (COMA) recommended a reduction in the intake of fat, particularly saturated fat. Since then there has been absolutely no change in the nation's average fat intake. There has been an increase in the consumption of polyunsaturated fat (probably largely as a result of major commercial advertising campaigns) so that on average it now approaches the level recommended by COMA. This chapter discusses evidence linking diet and CHD and its antecedents, particularly hyperlipidaemia, and then examines the latest recommendations from COMA (1991) in the light of this.

It is a fact universally acknowledged that CHD rates vary enormously throughout the world and that when people from regions of low CHD prevalence move to live in regions of high prevalence they assume a higher CHD risk. The major reason for this geographical variation in CHD is nutritional. CHD seems to follow northern European cuisine wherever it has travelled. Thus in northern Europe itself, North America, South Africa, Australia and New Zealand we find the highest rates with countries such as Poland, the former East Germany and the former Soviet Union showing the most rapidly rising levels as they both introduce food production and importation policies similar to those of other northern European countries. De Langen first observed the influence of the northern European diet on CHD when he compared the prevalence of CHD in Europeans, Javanese stewards on Dutch ships and Javanese not adopting a Western diet (de Langen, 1918). Since then there have been many similar studies, most significantly the Seven Countries Study (Keys, 1970). This was notable not only for its scale and design, but also because it included countries in southern Europe as well as Japan. This is important because the Mediterranean countries and Japan have low CHD rates, but do not have diets which are unattractive or which lack essential nutrients. It is one thing, for example, to point out that rural Africa or China have escaped the epidemic of CHD, but quite another to suggest that the richest nations of the world should adopt the tedious, often malnutritious, diet of the poorest.

In the Seven Countries Study the correlation between total fat intake and CHD rate was not as close as that between CHD and the ratio of polyunsaturated fat (PUFA) and saturated fat (SFA). This, therefore, suggests that even if we are not able to influence total fat consumption, there may be advantages to changing the type of fat we eat. We should not, however, lose sight of the fact that the Japanese—whose CHD rates are lower than Mediterranean Europe—not only have a diet with an even higher ratio of PUFA to SFA, but also a much higher proportion of their dietary energy in the form of carbohydrate.

Fatty acid biochemistry (Durrington, 1989)

Fatty acids comprise a hydrocarbon chain terminating usually at one end in a methyl group and at the other in a carboxyl group. They are found in structural lipids such as phospholipids and in cholesteryl esters. In the form of triglycerides they constitute the principal energy store in mobile animals. Pure fat yields 9 cal (38 mJ) per gram and pure carbohydrates 4 cal (17 mJ) per gram. The difference is due to the presence of more oxygen atoms in carbohydrate— unnecessary in an energy store for an aerobic environment. In practice, however, a gram of adipose cells stores almost 8 cal (34 mJ) whereas a gram of liver or of wheat will contain substantially less than 1 cal (4.2 mJ). This is because triglycerides are intensely hydrophobic and eschew water so that the adipose cell typically consists of a central droplet of triglyceride with its surrounding cytoplasm occupying only some 15% of the cell. Carbohydrate, even in the form of glycogen or starch, remains osmotically active and only comparatively small amounts can be stored in an ocean of cytoplasm. Plants and sessile animals may utilize carbohydrates as an energy store, because weight and its effects on mobility are unimportant, but even plants tend to use fat as an energy store in their seeds where excess weight will hamper dispersion. Hence olives, maize, sunflower seeds, coconuts and other nuts and seeds are important sources of nutritional fats.

The fatty acid hydrocarbon chain may contain no double bonds (a saturated fatty acid) or may do so (an unsaturated fatty acid). Fatty acids with one double bond are called monounsaturated and those with more than one, polyunsaturated.

The double bonds in a fatty acid link two carbon atoms, each of which is bonded to a single hydrogen atom. The single hydrogen atoms may lie on opposite sides of the double bond (trans isomer) or on the same side (cis isomer). Most natural fatty acids are cis isomers. However, trans isomers are formed in the gut of ruminants (thus they enter the diet in dairy products) and in the manufacture of margarine. The properties of cis unsaturated fatty acids are very different from those of trans isomers and of SFAs. This is because the asymmetrical disposition of hydrogen atoms in a cis double introduces a bend into their hydrocarbon chain whereas the chains of trans isomers and SFAs are

	Frequently used name	Melting point
Saturated		
C12:0	Lauric acid	44
C14:0	Myristic acid	54
C16:0	Palmitic acid	63
C18:0	Stearic acid	70
Unsaturated		
Omega 9		
C18:1 cis	Oleic acid	11
C18:1 trans	Elaidic acid	45
Omega 6		
C18:2	Linoleic acid	−5
Omega 3		
C18:3	Linolenic acid	−11
C20:5	Eicosapentaenoic acid (EPA)	−50
C20:6	Docosahexaenoic acid (DHA)	−54

Table 13.1: Major dietary fatty acids.

straight. Fatty acids which are trans or saturated lie readily side by side, whereas their cis relatives do not pack easily together and occupy more space. This means that the freezing point of unsaturated fatty acids is much lower than saturated and trans fatty acids of similar size (Table 13.1). Cold-blooded animals and plant tissues can contain only those fatty acids which remain liquid at the temperatures of their environment. Thus fish which live in cold waters, such as cod and halibut, contain highly polyunsaturated fatty acids such as eicosapentaenoic and docosahexaenoic acid with five and six double bonds respectively. These they acquire from other fish in their diet, which have grazed on phytoplankton. Warm-blooded animals can have saturated fats throughout their body tissues with higher melting points, but those which have a cold environment whose skin temperature is similar to the ambient temperature, such as seals and whales, must have blubber, which contains highly unsaturated fats or it would lose its fluidity and become a rigid straitjacket. These fats are acquired from dietary phytoplankton directly or via other animals in their food chain which graze on it.

Fatty acid nomenclature

A commonly used classification of fatty acids is to describe them according to their chain length (eg C16, C18), then to add the number of double bonds after a colon (eg C16:0, C18:1). The position of the last of any double bonds present is shown by its distance from the terminal methyl group in terms of carbon atoms. The carbon of the terminal methyl group is always called the omega carbon (the last letter of the Greek alphabet: the alpha, beta, gamma etc, carbons are at the other end of the chain). This gives rise to three major series of unsaturated fatty acids: the omega 3, omega 6 and omega 9 fatty acids (Table 13.1).

Effect of different fatty acids in human diet on serum lipoproteins

Saturated fat

The dietary fatty acid with the greatest influence on serum cholesterol levels are the SFAs with chain length 12–16 (Table 13.1) (Malmros and Wigand, 1957; Hegsted *et al.*, 1965; Keys *et al.*, 1965; Grundy, 1987; Durrington, 1989) These all raise the cholesterol and their exclusion from the diet lowers serum cholesterol and frequently also triglycerides. Trans fatty acids probably also raise serum cholesterol. Stearic acid (C18:0) unlike the other saturated fatty acids is neutral with regard to its effects on serum lipids, probably because it does not achieve high levels in the circulating lipids due to its conversion to oleic acid (C18:1).

Many people in Britain eat far more saturated fat than is good for them (on average 50% of the British diet is saturated and 5% trans fatty acids). When this is part of a diet which is already overendowed with energy, there is no nutritional reason for substituting any other energy source. However, in the non-obese energy must be substituted. There are even those who would recommend that, if a decrease in overall fat is not achievable, less harmful energy sources should nonetheless replace saturated fat even in the obese. A major debate has centred on whether monounsaturated fat, PUFA or carbohydrate should replace SFA in the diet.

Carbohydrate

The present balance of evidence would be that substitution of SFA with carbohydrate decreases the serum cholesterol less than when PUFA or monounsaturated fat is substituted (Grundy, 1987; Mensink and Katan, 1987). Carbohydrate also leads to a rise in serum triglycerides and to a decrease in high-density lipoprotein (HDL) cholesterol. It should, however, not be forgotten that those countries with the lowest rates of CHD subsist on a diet in which a much higher proportion of dietary energy is derived from carbohydrate and substantially less from fats, and that in Britain the major dietary change this century paralleling the rising CHD rate has been a decrease in carbohydrate intake in favour of fat. There is also evidence that diabetes is less common in nations subsisting on a high-carbohydrate/low-fat diet (WHO, 1985) and that the adoption of such a diet improves glucose tolerance, whereas a high-fat diet makes it worse (Himsworth, 1935)

Polyunsaturated fats

Linoleic acid lowers serum cholesterol and frequently also triglycerides (Chait *et al.*, 1974; Durrington *et al.*, 1977; Sommariva *et al.*, 1978; Grundy, 1987) when substituted for dietary saturated fat. Some authors have suggested that linoleic acid may lower serum HDL cholesterol slightly (Shepherd *et al.*, 1978; Grundy, 1987). Linoleic acid (in corn oil, sunflower seed oil, margarine etc) has been widely adopted in the diet in Britain and this is one of the few nutritional changes of recent years. This should not be viewed without some misgivings. There are no natural populations, in whom the principal oils consumed are rich in linoleic acid, so we cannot judge its long-term safety from international mortality statistics (as we can with carbohydrate or olive oil). Linoleic acid, like other PUFAs can be shown in experiments to decrease resistance to infection or neoplasia (Bennett *et al.*, 1987). Furthermore, fatty acids with double bonds are susceptible to oxidation and this susceptibility seems to increase with increasing numbers of double bonds. Low-density lipoprotein (LDL) from people on a linoleic acid-rich diet oxidizes more readily than that from people taking a diet rich in monounsaturated fat (Reaven *et al.*, 1991; Bonanome, 1992). Oxidation of LDL is believed to be important in the initiation of atheroma.

Fish oil (usually cod liver or halibut liver oil) containing EPA and DHA lowers serum triglycerides (Sanders, 1990). Generally it has no effect on total cholesterol or HDL cholesterol. In patients with marked hypertriglyceridaemia serum cholesterol may decrease. This is, however, due to a reduction in VLDL cholesterol and LDL cholesterol tends to rise. Like other fat, highly polyunsaturated fats produce a decline in glycaemic control in diabetes (Glauber *et al.*, 1988; Kasim *et al.*, 1988; Schectman *et al.*, 1988). Fish oil was associated with a decrease in myocardial reinfarction in one large trial (Burr *et al.*, 1989). Any beneficial effects it may have, however, require further evaluation and may have little to do with its action on lipids, but result from its effects on platelets. It should thus be evaluated alongside aspirin. There is no objection to fish in the diet. There are, however, no adequate dietary data about large amounts of highly polyunsaturated fats in the diet. The story that Eskimos do not get CHD is seriously flawed since the statistics are not supported by post-mortem studies and accounts of the physical fitness of Eskimos are highly anecdotal. Death due to infection was common amongst Eskimos and so also were deaths due to accidents and drowning. These days, few Eskimos maintain their traditional way of life, and stories of their healthiness must remain a romantic notion.

Monounsaturated fats

Traditionally olive oil, which is rich in oleic acid, has been a major constituent of the diet of Mediterranean countries. CHD mortality rates are much lower in these countries than in northern Europe, although total fat intake does not vary greatly. There do not appear to be any untoward effects of dietary oleic acid as judged by other causes of death in Mediterranean countries. Oleic acid was originally considered by Keys *et al.* (1965) and Hegsted *et al*, (1965) to be less effective than linoleic acid in decreasing serum cholesterol. This view dominated thinking in this area for many years, although it was not held by all of their contemporaries (Malmros and Wigand, 1957). Recently Grundy (1987) and Mensink and Katan (1987) have re-examined the issue and there seems little doubt that oleic acid is about as effective as linoleic acid in lowering total and LDL cholesterol. In addition it generally lowers serum triglycerides and appears not to lower HDL cholesterol.

The low-erucic acid rape-seed oil now available cheaply throughout Europe is rich in oleic acid. It seems to have the same effect when substituted for saturated fat as does olive oil (Valsta *et al.*, 1992).

Recommendations for the British diet

The Committee on the Medical Aspects of Food Policy recommend the following:

1 Total fat should be reduced to 30% of dietary energy. This might decrease the average Briton's energy intake by 10% (which might be desirable), but would more likely have the effect of increasing carbohydrate intake, which would still be an advantage.
2 Saturated fat should be 10% of dietary energy and trans fatty acids less than 2%. This should about halve the average intake of saturated fat and would be a good thing. But what is to replace it?
3 Cis-polyunsaturated fatty acids (mostly linoleic acid) should be held below 10%. They have already increased to around 8% on average. This reviewer would support the advice that they should not go above 10%.

| | % Fatty acids | | |
	Saturated	Oleic	Linoleic
Spreads			
Polyunsaturated margarine	18	20	50
Butter	69	28	3
Cooking fats			
Sunflower oil	12	25	63
Corn oil	12	30	54
Beef fat	51	39	2
Lard (pork)	39	45	10
Rape-seed oil	7	62	31
Olive oil	14	76	9

Table 13.2: The percentage of fatty acids.

4   Cis-monounsaturated fatty acids should remain at their present level of 12%. Here there is a major problem. The COMA report, perhaps tending to cling to the old Keys dogma, does not believe there is yet sufficient evidence to recommend an increase in monounsaturates. As we have seen there are advantages to at least maintaining our present intake of oleic acid. However, the other recommendations of COMA will probably not permit this. At present 30% of our total fat intake is monounsaturated. Most of this comes from meat and dairy products since foods rich in saturated fats are also rich in oleic acid (Table 13.2). If we cut our intake of these foods in order to decrease our saturated fat intake we shall also decrease dietary oleic acid. This is not replaced by eating more polyunsaturate-rich fats (Table 13.2) (Durrington *et al.*, 1977) nor, of course, by eating more carbohydrate. Only by increasing consumption of olive oil or rape-seed oil can our oleic acid levels be maintained.

Dietary cholesterol

One often hears doctors and patients speak of a 'low-cholesterol diet'. Foods are also frequently labelled as low in cholesterol. Both these practices reflect a lack of awareness that our daily diet contains less than half a gram of cholesterol and that the effect of halving this would be to have little impact on serum cholesterol (approximately 0.2 mmol/l reduction) (Keys, 1984). In any case, the decrease in saturated fat recommended by COMA would have the effect of reducing cholesterol intake, because cholesterol is often present in foods rich in SFA, so there is no need to make this a primary aim of diet. The primary aim should be to avoid excess energy intake and to decrease saturated fat intake.

References

Bennett M *et al.*, (1987) Dietary fatty acid effects on T cell-mediated immunity in mice infected with Mycoplasma pulmonis or injected with carcinogens. *American Journal of Pathology.* 126:103–113.

Bonanome A *et al.* (1992) Effect of dietary monounsaturated and polyunsaturated fatty acids on the susceptibility of plasma low density lipoproteins to oxidative modification. *Atherosclerosis.* 12:529–33.

Burr M L *et al.* (1989) Effects of change in fat, fish and fibre intakes on death and myocardial reinfarction: Death and Reinfarction Trial (DART). *The Lancet*, **ii**: 757–60.

Chait A *et al.* (1974) Reduction of serum triglyceride levels by polyunsaturated fat. Studies on the mode of action and on very low density lipoprotein composition. *Atherosclerosis.* 20:347–60.

COMA (1991) *Report of the Panel on Dietary Reference Values of the Committee on Medical Aspects of Food Policy 41. Dietary reference values for food energy and nutrients for the United Kingdom.* Department of Health Report on health and social subjects. HMSO, London.

de Langen CD (1918) Cholesterine metabolism and pathology of races. *Meded. burg. geneesk. Dienst. Ned-Indie.* **1**:1–35.

Durrington PN *et al.* (1977) The effect of a low-cholesterol, high-polyunsaturated diet on serum lipid levels, apolipoprotein B levels and fatty acid composition. *Atherosclerosis.* **27**:465–75.

Durrington PN (1989) *Hyperlipidaemia: diagnosis and management.* John Wright, London.

Glauber H *et al.* (1988) Adverse metabolic effect of omega-3 fatty acids in non-insulin-dependent diabetes mellitus. *Annals of Internal Medicine* **108**:663–8.

Grundy SM (1987) Dietary therapy of hyperlipidaemia. *Baillieres Clinical Endocrinology and Metabolism,* **1**:667–98.

Hegsted DM *et al.* (1965) Quantitative effects of dietary fat on serum cholesterol in man. *American Journal of Clinical Nutrition* **17**:281–95.

Himsworth HP (1935) The dietetic factor determining the glucose tolerance and sensitivity to insulin of healthy man. *Clinical Science.* **2**:67–94.

Kasim SE *et al.* (1988) Effects of omega-3 fish oils on lipid metabolism, glycemic control, and blood pressure in type II diabetic patients. *Journal of Clinical Endocrinology and Metabolism.* **67**:1–5.

Keys A *et al.* (1965) Serum cholesterol response to changes in the diet. IV. Particular saturated fatty acids in the diet. *Metabolism.* **14**:776–87.

Keys A (1970) Coronary heart disease in seven countries. *Circulation.* **41** (Suppl. 1): 11–211.

Keys A (1984) Serum cholesterol response to dietary cholesterol. *American Journal of Clinical Nutrition.* **40**:351–9.

Malmros H and Wigand G (1957) The effect on serum cholesterol of diets containing different fats. *The Lancet.* **ii**:1–8.

Mensink RP and Katan MB (1987) Effect of monounsaturated fatty acids versus complex carbohydrates on high-density lipoproteins in healthy men and women. *The Lancet.* **i**:122–5.

Reaven P *et al.* (1991) Feasibility of using an oleate-rich diet to reduce the susceptibility of low-density lipoprotein to oxidative modification in humans. *American Journal of Clinical Nutrition.* **54**:701–6.

Sanders TAB (1990) Polyunsaturated fatty acids and coronary heart disease. *Baillieres Clinical Endocrinology and Metabolism.* 4:877–94.

Schectman *et al.* (1988) Effect of fish oil concentrate on lipoprotein composition in NIDDM. *Diabetes.* 37:1567–73.

Shepherd J *et al.* (1978) Effects of dietary polyunsaturated and saturated fat on the properties of high density lipoproteins and the metabolism of apolipoprotein AI. *Journal of Clinical Investigations.* 61:1582–92.

Sommariva D *et al.* (1978) Low-fat diet versus low-carbohydrate diet in the treatment of type IV hyperlipoproteinaemia. *Atherosclerosis.* 29:43–51.

Valsta LM *et al.* (1992) Effects of a monounsaturated rapeseed oil and polyunsaturated sunflower oil diet on lipoprotein levels in humans. *Arteriosclerosis.* 12:50–7.

WHO (1985) *Report of a WHO Study Group. Diabetes mellitus. World Health Organization Technical Report Series 727.* WHO, Geneva.

14

Lipoprotein Lp (a) and the Apolipoproteins

AF WINDER

The apolipoproteins—the protein components of the lipoproteins—are the vehicles facilitating the transport of predominantly water-insoluble lipids in plasma. However, they are more than inert carriers of lipid: they can modulate the activity of plasma and intracellular enzymes and transport processes of lipoprotein metabolism, and they are the components involved in the interaction of lipoproteins with cell surface receptors. Individual apoproteins can also serve as markers for specific lipoproteins of clinical interest. Their structure and expression is under genetic control, and variation in structure and expression leads to a wide spectrum of effects on lipoprotein metabolism.

Classification and nomenclature of the apolipoproteins

The plasma globulins may be conveniently classified according to their elec-trophoretic mobility in alkaline buffer systems as alpha, beta and gamma globulins. Such separations can also be stained for lipid to reveal the lipopro-teins located in the alpha, beta and pre-beta positions and can thus be so classified. On this basis, the main and characteristic protein of alpha lipoprotein was defined as apo(lipoprotein) A, that of beta-lipoprotein as apo B, and (for convenience) that of pre-beta lipoprotein as apo C. As with that for vitamins, this tidy system then had to be extended to include further heterogeneity as apo A-I, A-II etc, and further components such as forms of apo D and apo E not predominating in any specific lipoprotein. Information on the major apo-proteins may be summarized as follows.

Apo A. Two major fractions, A-I and A-II, are released from intestine and liver. Apo A-I may be active in the mobilization of cholesterol from intracellular stores to the cell surface as a requirement for reverse cholesterol transport, and in the activation of the enzyme lecithin:cholesteryl acyltransferase (LCAT) which circulates in association with high-density lipoprotein (HDL) in plasma, and catalyses the esterification of cholesterol also necessary for that transfer process.

Apo B. The full apo B form (100% thus B-100) is secreted by liver in very low-density lipoprotein (VLDL), in Lp(a) and in some circumstances in LDL. Intestine expresses 48% of the full sequence, hence apo B-48, in chylomicrons, and various truncated forms (eg B-89) may circulate in forms of homozygous familial hypobetalipoproteinaemia because of defects in the gene structure, and form as artifacts from breakdown of apo B-100 on storage. Specific regions of apo B-100 bind to the high-affinity cell surface receptor in the process of LDL uptake into cells.

Apo C. The main components C-I, C-II and C-III are synthesized mainly in liver and circulate in VLDL and HDL, with further transfer intravascularly into chylomicrons. Apo C-II is a major co-factor in the activation of lipoprotein lipase.

Apo D. A further trace apoprotein in HDL.

Apo E. Arising mainly from liver, and macrophages, but apo E mRNA is also found elsewhere (eg the brain) and other sites could therefore also be involved in its synthesis and secretion. Considering E-3 as a base form, amino-acid substitutions at each of two sites gives E-2 and E-4 variants: codominant genes are inherited from each parent and thus six apo E patterns arise: E-2/E-2; E-3/E-3; E-4/E-4; E-2/E/3; E-3/E-4 and E-2/E-4. There are also other rare forms with structural changes at other sites than the E-2/3/4 series, discussed below. Interaction between lipoprotein particle surface apo E and cell receptors is involved in the clearance of chylomicron remnants by liver and of VLDL and large HDL-1 particles by liver and probably more generally (Mahley *et al.*, 1984; Davignon *et al.*, 1988).

Apo(a)

This large glycoprotein is apparently secreted intact from liver in a complex with LDL as lipoprotein (a) [Lp(a)], without the intravascular maturation normally affecting LDL (Utermann, 1989). Traces of apo(a) also circulate in triglyceride-rich particles. Disulfide bridges are involved in the attachment to LDL, and in organization of the structure into a number of coiled repeats known as kringles. The structure has substantial structural homology to other components affecting thrombosis and thrombolysis in plasma, particularly plasminogen, except that the fourth structural component of plasminogen, kringle 4, is repeated many times in Lp(a), between 10 and 44 repeats being described at present. Lp(a) is codominantly expressed as with apo E, and two parental forms are expressed in plasma, although these are occasionally the same form in a homozygote. More sensitive methods of measurement suggest that an earlier reported null form is an artifact, and that some material is always present in plasma. The larger apo(a) structures are generally but not exactly associated with lower electrophoretic mobility and below-average levels in plasma. Substantial racial variation is reported (Parra *et al.*, 1987), also showing that component size is not the only determinant of level in plasma. Levels in plasma vary considerably between individuals and populations: present information suggests that they are under substantial genetic control, expressed through rates of production rather than metabolism. Liver transplantation alters the molecular form of Lp(a) to that of the donor, supporting direct release from liver of Lp(a) as a preformed LDL-apo(a) complex.

Measurement in clinical diagnosis and management

Three different areas of application arise.

- Qualitative approaches, to establish the presence or absence of specific normal or variant components in plasma or tissues, as in arterial wall.
- Quantitative approaches may also be applied to such components, particularly when the apolipoprotein is a marker for a specific normal or variant lipoprotein and levels are of clinical or pathological interest.
- Aspects of gene expression are also of growing interest, considering through restriction fragment-linked polymorphisms (RFLPs), expression of mRNA, and direct gene sequencing, how variation in the synthesis and turnover of the structurally normal apolipoproteins is controlled in normal and pathological states.

Qualitative approaches

Qualitative approaches can be less technically demanding than those involving direct measurement, although such direct measurement may be required to investigate any abnormal result. These are several current applications.

Apo A-I and HDL in plasma. Premature coronary heart disease (CHD) may be associated with low or very low levels of HDL and apo A-I, and sometimes this is associated with structural variants of apo A-I (Schaefer, 1984). Some variants (often named after their place of discovery, eg apo A-I Marburg) are charge shift mutations and can therefore be identified by isoelectric focusing analysis as bands locate in different positions to those for normal samples (Assmann *et al.*, 1987). VLDL which has been separated from plasma by flotation, removed, mixed with 0.15M saline and washed free of plasma proteins by reflotation and then delipidated by organic solvent extraction (the whole process taking at least 48 hours) is convenient starting material for all apolipoprotein qualitative studies as most components of current interest are present. Corneal clouding may be associated with major deficiency of apo A-I and HDL in plasma as in Tangier disease, familial LCAT deficiency and Fish-Eye disease (Schaefer, 1984). Complete or near complete HDL deficiency is revealed by simple HDL-cholesterol assay and agarose or similar electrophoresis, and can be confirmed by immunoelectrophoresis against anti-apo A-I antibody. Further specific tests (eg LCAT assay) may then confirm the diagnosis. At least one form of Fish-Eye disease, which involves restricted LCAT activity and tissue accumulation of free cholesterol, arises through a structural variant of A-I affecting interaction of LCAT with HDL components (Assmann *et al.*, 1990). Tangier disease seems to involve a normal apo A-I gene structure but very rapid turnover of HDL, with insignificant circulating levels of mature HDL and apo A-I in plasma, and tissue accumulation of cholesterol esters. The essential genetic fault remains obscure.

The apo A-I/C-III/A-IV genes are organized as a cluster on the short arm of chromosome 11 and various major deletions within this cluster are described, with major HDL deficiency and associated vascular disease (Schaefer, 1984).

Hypertriglyceridaemia. Homozygous autosomal recessive deficiency of apo C-II with defective activation of lipoprotein lipase is rare but can present with major hyperchylomicronaemia and pancreatitis (Breslow, 1988; Bhatnagar and Durrington, 1991). The diagnosis can be pursued by isofocusing analysis of washed delipidated VLDL. Apo E-2/E-2 homozygotes (about 1.3% of the UK population), and some other rare variant forms also with impaired interaction with liver receptors, can in occasional cases express with mixed lipaemia through delayed clearance of chylomicron remnants and VLDL, particularly when a further problem of lipid overload or delayed clearance (such as alcoholism or hypothyroidism) is also present. Expression may sometimes involve the full-blown clinical syndrome of familial (Type III) dysbetalipoproteinaemia with claudication and CHD, soft-tissue xanthomas and in about 50% of cases the striking linear palmar crease xanthomas (Breslow, 1988; Davignon *et al.*, 1988). Chylomicron remnants are lipid-rich and are within the VLDL density range, but have the electrophoretic mobility of LDL. Thus floated VLDL prepared for apolipoprotein analysis shows two bands on electrophoresis—normal pre-beta VLDL and a further 'floating beta' band, the chylomicron remnants. This is a simple screening test for the remnants, particularly as the rare variant forms causing this syndrome are also then identified. Apo E-2/3/4 status can be defined by electrofocusing and immunoblotting of native plasma (Assmann *et al.*, 1987), and oligonucleotide probe approaches after gene amplification by PCR are also now well defined (Houlston *et al.*, 1989). The problem is that the rare variant forms have structures different from apo E-2, 3 and 4, and the structural changes involve sites not targeted by the probes defining the E-2, 3, 4 variation. Charge shift and isofocusing is also not generally helpful as overall charge may be the same as that of a common variant. Thus rare variants focusing in the E-2 position but of different structure are defined as apo E-2*, E-2** etc. Also, when the structures of some rare variant forms are overloaded with lipid, the second process generally required to induce clinical expression of apo E variants, interaction with apo E receptors can be so impaired that a single dose of the gene and thus dominant expression is associated with major dyslipidaemia. Until the exact prevalence of these apparently rare forms and appropriate methodology is established they cannot be ignored, and at present the identification of floating beta material remains the most secure diagnostic first screening test in the definition of apo E-related dyslipidaemias. This does seem worthwhile in view of the sometimes startling clinical as well as biochemical response to early treatment, with attention to other associated lipid disorders, diet and sometimes drugs.

The common apo E types may also influence cardiovascular risk, perhaps through relationships with levels of Lp(a), and responses to diets and to lipid-lowering drugs (Davignon *et al.*, 1988).

Apo B. In abetalipoproteinaemia all apo B lipoproteins—chylomicrons,

VLDL and LDL—are not expressed in plasma, with associated steatorrhoea, ataxia, peripheral neuropathy, retinal degeneration, myopathy and acanthocytosis (Breslow, 1988); simple electrophoresis of plasma may reveal the diagnosis. The apo B gene in intestine and liver is apparently of normal structure, and as mRNA can also be detected there may be some defect of assembly or secretion (Talmud et al., 1988). Heterozygotes are clinically and biochemically unaffected, in contrast to the various forms of hypobetalipoproteinaemia, in which defects arise in the apo B structure (Collins et al., 1988). Truncated forms of apo B (eg B-89) may be found in plasma when the residual normal gene is sufficient to allow expression. Size can be defined by SDS-gel electrophoresis. Defects can also be identified through direct analysis of the gene; all cases so far defined have shown mutations within the coding sequence of the apo B-100 gene. Hypobetalipoproteinaemia can also arise secondarily, eg to hepatic necrosis or hyperthyroidism.

One form of clinical familial hypercholesterolaemia—familial defective hyperbetalipoproteinaemia—arises because of structural variation at amino-acid 3500, in the region of apo B-100 binding to the high-affinity cell surface receptors. Heterozygotes express normal and defective apo B-100, circulating LDL being enriched with the slowly cleared defective material. An oligonucleotide gene probe approach is also developed for this diagnosis (Tybjaerg-Hansen et al., 1990). Assays for this diagnosis based upon receptor uptake of LDL must use the patients own defective LDL, not the pooled normal material appropriate for definition of receptor defects. Other minor and apparently common structural variants of apo B-100 also have some slight influence on cardiovascular risk, in some cases independent of effects on gross levels of lipids in plasma. Effects on production or turnover of the apo B-100-containing lipoproteins could be involved (Hegele et al., 1986; Talmud et al., 1987).

Quantitative approaches

The atherogenic lipoprotein LDL is associated with around 70% of the cholesterol but 90% of the apo B-100 in plasma. However, it has been difficult to establish that apo B levels are a closer marker for cardiovascular risk than cholesterol, perhaps because methods of measurement have been inadequate, but this relationship is now coming out. Thus high apo B and low apo A-I have been shown to be closer markers for the presence of coronary artery disease (CAD) in middle-aged men than other lipid-related variables (Genest et al., 1990). The inverse relationship between risk and levels of HDL and the associated apo A-I, and particularly with the sub-fraction of HDL particles that contain A-I only, may arise through involvement of apo A-I in mobilisation of cholesterol from intracellular pools as an early necessary step in reverse cholesterol transport (Fruchart and Ailhaut, 1992). However, the value of apoprotein data in prospective prediction of risk, as outcome, is not yet well defined. Accelerated CVD is also associated with delayed clearance of VLDL and thus impaired maturation of LDL, with persistence of small dense apo B-enriched LDL particles as hyperapobetalipoproteinaemia. Finally, qualitative analyses suggesting major deficiency states as in abetalipoproteinaemia or Tangier disease may then proceed to confirmation by direct quantitative analysis of apo B-100 or apo A-I.

Lipoprotein Lp(a)

The distribution of Lp(a) levels within populations is markedly skewed, and above-median levels can be associated with premature coronary and cerebrovascular disease. Three problems arise in the evaluation of these associations: *analytical*, in the measurement of Lp(a); *pathophysiological*, in defining the adverse processes involved; and *therapeutic*, in defining appropriate management of patients.

Methods for measurement can be directed at apo(a) after dissociation from LDL, or at the intact particle. Immunological methods can involve antibody directed at different regions of the apo(a) sequence, and different reagents give widely differing results. Potential cross-reactivity with plasminogen has been overcome, but the widely varying structures involved in apo(a) within populations further complicates the calibration of all assays for which there are as yet no established quality assurance schemes. Some published data are thus rather qualitative, and comparison of data between centres and derived from different assays is not secure. As for pathogenesis, Lp(a) can be detected in arterial wall (Rath *et al.*, 1989), and is also subject to oxidative change which could facilitate uptake into cells (Sattler *et al.*, 1991). The association with premature vascular disease increases when levels in plasma exceed about 30 mg/dl. Some patients have levels up to 1000 mg/dl, but the generally low levels in comparison with LDL suggests that adverse effects are unlikely simply to express cell uptake and atherogenesis. The structural homology with plasminogen has excited interest in possible antithrombolytic effects (Scott, 1989). Lp(a) can bind to plasminogen receptors and to fibrin and fibrin fragments, and compete with tissue-type plasminogen activator tPA, consistent with impairment of plasmin production and of fibrinolysis. However these *in vitro* observations are not confirmed *in vivo*. High Lp(a) levels have not obviously impaired the effects of thrombolytic therapy, and mechanisms of effect remain to be defined: Lp(a) levels could be a consequence rather than a cause of accelerated arterial disease. In treatment, the failure of statin drugs to control Lp(a) levels in plasma is unexpected and unexplained as Lp(a) is released from liver as an LDL-related complex from liver and LDL synthesis does respond. Nicotinates can reduce levels through undefined mechanisms (Carlson *et al.*, 1989), and this could explain why nicotinate treatment has produced clinical cardiovascular benefit greater than that expected from the effects on gross plasma lipids alone. Exogenous gonadal steroids may also reduce Lp(a) levels, possibly through effects on hepatic synthesis, and lesser effects may also arise with equine hormonal replacement preparations, although clinical indications are not defined. Families with premature coronary disease may be affected because of associated elevation of Lp(a) levels (Durrington *et al.*, 1988), and elevation is also associated in some but not all surveys with particularly severe expression in heterozygous familial hypercholesterolaemia (Seed *et al.*, 1990). The overall data on premature vascular disease and inter-racial variation is consistent with an effect of Lp(a) as a conditional risk factor for premature disease, with markedly enhanced but still variable expression in the presence of co-existing excess of LDL. It follows, therefore, that levels of LDL and Lp(a) can be useful in the evaluation of overall prognosis, and, deciding on active treatment; but decisions will rarely, if ever, be taken on the basis of Lp(a) levels alone, although cases of premature coronary disease with elevation of Lp(a) level as the only obvious risk association are reported (Rader and Brewer, 1992).

Aspects of gene expression

Apolipoproteins may be substantially or even completely deficient in plasma, but investigation of the gene or its product when present shows that the product and/or its coding sequence is of normal structure, or present in normal precursor immature form. Defects are of gene expression, located outside the coding sequence, and may be approached through a search for linkage to restriction sites outside that sequence, together with direct sequencing of the flanking regions around the gene. Polymorphisms around the A-I/C-III/A-IV gene cluster and their association with hypertriglyceridaemia and low circulating levels of HDL and apo A-I in families with premature coronary disease have been investigated in particular detail (Ordovas *et al.*, 1991). Gene expression may be controlled from sites distant from the coding sequence. Thus, in abetalipoproteinaemia, the mutations involved are not within or apparently even close to the normal apo B gene, as various direct and linkage studies have shown that transmission of the apo B gene within affected families does not correlate with the clinical picture (Talmud *et al.*, 1987).

Such gene marker associations with clinical outcome may lead to improved recognition of families and individuals at risk, pending identification of the processes involved in clinical expression.

Summary

Levels of gross lipids in plasma as triglycerides and total (HDL) cholesterol have general associations with the expression of CVD but low predictive power for individual clinical outcome. Interest in the determination of specific apolipoproteins has arisen in the hope that such predictive power is increased, through their involvement as markers of specific potentially protective or atherogenic lipoproteins such as LDL and lipoprotein Lp(a) with structural homology with plasminogen and thus possible antithrombolytic activity, and for their activation of specific steps in lipoprotein metabolism such as chylomicron clearance or reverse cholesterol transport. Some potentially attractive applications are however limited by difficulties affecting analytical performance and calibration of currently available apolipoprotein assays, and uncertainty as to how to target any potential therapeutic approach.

References

Assmann G *et al.* (1987) Analytical procedures for the detection and characterization of apolipoprotein mutants. *American Heart Journal.* 113:598–603.

Assmann G *et al.* (1990) Clinical, biochemical and genetic heterogeneity of lecithin: cholesterol acyltransferase syndromes. In: Carlson LA (ed.) *Disorders of HDL.* London. Smith-Gordon, pp. 169–175.

Bhatnagar D and Durrington PN (1991) Clinical value of apolipoprotein measurement. *Annals of Clinical Biochemistry.* 28:427–37.

Breslow JL (1988) Apoprotein genetic variation in human disease. *Physiological Review.* 68:85–132.

Carlson LA *et al.* (1989) Pronounced lowering of serum levels of lipoprotein Lp(a) in hyperlipidaemic subjects treated with nicotinic acid. *Journal of Internal Medicine.* 226:271–6.

Collins DR *et al.* (1988) Truncated variants of apolipoprotein B cause hypobetalipoproteinaemia. *Nucleic Acids Research.* 16:8361–75.

Davignon J *et al.* (1988) Apolipoprotein E polymorphism and atherosclerosis. *Arteriosclerosis.* 8:1–21.

Durrington PN *et al.* (1988) Apolipoprotein (a), A-I and B and parental history in men with early onset ischaemic heart disease. *The Lancet.* i:1070–3.

Fruchart JC and Ailhaut G (1992) Apolipoprotein A-containing particles: physiological role, quantification, and clinical significance. *Clinical Chemistry.* 38:793–7.

Genest JG *et al.* (1990) Plasma apolipoprotein A-I, A-II, B, E and C-III containing particles in men with premature coronary artery disease. *Atherosclerosis.* 90:149–57.

Hegele RA *et al.* (1986) Apolipoprotein B-gene DNA polymorphisms associated with myocardial infarction. *New England Journal of Medicine.* 315:1509–15.

Houlston RS *et al.* (1989) Apolipoprotein E genotypes by polymerase chain reaction and allele-specific oligonucleotide probes. *Human Genetics.* 83:364–8.

Mahley RW *et al.* (1984) Plasma lipoproteins: apolipoprotein structure and function. *Journal of Lipid Research.* 25:1277–94.

Ordovas JM *et al.* (1991) Restriction fragment length polymorphisms of the apolipoprotein A-I, C-III, A-IV gene locus. *Atherosclerosis.* 87:75–86.

Parra H-J *et al.* (1987) Black-white differences in serum Lp(a) lipoprotein levels. *Clinica Chimica Acta.* 167:27–31.

Rader DJ and Brewer HB Jr (1992) Lipoprotein (a). Clinical approach to a unique atherogenic lipoprotein. *Journal of the American Medical Association.* **267**:1109–12.

Rath M *et al.* (1989) Detection and quantification of lipoprotein (a) in the arterial wall of 107 coronary bypass patients. *Arteriosclerosis.* **9**:579–92.

Sattler W *et al.* (1991) Oxidation of lipoprotein Lp(a). A comparison with low-density lipoproteins. *Biochimica Biophysica Acta.* **1081**:65–74.

Schaefer EJ (1984) Clinical, biochemical and genetic features in familial disorders of high density lipoprotein deficiency. *Arteriosclerosis.* **4**:303–12.

Scott J (1989) Lipoprotein (a). Thrombogenesis linked to atherogenesis at last? *Nature.* **341**:22–3.

Seed M *et al.* (1990) Relation of serum lipoprotein (a) concentration and apolipoprotein (a) phenotype to coronary heart disease in patients with familial hypercholesterolemia. *New England Journal of Medicine.* **322**:1494–9.

Talmud PJ *et al.* (1987) Apolipoprotein B gene variants are involved in the determination of serum cholesterol levels: a study in normo- and hyperlipidaemic individuals. *Atherosclerosis.* **67**:81–9.

Talmud PJ *et al.* (1988) Genetic evidence from two families that the apolipoprotein gene is not involved in abetalipoproteinaemia. *Journal of Clinical Investigation.* **82**:1803–6.

Tybjaerg-Hansen A *et al.* (1990) Familial defective apolipoprotein B-100: detection in the United Kingdom and Scandinavia, and clinical characteristics of ten cases. *Atherosclerosis.* **80**:1235–42.

Utermann G (1989) The mysteries of lipoprotein (a). *Science.* **246**:904–10.

15

The Role of Antioxidant Nutrients in Disease

ANTHONY T DIPLOCK

Increased interest in the free radical theory of disease causation during the past 15 years has led to a very large upsurge in attention to the possibility that the aetiology of a number of diseases involves, at least at some stage, the intervention of free radical-initiated or -mediated processes. From this basis a further major field has developed, namely investigation of the possibility that those dietary agents which have become known as the 'antioxidant nutrients' (eg vitamins A, C, and E), may have a prophylactic or even curative role in the disease process. The fact that serious killer diseases, particularly cardiovascular and cerebrovascular disease and certain forms of cancer, are considered to involve free radicals at some point in their development, has turned a spotlight on the possibilities, in public health terms, of disease prevention by simple and inexpensive means. The attractiveness to governments of such possibilities has only just begun to have an impact, but it is already clear from the advice given by the World Health Organization (ie to increase intake of fresh fruits and green vegetables that contain the nutrients in question as well as other necessary items) that such advice will become of increasing importance.

Animals depend upon molecular oxygen for the life-supporting action of respiration, which is generally regarded as a benign process providing the mechanism for the release of energy in a packaged form for driving essential bodily functions. The possibility that this process also may produce harm is often overlooked. In fact, the addition of four electrons to molecular oxygen to form water is highly hazardous because the intermediates are very reactive compounds, usually free radicals that are potentially damaging to living cells.

A free radical is defined as any chemical species that has one or more unpaired electrons. The formation of such products, and metabolites derived from them, is controlled very precisely in mammalian cells by a series of protective mechanisms. These can be identified as a first line of defence that depends on enzymes that contain, and depend functionally upon, the minerals manganese, copper, zinc and selenium. A second line of defence is provided by vitamin E, which is generally thought to function in close concert with vitamin C, and a third line of protection that involves again the selenoenzymes. β-carotene also has emerged as a rather unexpected contributor to this protective mechanism although the precise nature of this protection is unclear at present. These protective substances are required in small amounts in the diet and it follows that, if diets are lacking in these 'antioxidant nutrients', then there is a possibility that free radical-initiated or -mediated reactions will lead to pathological effects. This concept lies at the centre of the current intense worldwide effort devoted to studies in this area.

The reduction of molecular oxygen to water can proceed stepwise: the addition of one electron (of the four) results in the formation of the superoxide anion radical $(O_2^{\cdot-})$ which is only moderately reactive. When a further electron is added, the peroxyl anion so formed (O_2^{2-}) combines at once with protons from solution to form H_2O_2. The major potential problem for living cells is the production of the highly reactive species, the hydroxyl radical $OH^{\cdot}$. This reaction is catalysed by either iron or copper which may exist free in the system in sufficient, albeit very small, quantities. These metals are highly effective in carrying out this catalysis. This process, for iron, involves the reduction of Fe^{3+} to Fe^{2+} by $O_2^{\cdot-}$ and the subsequent reduction of hydrogen peroxide by Fe^{2+} to the $OH^{\cdot}$ radical. The enzymic mechanism that modulates this reaction involves superoxide dismutases, which contain either manganese or copper and zinc, and the selenoenzyme, glutathione peroxidase, which catalyzes the reduction of H_2O_2 to water. The removal of the reactants therefore prevents the formation of significant amounts of the OH radical by the Fenton reaction $(Fe^{2+} + H_2O_2 \rightarrow Fe^{3+} + OH^- + OH^{\cdot})$.

Targets for attack

Among the targets for attack by the hydroxyl radical are DNA, protein and the polyunsaturated fatty acid residues of membrane phospholipids. In terms of possible pathogenesis, these targets are clearly fundamental to the cellular economy. There is much evidence of the damage that can be caused by free radicals to DNA. The possibility that this may be a major factor in mutagenesis and carcinogenesis is of great interest, and evidence already exists that in animals free radical reactions are involved in some of the events that lead to cancer. The attack by free radicals on proteins (enzymes) has received less attention, but it is clear that modifications to constituent amino acid structure take place, which, if they affect amino acids close to the active site of the protein, may have severely detrimental consequences.

The greater part of the work in this area has been concerned with free radical damage to membrane polyunsaturated fatty acids (PUFA), and here we have a clear picture of the events that occur. Attack by a radical involves the initial formation of a carbon-centered radical (which we will arbitrarily designate as $L^{\cdot}$) which immediately undergoes conjugation of the double bond system. Attack by this radical on molecular oxygen results in the formation of PUFA radical $LOO^{\cdot}$. In the presence of adequate amounts of vitamin E, the peroxyl radical is quenched to LOOH with formation of the vitamin E radical; this probably interacts with vitamin C to reform the vitamin E molecule which can be used for further cycles of lipid peroxyl radical quenching. When vitamin E is not present in adequate amounts, such as would occur in dietary deficiency, the peroxyl radical attacks a further molecule of PUFA in the vicinity so that chain reactions of lipid peroxidation become established. The consequence is disturbance of the highly ordered structure of the membrane that may lead to pathological damage to the tissue concerned. The LOOH that is formed by this process may be attacked by iron so that either the PUFA radical LOO˙ or the alkoxy radical LO˙ may be formed. This consequence is avoided because phospholipase A_2 will cause cleavage of the LOOH from the membrane so that the resultant free fatty acid can act as substrate for the selenoenzyme glutathione peroxidase which catalyzes its reduction to a harmless hydroxy acid; glutathione peroxidase thus has a dual function in protecting cells from free radical-induced damage.

There is a considerable potential for involvement of free radical-mediated events in the pathology of disease. Indeed there has been a remarkable catalogue of diseases in which such pathogenesis may be involved. At present there is much speculation, and hypotheses have highlighted several key questions. The possibility that free radical events are involved in the disease process implies that those agents, the antioxidant nutrients that modulate the free radical reactions, may have a preventive role for the disease in question. This leads to series of questions: (1) Is there evidence of an inverse relationship between disease risk and blood or tissue level of some or all of the antioxidant nutrients? (2) Can it be shown that a low level of intake of a nutrient is associated statistically with a higher subsequent risk of disease? (3) Can the blood levels required to provide the lowered risk of disease be defined? (4) What level of dietary intake of antioxidant nutrients is required to provide optimal protection against disease?

These questions can be answered only partly, and the evidence that enables these partial answers is largely epidemiological. Ideally, three levels of evidence should be available to prove that an enhanced level of a nutrient may lead to a lower subsequent risk of disease. First, it must be shown that in a cross-cultural epidemiological study there is a statistically proven association between low levels of intake of a nutrient in a sample population, demonstrated by low plasma levels of that nutrient and high risk of disease. Secondly, it must be shown in prospective trials, with a high level of statistical certainty, that there is a correlation between a low initial serum level of the nutrient and high subsequent risk of disease in individuals in the same study group. Thirdly, and most convincingly of all, intervention trials must demonstrate that a supplement of the nutrient to the diet of a sample population then leads, in the absence of any other intervention, to a lowered incidence of the disease as compared to a similar group to whom only a placebo is administered. The trials should be conducted under rigorous double-blind conditions. At the present time there is ample evidence of the first and second kinds, both for some forms of cancer and for CVD, that demonstrates that low levels of intake of vitamin C, vitamin E and β-carotene may be associated with an increased risk of disease. Also, a number of other prospective trials are being reported that demonstrate the same trends. There is as yet little evidence from intervention trials although several large trials are now in progress or are about to be started.

Cancer

With respect to cancer, intake of low amounts of vegetables, fruits and carotenoids was shown to be associated consistently with increased risk of lung cancer, and low levels of β-carotene in plasma are associated consistently with an increased incidence of lung cancer. Furthermore, both prospective and retrospective studies have suggested that intake of high amounts of vegetables and fruits may reduce the risk of a range of other cancers, it is presumed in these studies that the protective nutrients are some or all of the antioxidant nutrients.

In a study of 26 000 volunteers in Washington County, Maryland (Comstock *et al.*, 1991), prediagnostic serum samples of 436 subsequent cancer cases at nine cancer sites were compared with 765 matched control subjects. Serum β-carotene levels showed a strong protective association with lung cancer and weaker but significant associations for other sites. Serum vitamin E had a protective association with lung cancer but not with other sites whereas lycopene (a carotenoid occurring in some ripe fruits) was strongly associated with pancreatic cancer, and with cancer of the bladder and rectum.

In a study in Basel, Switzerland (Gey *et al.* 1987), statistically significantly lower mean carotene levels were found for all cancers, including bronchus cancer and stomach cancer as compared to matched healthy controls. In reviewing the evidence with respect to vitamin C, Block (1991) recently concluded that '*epidemiologic evidence of a protective effect of vitamin C for nonhormone cancers is very strong. Of the 46 such studies in which a dietary vitamin C index was calculated, 33 found statistically significant protection.*'

In a study in Finland (Knelt *et al.*, 1991), vitamin E was shown to confer protection in 766 cases, compared to 1419 control subjects, against cancer in certain sites. Strongest correlations were found for some gastrointestinal cancers and for the combined group of cancers unrelated to smoking.

The potential for prevention of oral cancer by β-carotene has been explored in some detail; the use of retinoids for this purpose is limited by their toxicity, and β-carotene and other carotenoids with their very low toxicity therefore have been investigated carefully as putative chemopreventive agents. In an intervention trial with vitamin A and β-carotene among fishermen in Kerala, India, who chewed tobacco-containing betel quids daily throughout the three-year study, Stich *et al.* (1991) studied the frequency of oral leukoplakia (a condition, often considered precancerous, in which thickened white patches of epithelial cells occur on the mucous membrane). Vitamin A administration resulted in complete remission of leukoplakia in 57% of cases and a 96% reduction in the incidence of micronucleated cells, β-carotene induced remission in 15% of cases and caused 98% reduction of micronucleated cells; the protective effect of these treatments could be maintained by the administration of a much lower maintenance dose during an eight-month follow-up period.

The data summarized above are remarkable in their consistency in promoting the argument for the antioxidant nutrients as chemopreventive agents of cancer in certain specifically identified sites.

Cardiovascular disease

With regard to CVD, the large body of evidence for a preventive role of the antioxidant nutrients in the etiogenesis of atherosclerosis with its subsequent association with cardiovascular and cerebrovascular disease will be summarized by reference to two key studies.

The best example of a cross-cultural study is the European cross-sectional trial based on the North-South gradient with respect to ischaemic heart disease (Gey et al., 1991). In this study, groups of approximately 100 healthy men, 40 –59 years of age, were chosen in three general areas defined by their ischaemic heart disease mortality statistics. The study populations were representative of: (1) high incidence of ischaemic heart disease (410–414 deaths/year/100 000 males 40–59 years); (2) modeate incidence of ischaemic hert disease (approximately 250 deaths/year/100 000 males); and (3) low incidence of ischaemic heart disease (<130 deaths/year per 100 000 males).

It was found that for vitamin C, mean plasma levels less than 22.7 µmol were found in those regions that had a moderate to high risk of disease, whereas plasma levels in excess of this level tended to be found in those areas of low risk. Similarly for vitamin E, mean plasma levels lower than 25 µmol were associated with high risk of coronary heart disease, whereas, with a high degree of statistical certainty, plasma levels above this value were associated with a lower risk of disease. While there was inevitably some overlap in the data, which made the statistical association with respect to vitamin C rather low, in the case of vitamin E the level of statistical certainty was very convincing.

In a major case control study conducted in Edinburgh, Scotland, Riemersma et al. (1991) studied the possible association of risk of angina pectoris with low plasma concentration of vitamins A, C, and E and β-carotene. The population sampled was 6000 men ages 35–54; among these, complete antioxidant nutrient data were obtained in 110 cases of angina and 394 matched control subjects. No correlation was found between vitamin A levels in the two groups, but highly significant correlations were found for β-carotene, vitamin C and cholesterol standardized vitamin E.

Much other evidence exists in the literature which, taken together, begins to make an overwhelming case for the existence of a relationship between high blood level of antioxidant nutrients and a lowered incidence of disease. In the interim, while the results of intervention trials are awaited, some progress may be made in attempting to quantitate the likely optimal intake of these nutrients for disease prevention. In the epidemiological trials referred to, common practice is to divide the risk of disease into quartiles or quintiles; if the blood level of nutrients found in subjects in the lowest quartile or quintile of disease risk is taken, it is possible to make some calculations as to the likely level of intake of the nutrient that might be needed to achieve this blood level. When this is done, it becomes apparent that the levels of required intake of vitamins E and C for prophylaxis, based on epidemiological data, are three to five times above the recommended daily allowance.

References

Block G (1991) Vitamin C and cancer prevention: the epidemiologic evidence. *American Journal of Clinical Nutrition.* **53**:270–82S.

Comstock GW, Helzlsouer KJ and Bush TL (1991) Prediagnostic serum levels in carotenoids and vitamen E as related to subsequent cancer in Washington County, Maryland. *American Journal of Clinical Nutrition.* **53**:260–4S.

Gey KF, Brubacher GM and Stahelin HB (1987) Plasma levels of antioxidant vitamins in relation to ischemic heart disease and cancer. *American Journal of Clinical Nutrition.* **45**:1368–77.

Gey KF, Puska P, Jordan P and Moser UK (1991) Inverse correlation between plasma vitamin E and mortality from ischemic heart disease in cross-cultural epidemiology. *American Journal of Clinical Nutrition.* **53**:326–34S.

Knekt P *et al.* (1991) Vitamin E and cancer prevention. *American Journal of Clinical Nutrition.* **53**:283–6S

Riemersma RA *et al.* (1991) Risk of angina pectoris and plasma concentrations of vitamins A, C, and E and carotene. *The Lancet.* **337**:1–5.

Stich HF *et al.* (1991) Remission of precancerous lesions in the oral cavity of tobacco chewers and maintenance of the protective effect of beta-carotene or vitamin A. *American Journal of Clinical Nutrition.* **53**:298–304S.

This article has been reproduced with the kind permission of *INFORM*, American Oil Chemists' Society.

16

Sodium and Potassium: Blood Pressure and Stroke

KAY-TEE KHAW

Although there is little new about the hypothesis that high dietary sodium and low dietary potassium may be aetiologically related to raised blood pressure and increased risk of cardiovascular disease (CVD), the debate still continues over whether dietary recommendations to reduce dietary sodium intake or to increase dietary potassium intake are warranted, either for hypertensives or for the general population. This debate is exemplified by the numerous reviews, statements of opinion and often acrimonious correspondence published in both the medical literature and the popular media. The arguments revolve around several issues which will be addressed separately.

Aetiological association: This is the question of whether dietary sodium and potassium intake are causally related to blood pressure levels

Genetic susceptibility: Recommendations to the whole community or even to hypertensives may not be justified if only a small proportion of the population is genetically susceptible to the effects of sodium or potassium.

Clinical relevance: Even if a causal association exists between dietary sodium and potassium and blood pressure, the magnitude of the relationship is clinically trivial.

Feasibility and safety: There are potentially adverse effects, and questions of the feasibility of reducing dietary sodium and increasing dietary potassium intake, which may outweigh any potential benefits.

Aetiological association

The abundant evidence that a causal association exists between high dietary sodium, low dietary potassium and raised blood pressure has been extensively reviewed elsewhere (Langford, 1983; MacGregor, 1983; INTERSALT Cooperative Research Group, 1988; Cutler *et al.*, 1991 *a, b*; Elliott, 1991; Frost *et al.*, 1991; Law *et al.*, 1991 *a, b*; Stamler 1991). This includes experimental and clinical studies, ecologic evidence, correlations within populations, migration studies, and randomized double-blind controlled trials. While it has been suggested that the evidence is not fully consistent, in that some individual trials have demonstrated no significant effect of changing sodium and potassium intake on blood pressure, and some population studies have shown no correlations between individuals, these can arguably be attributed to lack of power in the studies and interaction with other factors which also influence blood pressure. Nevertheless, meta-analyses indicate that significant associations exist (Cutler *et al.*, 1991*b*; Frost *et al.*, 1991; Law *et al.*, 1991*a, b*), and most would agree that the criteria for causality—including biological plausibility, time sequence, consistency and dose response—have been amply satisfied. On balance, few researchers would deny a causal relationship, at least in some circumstances, between high sodium and low potassium intake and raised blood pressure.

Genetic susceptibility

It is suggested that susceptibility to hypertension—and notably to the hypertensive effect of sodium—is genetically determined, and affects only a small subset of the population, perhaps less than 10%. Thus recommendations to change dietary sodium intake would be irrelevant to most people in the general population. The early Platt-Pickering debate centred on the question of whether hypertension is a separate entity or the tail-end of a continuum in the population. There is no evidence from either population-based data or trials to support the notion of a separate genetic subset who are particularly susceptible to sodium. Where population studies have shown correlations between dietary sodium or potassium and blood pressure, these have been apparent over the whole range of blood pressure and of dietary sodium and potassium intake, not just in hypertensives (INTERSALT Cooperative Research Group, 1988; Khaw and Barrett-Connor, 1988). The strongest evidence against the notion of a genetically separate subset lies both in the international comparisons of blood pressure distributions in different communities, and in migrant studies. Data from these studies indicate that sodium and potassium intake are in fact related to blood pressures of the whole population. INTERSALT, the largest study of populations ever undertaken to examine sodium, potassium and blood pressure (10 079 adults in 52 population samples in 32 countries), found that the higher the population average sodium intake (as measured from 24-hour sodium excretion) the higher the population average blood pressure. From this, Rose and Day (1990) demonstrated that the prevalence of hypertension is related to where the population mean and distribution lies. There is no evidence of any bimodality in populations that have either high or low mean blood pressures. Poulter *et al.* (1990), in studies of the Luo in Kenya has shown that when migrants from the rural population (where mean blood pressures and sodium intake and are low) move to Nairobi (where mean blood pressures and sodium intake as higher), the whole blood pressure mean and distribution shift upwards so that there is not only a greater prevalence of hypertensives, arbitrarily defined as systolic blood pressure greater than 140 mmHg, but also a lower prevalence of persons with low blood pressure, arbitrarily defined as less than systolic 100 mmHg.

There is clearly genetic variability in susceptibility to hypertension or to the effects of sodium, but—as with any other physiological variable—this appears to be evenly distributed in the population. In the migrant studies, the whole population, even those at the low end of the distribution, is susceptible to the hypertensive environmental circumstances in Nairobi and there is no evidence of any bimodality.

Clinical relevance

A third line of argument against dietary changes is that the magnitude of the sodium and potassium and blood pressure relationship is clinically trivial. Based on trials and population studies, reduction in daily sodium intake or increase in potassium intake by 40 mmol/d is associated with a 2–6 mmHg reduction in systolic blood pressure (Frost *et al.*, 1991; Law *et al.*, 1991 *a*, *b*). Clinicians might argue that such reductions are not worthwhile. Nevertheless, the notion that the blood pressure of everyone in the whole population may be affected to some degree by dietary sodium and potassium intake has profound implications for public health. CVD risk increases continuously with increasing blood pressure across the whole blood pressure range. Rose (1981, 1985) has shown that the majority of cardiovascular events in the population attributable to raised blood pressure occur not in the small numbers of those at extremely high risk but in the large numbers of those in the centre of the population distribution. Thus a small shift downwards in the whole population mean and distribution of blood pressure may have a considerable impact on CVD both by lowering risk (even if by a small amount) in the large numbers of persons exposed to the risk, and by decreasing the prevalence of hypertensives. This is the now well recognized population strategy for prevention. A 2 mmHg reduction in population mean blood pressure could theoretically result in a 5% reduction in ischaemic heart disease (IHD) and an 11% reduction in stroke mortality, and an 8 mmHg reduction in mean blood pressure could result in a 15% reduction in IHD and a 35% reduction in stroke mortality. It is notable that clinical trials of pharmacologic treatment of hypertension show a similar order of magnitude of blood-pressure reduction and cardiovascular events.

While there are no long-term randomized trials of the effects of changing dietary sodium and potassium on clinical events such as stroke or IHD, there are observational data to suggest that these estimates of the potential magnitude of dietary effect are not unrealistic. Sasaki (1962) reported approximately twofold differences in stroke rates in two different provinces in Japan which were related to differences in mean blood pressures and in dietary sodium/potassium intake. Several prospective population studies have reported an inverse relationship between stroke incidence or mortality and either dietary potassium intake or the intake of potassium-rich foods such as fruit and vegetables. In one such study, the magnitude of the association was a 40% reduction in stroke mortality associated with a daily increase of 10 mmol dietary potassium (Khaw and Barrett-Connor, 1987). It is notable that in these studies the effect was apparent across the whole population, even in those not classified as hypertensive. Even in England and Wales, there is a threefold regional variation in hypertension and stroke mortality, and regional stroke rates are inversely correlated with regional fruit and vegetable intake (Acheson and Williams, 1983).

Feasibility and safety

A major concern about any dietary recommendations must be feasibility and safety. This requires some estimates of feasible dietary changes, how they might be achieved, and their potential benefits and risks.

The international variation in average daily dietary sodium and potassium intake in different communities is enormous, ranging from 10–400 mmol/d dietary sodium and 20–120 mmol/d dietary potassium. Most primitive societies consume very low-sodium and high-potassium diets in contrast to the opposite in more modern communities. The main reason for this is food processing. In its natural form, most food is low in sodium and high in potassium but as it is processed, sodium tends to be added and potassium leached out. Since the large proportion of sodium in western diets comes not from added table salt (which contributes only about 10–30% of the total) but from processed food, simply reducing the intake of processed food and increasing the intake of fresh food, notably fresh fruit and vegetables, can have a considerable impact on dietary sodium and potassium intake (Khaw, 1986). There is no evidence that reducing our current average sodium intake by 20–50% daily from current western levels of 120–200 mmol/d to 70–100 mmol/d is likely to be harmful in any way, except in circumstances (such as absence of refrigeration) where salted food is the only method of food preservation. However, there is considerable evidence that reducing sodium might be beneficial for CVD. It is only in circumstances when salting is the only available means of preserving food that concerns about malnutrition or food poisoning might arise, but these are hardly conditions that pertain in most western countries. Similarly, while there may be concerns about the potential side-effects such as gastrointestinal upset or cardiac toxicity, associated with large doses of potassium salts, such as with salt substitutes, there is no evidence at all of any dangers associated with considerably increasing our intake of fruit and vegetables and much evidence that this may be beneficial not just for CVD but also for other chronic diseases such as cancer (Colditz *et al.*, 1985).

As Austin Bradford Hill has suggested: '*All scientific work is incomplete— whether it be observational or experimental. All scientific work is liable to be upset or modified by advancing knowledge. That does not confer upon us a freedom to ignore the knowledge we already have, or to postpone the action that it appears to demand at a given time.*'

We can hardly be complacent about the current high rates of CVD. There are undoubtedly many other factors, known and as yet unknown, that influence blood pressure. These may include other dietary variables such as alcohol, calcium and magnesium intake, and other behavioural variables such as physical activity or stress. Nevertheless, these do not contradict or negate the accumulated evidence for the role of sodium and potassium nor, as Stamler (1991) has suggested, can they responsibly be used to justify our modern high salt intake. There is no evidence that a 20–50% reduction of current high western levels of sodium intake by decreasing processed food intake, or increasing fresh fruit and vegetable (and hence dietary potassium) intake by one or two servings a day is harmful in any way and considerable evidence that such dietary changes may be beneficial not only for CVD but for other health endpoints as well (National Research Council, Food and Nutrition Board, 1989).

Summary

The debate over dietary recommendations to the community to reduce dietary sodium or increase potassium intake continues. Based on abundant clinical, experimental and epidemiological evidence, there is now little argument that high dietary sodium intake or low potassium intake are aetiologically related to raised blood pressure. The controversy focuses on two main issues: clinical relevance (based on the arguments of variable individual susceptibility and small magnitude of effect) and safety. Reduction of dietary sodium intake or increase of dietary potassium intake of 20 mmol/d is associated with approximately 2 mmHg reduction in blood pressure. While clinically trivial in individuals, if applied over the whole population the public health consequences may be considerable; such a reduction in population mean is associated with a 10% reduction in prevalence of hypertension and estimated 5–10% reduction in CVD. Epidemiological data indicate such estimates are not unrealistic; in prospective studies, an increase of 10 mmol potassium intake daily is associated with 40% decrease in stroke mortality; the large geographical and secular variations in CVD are also consistent with these estimates. There is no evidence that a modest 20–50% reduction of current high western levels of sodium intake of around 120–200 mmol/d, achievable by reduction in processed food intake, or increasing the intake of fresh fruit and vegetables (and hence dietary potassium) by one to two servings a day is harmful in any way and considerable evidence that such dietary changes may be beneficial not only for CVD but for other health endpoints including cancer.

References

Acheson RM and Williams DRR (1983) Does consumption of fruit and vegetables protect against stroke? *The Lancet.* i:1191–3.

Colditz GA *et al.* (1985) Increased green and yellow vegetable intake and lowered cancer deaths in an elderly population. *American Journal of Clinical Nutrition.* **41**: 32–6.

Cutler JA *et al.* (eds) (1991*a*) National Heart, Lung and Blood Institute workshop on salt and blood pressure. *Hypertension.* **17**:(Suppl.I):1–22.

Cutler JA *et al.* (1991*b*) An overview of randomized trials of sodium reduction and blood pressure. *Hypertension.* **17**(Suppl.I):27–33.

Elliott P (1991) Observational studies of salt and blood pressure. *Hypertension.* **17**(Suppl.I):3–8.

Frost CD *et al.* (1991) By how much does dietary salt reduction lower blood pressure? II. Analysis of observational data within populations. *British Medical Journal.* **302**:815–18.

INTERSALT Cooperative Research Group (1988) INTERSALT: an international study of electrolyte excretion and blood pressure. Results for 24 hour urinary sodium and potassium excretion. *British Medical Journal.* **297**:319–28.

Khaw KT (1986) Feasibility of changing potassium intake in the general community. *In*: Whelton A *et al.* (eds) *Potassium in cardiovascular and renal medicine.* Marcel Dekker, New York. pp. 417–24.

Khaw KT and Barrett-Connor E (1987) Dietary potassium and stroke-associated mortality. A 12 year prospective population study. *New England Journal of Medicine.* **316**:235–40.

Khaw KT and Barrett-Connor E (1988) The association between blood pressure, age and dietary sodium and potassium: a population study. *Circulation.* **77**:53–61.

Langford HG (1983) Dietary potassium and hypertension: epidemiologic data. *Annals of Internal Medicine.* **98**:770–2.

Law MR *et al.* (1991*a*) By how much does dietary salt reduction lower blood pressure? I. Analysis of observational data among populations. *British Medical Journal.* **302**:811–15.

Law MR *et al.* (1991*b*) By how much does dietary salt reduction lower blood pressure? III. Analysis of data from trials of salt reduction. *British Medical Journal.* **302**:819–24.

MacGregor GA (1983) Sodium and potassium and blood pressure. *Hypertension.* **5** (Suppl. III):79–84.

National Research Council, Food and Nutrition Board (1989) *Diet and health: implication for reducing chronic disease risk.* National Academy Press, Washington DC.

Poulter N *et al.* (1990) The Kenyan Luo Migration Study: observations on the initiation of a rise in blood pressure. *British Medical Journal.* **300**:967–72.

Rose G (1981) Strategy of prevention: lessons from cardiovascular disease. *British Medical Journal.* **282**:1847–51.

Rose G (1985) Sick individuals and sick populations. *International Journal of Epidemiology.* **14**:32–8.

Rose G and Day S (1990) The population mean predicts the number of deviant individuals. *British Medical Journal.* **301**:1031–4.

Sasaki N (1962) High blood pressure and the salt intake of the Japanese. *Japanese Heart Journal.* **3**:313–24.

Stamler J (1991) Blood pressure and high blood pressure: aspects of risk. *Hypertension.* **18**(Suppl.I):95–107.

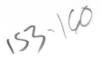

17

Is Obesity an Independent Risk Factor?

JS GARROW

For more than a decade it has been acknowledged in developed countries that obesity is one of the most important public health problems of our time, mainly because obese people are more liable to heart disease, hypertension, stroke, non-insulin-dependent diabetes and some sex-hormone-sensitive cancers (Garrow, 1988). Mortality from these causes increases significantly if Quetelet's Index (QI—weight/height^2; kg/m^2) exceeds 30. Recently it has been shown that although there is little increased mortality in the range QI 25–30, there is a significantly increased risk of disability, mainly from musculoskeletal and cardiovascular diseases (Rissanen *et al.*, 1991). However there is less consensus about the extent to which obesity is a prime cause of these diseases, or merely a marker which indicates the people who are at high risk.

Opinions about the epidemiology of cardiovascular disease (CVD) were greatly influenced by the Seven Countries Study of Keys *et al.* (1984). Concerning the aetiological role of obesity, they wrote: '*The risk of all causes or of coronary heart disease death did not increase with increasing body weight in any of the regions of the study.*' Indeed they noted that the only region in which QI (BMI as they called it) was significantly related to all causes of death was southern Europe, and here increasing weight was associated with decreasing mortality. This finding greatly influenced the Committee on Medical Aspects of Food Policy (1984), whose panel on diet and CVD wrote that being overweight '*is associated with an increased risk of hypertension, increased plasma cholesterol and diabetes mellitus. Most studies have shown no residual effect of weight on risk once age, sex, and the above risk factors have been taken into account.*' In other words, obesity itself was harmless: the increased mortality merely reflected risk factors associated with obesity.

In my view, this was a most unfortunate misapplication of the results of multiple regression analysis. The logical error becomes obvious if we consider another hypothetical example. Suppose that a committee were to review the evidence concerning death and injury sustained as a result of falling. They might note that the risk was affected by the presence of hard or sharp objects on the surface onto which the victim fell, the part of the body which took the first impact, and the velocity at which the body hit the ground. They might further conclude that, if the above risk factors were taken into account, there was no residual risk associated with the height from which the victim fell. This may be true, but of course the height from which the victim falls is a very powerful determinant of the velocity with which the body hits the ground, so it is unwise to assure people that jumping off high buildings is in fact a safe procedure.

To determine the role of obesity in causing CVD it is necessary to examine the data from which Keys *et al.* (1984) drew their conclusions, the strength of the association between obesity and the risk factors which they identified, and also the evidence of obesity causing an extra risk of CVD, even when the classic risk factors have been allowed for. Cigarette smoking is an important confounding factor. Then we may review the evidence for mechanisms by which increasing obesity may increase the risk, and decreasing obesity decrease the risk, of CVD.

The Seven Countries Study

Keys *et al.* (1984) recruited 12 225 men aged 40–59 years; 646 showed evidence of CVD at entry, so they were removed from the prospective study. Of the remaining 11 579 men, 2315 worked on the US railroads; 2379 lived in 'northern Europe' (west and east Finland and The Netherlands), 5885 lived in 'southern Europe' (Italy, Yugoslavia and Greece) and 1000 lived in Japan. After 15 years there had been 2289 deaths, of which 618 (27%) were from coronary heart disease (CHD). The CHD death rate/10 000 varied widely between regions: the highest was East Finland (1202) and the lowest was Crete (38). The average rate for northern Europe was 843, for the US was 773, for southern Europe 313, and for Japan 144. On univariate analysis the correlation between five risk factors and CHD deaths was 0.87 for serum cholesterol, 0.66 for systolic blood pressure, 0.43 for BMI, -0.11 for cigarettes smoked per day, and -0.26 for physical activity. It will be noted that BMI was the third strongest predictor of CHD death, and that cigarette smoking appeared at this stage to have a slight *protective* effect. Of course this result reflects confounding variables: if smoking is common in southern Europe and Japan, where CHD death rate is low, it will appear to have a protective effect. On multiple regression, cholesterol and blood pressure remained significant predictors of CHD death, and cigarette smoking and (of course) age were also significant predictors. However obesity did not enhance ability to predict which men would die of CHD when age, cholesterol, blood pressure and smoking had already been considered in the multiple regression equation. Keys *et al.* (1984) did not consider the possibility that obesity was itself contributing to raised cholesterol and blood pressure: that obesity was a *cause* of heart disease, and that increased blood pressure and cholesterol were among the mechanisms by which obesity had this effect. Of course, if obesity had a large effect on CVD risk, independent of age, cholesterol, blood pressure and smoking, this would have been revealed in the analysis of Keys *et al.* (1984) It is therefore pertinent to consider the strengths of the associations between obesity and these risk factors.

Associations between obesity and age, cholesterol, blood pressure and smoking, and the residual effect of obesity on CVD

In general there is a positive association between obesity and age, but this is not marked among men over the age of 45 years, as was the case with the subjects of Keys *et al.'s* study. Longitudinal studies have shown an inverse relationship between body weight and smoking: smokers tend to have a lower weight, and to gain some weight if they stop smoking. However, both smoking and obesity are associated with lower socio-economic status. We can therefore assume that correlations between obesity and age, or smoking, are unlikely to have affected the results of multiple regression much. However when we consider blood pressure and serum lipids the situation is very different. Many studies have shown—in both men and women, in adults aged 18–30 years or 45–65 years, and among black and white populations—that obesity (measured by skinfold thickness) is highly positively correlated with blood pressure, total cholesterol, low-density lipoprotein cholesterol, triglycerides, blood glucose and insulin, and is negatively correlated with the protective high-density lipoprotein cholesterol (Folsom *et al.*, 1991). Of course, if obesity was perfectly correlated with these factors, it would be impossible to show that obesity had any primary role in causing CVD, since in the regression equation any effect of obesity would already have been 'explained' by the other risk factors. However, even when due allowance has been made for age, systolic blood pressure, cholesterol, cigarettes smoked per day, impaired glucose tolerance and left ventricular hypertrophy, if the follow-up period is extended to eight years for men and to 14 years for women, relative weight does still show a small but significant association with CVD (Hubert *et al.*, 1983). On more prolonged follow-up the association of obesity and CVD becomes stronger, even when all the above risk factors have been allowed for.

Confounding effects of obesity and cigarette smoking

The effect of cigarette smoking on the multiple regression analyses of the Seven Countries Study has already been mentioned. The Whitehall Study on deaths from stroke (Shinton *et al.*, 1991) provides another good example of cigarette smoking obscuring the effect of obesity on CVD. When the men aged 40–64 years are divided into quintiles of QI, there is no obvious relation between the death rate from stroke and obesity status. When the data are broken down to smokers, ex-smokers and non-smokers however, there is a clear and statistically significant trend for increased stroke mortality with increasing obesity among non-smokers, but this is confounded by the high stroke mortality among thin smokers.

Mechanisms for obesity to cause CVD

It has now been clearly shown in animal studies that the metabolic abnormalities which are seen in obese animals arise primarily as a result of decreased sensitivity of peripheral tissues to the action of insulin (Jeanrenaud, 1991). This in turn has profound effects on the pattern of substrate utilization, and of 'counter-regulatory' hormone secretion. That this is true also in man was shown by the studies of experimental obesity in volunteers conducted by Sims *et al.* (1973): normal young men with no personal or family history of obesity or diabetes were overfed for six months so they increased their body weight by 21%, of which 73% was fat. They then showed significantly increased fasting insulin, glucose, triglyceride, cholesterol and aminoacid concentrations, and decreased oral and intravenous glucose tolerance; these are all changes of the type which characterize the non-insulin-dependent diabetic. They did not become frankly diabetic, but their QI at maximum weight was only about 28 kg/m^2. The overfeeding was then stopped, they lost weight, and the insulin insensitivity reverted towards normal. It is unreasonable to ask for a more convincing demonstration that obesity causes (and is not merely associated with) insulin insensitivity.

The consequences of insulin resistance and hyperinsulinaemia have been widely debated (Modan *et al* 1985: see also Chapter 5). The most obvious association is with non-insulin-dependent diabetes, which is certainly much more prevalent among obese people than lean ones when allowance has been made for age, sex and ethnic background (Bonham and Brock, 1985), and the association of diabetes with both peripheral and coronary artery disease is also well established. Obesity is associated with hypertension, perhaps through the action of hyperinsulinaemia, although the mechanism of this association is not entirely clear. Patients who have insulin-secreting tumours removed do not show a significant fall in blood pressure after the operation, but the hypertension could have been initiated by the hyperinsulinaemia and then sustained by other mechanisms. Obesity is associated with left ventricular hypertrophy (Lauer *et al.*, 1991) which may be explained by the combination of hypertension and the increased cardiac output which is required in the obese state. The association between obesity and the unfavourable plasma lipid profile, which has already been discussed, is to be expected in view of the greatly increased cholesterol flux in the obese person (Whiting *et al.*, 1984).

The effect of weight loss on mortality and on cardiovascular risk factors

It would not be practicable or ethical to conduct a trial in which the mortality of a randomly selected group of obese people who lost weight was compared with that of a control group who remained obese. However, anecdotal evidence strongly favours the hypothesis that weight loss in obese people improves life expectancy: this has been the experience of life insurance companies among formerly overweight clients who achieved normal weight to obtain life insurance at normal rates (Dublin, 1953).

The effect of weight change on cardiovascular risk factors is well documented. In the Framingham population, people who lost weight between serial examinations showed a decrease in blood pressure, cholesterol, glucose and uric acid, while those who gained weight showed a worsening of these risk factors (Kannel and Gordon, 1975). In the normative ageing study, weight change was similarly associated with change in cardiovascular risk factors after controlling for the initial levels of the risk factor, age, weight and smoking status (Borkan et al., 1986). This is important evidence, since it argues strongly that the association between obesity and these risk factors is not just a coincidence, but that obesity really is an important and reversible risk factor for CVD.

Weight cycling and cardiovascular risk

It has been observed among populations both in the UK (Wannamethee and Shaper, 1990) and the USA (Lissner et al., 1991) that individuals who show large fluctuations in weight have a higher mortality rate and a greater risk of CVD than individuals who maintain a fairly constant weight. This observation has been interpreted by some people as an indication that obesity should not be treated. The argument goes thus: (1) obese people who lose weight always regain it, (2) it is worse to have a fluctuating weight than a constant one, so (3) it is better for obese people not to attempt weight loss.

There is some substance in this argument, although the premise is false. Weight regain is not inevitable, and it is not certain that the association between fluctuating weight and increased risk of CVD is a causal one. People who show large fluctuations in body weight may well have characteristics which predispose them to CVD, regardless of their weight fluctuations. However it should be noted that both starvation and overeating diminish insulin sensitivity, so alternating these two states could well aggravate the cardiovascular risks associated with obesity. I would agree that if the proposed treatment of obesity is to put the patient on a semi-starvation diet for a month or two, achieve rapid weight loss, and then imagine that the problem is solved, it would probably be better not to attempt treatment. Anyone who attempts to treat obese patients must be willing to invest quite a lot of work in helping the patient to lose weight at an appropriate rate and then to maintain this weight loss (Garrow, 1988). The fact that it is possible to treat obesity badly is not a good argument for not treating it at all.

Wider health implications of obesity

Obesity does not only affect CVD (Garrow, 1988, 1991). Figure 17.1 indicates important diseases (in black boxes) and lifestyle factors which contribute to the aetiology of these diseases (in white boxes). In this scheme obesity and cigarette

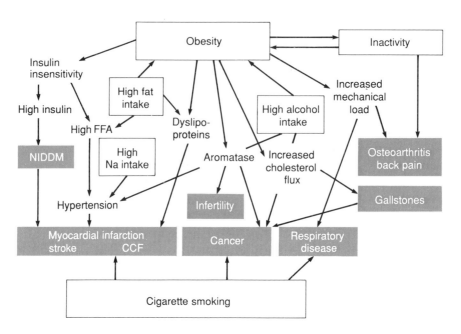

Figure 17.1: Important causes of death and disability (shown in black boxes) and lifestyle factors which dispose to them (in white boxes). Linking mechanisms are indicated by arrows. (Source: Garrow, 1991.)

smoking are shown as important and alterable lifestyle factors which make independent contributions to the risk of cardiovascular, respiratory and malignant disease. The contribution of obesity to CVD risk has already been discussed in some detail, but a high intake of sodium, fat and alcohol also contribute to the disease risk. Adipose tissue is an important store of the aromatase enzyme system, which converts androgens to oestrogens, and this probably explains the increased liability of obese people to certain sex-hormone-sensitive cancers. The contribution of the increased cholesterol flux arising from excess adipose tissue has already been mentioned in connection with atherogenic risks, but it is also a risk factor for gallstone formation, and for diseases of the biliary system. The increased mechanical load associated with obesity contributes to musculoskeletal diseases, especially osteoarthritis of weight-bearing joints, and decreases exercise tolerance. Another handicap of obese people, which is less easy to study quantitatively, is social discrimination: there is good evidence that, for a given level of ability and training, obese people are less socially successful than their leaner peers.

The view that obesity is harmless is not tenable in the light of the evidence that has accumulated over the past decade.

References

Bonham GS and Brock DB (1985) The relationship of diabetes with race, sex, and obesity. *American Journal of Clinical Nutrition*. **41**:776–83.

Borkan GA *et al.* (1986) Body weight and coronary heart disease risk: patterns of risk factor change associated with long-term weight change. *American Journal of Epidemiology*. **124**:410–19.

Committee on Medical Aspects of Food Policy (1984) *Diet and cardiovascular disease. DHSS Report on Health and Social Subjects No 28*. HMSO, London. p 32.

Dublin LI (1953) Relation of obesity to longevity. *New England Journal of Medicine*. **248**:971–4.

Folsom AR *et al.* (1991) Implications of obesity for cardiovascular disease in blacks: the CARDIA and ARIC studies. *Americal Journal of Clinical Nutrition*. **53**:1604–11S.

Garrow JS (1988) *Obesity and related diseases*. Churchill Livingstone, London. p. 329.

Garrow JS (1991) Importance of obesity. *British Medical Journal*. **303**:704–6.

Hubert HB *et al.* (1983) Obesity as an independent risk factor for cardiovascular disease: a 26-year follow-up of participants in the Framingham heart study. *Circulation*. **67**:968–77.

Jeanrenaud B (1991) Neuroendocrinology and evolutionary aspects of experimental obesity. In: Oomura Y *et al.* (eds), *Progress in obesity research 1990*. John Libbey, London. pp. 409–21.

Kannel WB and Gordon T (1975) Some determinants of obesity and its impact as a cardiovascular risk factor. In: Howard A (ed.) *Recent advances in obesity research*, 1. Newman Books, London, pp. 14-27.

Keys A *et al.* (1984) The Seven Countries Study: 2289 deaths in 15 years. *Preventive Medicine*. **13**:141–54.

Lauer MS *et al.* (1991) The impact of obesity on left ventricular mass and geometry. The Framingham Heart Study. *Journal of the American Medical Association*. **266**:231–6.

Lissner L *et al.* (1991) Variability of body weight and health outcomes in the Framingham population. *New England Journal of Medicine*. **324**:1839–44.

Modan M *et al.* (1985) Hyperinsulinaemia: a link between hypertension obesity and glucose intolerance. *Journal of Clinical Investigation*. **75**:809–17.

Rissanen A *et al.* (1991) Risk of disability and mortality due to overweight in a Finnish population. *British Medical Journal.* **301**:835–6.

Shinton R *et al.* (1991) Overweight and stroke in the Whitehall study. *Journal of Epidemiology and Community Health.* **45**:138–42.

Sims EAH *et al.* (1973) Endocrine and metabolic effects of experimental obesity in man. *Recent Progress in Hormone Research.* **29**:457–96.

Wannamethee G and Shaper AG (1990) Weight change in middle-aged British men: implications for health. *European Journal of Clinical Nutrition.* **44**:133–42

Whiting MJ *et al.* (1984) The cholesterol saturation of bile and its reduction by chenodeoxycholic acid in massively obese patients. *International Journal of Obesity.* **8**:681–8.

18

Smoking as a Risk Factor for Cardiovascular Disease

GODFREY FOWLER

Although over the last 30 years or so there has been a substantial decline in smoking prevalence in Britain and many other developed countries, especially among men, tobacco use is still increasing rapidly worldwide. In the UK, roughly a third of the adult population still smokes cigarettes: the latest available survey data show that in 1990, 31% of men and 29% of women were cigarette smokers (Table 18.1). These figures hide two important details: prevalence peaks in young adulthood in both men and women (Table 18.2), and there is a steep social-class gradient in both men and women, with a threefold increase from professional to unskilled manual males (Figure 18.1).

This chapter is concerned primarily with two basic questions: (1) what is the evidence that tobacco smoking causes cardiovascular disease (CVD)? (2) If there are benefits from stopping smoking, how quickly are they achieved?

Smoking as a cause of CVD

Tobacco smoking is a well known cause of lung cancer and respiratory disease but its contribution to CVD is less widely appreciated, at least by the public.

Although the relationship between smoking and diseases of the lungs (especially lung cancer) was established first (Doll and Hill, 1950; Wynder and Graham, 1950), the link with CVD also soon became apparent, the early results of the first cohort studies showing that death from coronary heart disease (CHD) was more common in smokers than non-smokers (Doll and Hill, 1956). From many prospective studies it is now clear that, in countries where CHD is common, CVD is the most important cause of smoking-related premature death. Although the relative risk of lung cancer in smokers, compared with non-smokers, is much greater than that of CHD, the absolute risk of CHD death is greater than that of death from lung cancer.

Numerous prospective studies have investigated the relationship between smoking and vascular disease. In the Seven Countries Study (Keys, 1970) there was no apparent relationship across countries between cigarette smoking and the incidence of ischaemic heart disease; the Japanese were the heaviest smokers, but had the lowest risk of CHD. Prospective studies within countries, however, have shown that where CHD is common because of elevated blood lipid levels, there is a clear relationship between smoking and CVD (Doll and Peto, 1976; Reid et al., 1976; Doll et al., 1980; Shaper et al., 1985.) This

	Men	Women
Current smokers	31	29
Ex-regular smokers	32	19
Never/occasional only smokers	37	52

Table 18.1: Percentage of men and women who smoked cigarettes in 1990. (Source: OPCS.)

Age (years)	Men	Women
16–19	28 (28)	32 (28)
20–24	38 (37)	39 (37)
25–34	36 (37)	34 (35)
35–49	34 (37)	33 (35)
50–59	28 (33)	29 (34)
≥ 60	24 (26)	20 (21)

Table 18.2: Percentage of cigarette smokers by age and sex in 1990 (1988 figures in brackets). (Source: OPCS.)

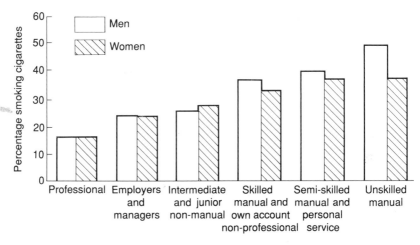

Figure 18.1: Cigarette smoking prevalence by sex and socio-economic group, Great Britain, 1990. (Source: OPCS Monitor 1991, SS91/3.)

Cause	Excess deaths per 100 000 smokers per year
Lung cancer	94 (19%)
Chronic bronchitis and emphysema	47 (10%)
Coronary heart disease	152 (31%)
Other cardiovscular diseases, including stroke	100 (21%)
Other diseases	92 (19%)
Total	485 (100%)

Table 18.3: Excess death rates (age-standardized) in male smokers attributable to various causes. (Source: Doll and Peto, 1976.)

relationship is well demonstrated by one of the earliest prospective studies, the British Doctors Study, initiated by Doll and Hill in 1951 (Doll and Peto, 1976; Doll *et al.*, 1980). Data from the 20-year follow-up of 34 000 male doctors, reported in 1976, showed that about half the excess mortality from smoking is from CVD, with about a third of the excess mortality from CHD alone (Table 18.3).

Interaction with other risk factors is important, and this interaction with the other major modifiable risk factors—blood pressure and cholesterol level—is well illustrated by the CHD mortality data from the follow-up of over one third of a million people screened for the Multiple Risk Factor Intervention Trial (Marmot, 1986; Martin, 1986).

Smoking contributes variably to the different types of vascular disease. Deaths from pulmonary heart disease and aortic aneurysm are most strongly associated with smoking, as is peripheral vascular disease (although this is not itself a major cause of cardiovascular death). The risk associated with primary pipe or cigar smoking is much lower than that for cigarette smoking (Doll and Peto, 1976; Shaper *et al.*, 1985) but switching from cigarettes to pipe or cigars appears not to be associated with significant reduction of risk. The number of deaths due to various types of vascular disease and the risks relative to non-smokers in current and ex-smokers in the British Doctors Study at follow-up in 1986 is shown in Table 18.4.

Generally speaking, the prospective studies have shown that the relative risk of death from CHD for smokers compared to non-smokers is roughly doubled for both men and women. But this relative risk varies with age, being substantially greater at a younger age but not much greater than that for non-smokers over the age of 65. Again this is illustrated by data from the British Doctors Study. As in many other prospective studies, there was also a clear dose response relationship, with the amount smoked being clearly related to risk (Figure 18.2). Cook *et al.* (1986), however, found that risk was related to duration of smoking rather than daily smoking habit (Figure 18.3). The

Type of circulatory disease	Pure cigarette smokers			Pure pipe smokers	Statistical significance of trend with cigarette smoking
	Ex	All current	25 or more	All current	
Pulmonary heart disease* (N = 58)	3.3	3.8	9.5	2.8	$P < 0.001$
Aortic aneurysm (N = 271)	2.0	4.3	5.7	3.2	$P < 0.001$
Myocardial degeneration (N = 803)	1.3	1.9	2.7	1.3	$P < 0.001$
Ischaemic heart disease (N = 5593)	1.2	1.6	1.8	1.1	$P < 0.001$
Cerebrovascular disease (N = 2267)	1.1	1.5	1.7	1.0	$P < 0.001$
Other cardiovascular disease (N = 1231)	0.9	1.2	1.4	0.9	$P < 0.05$

*Risk related to risk in non-smokers and light cigarette smokers combined, as no deaths occured in non-smokers.

Table 18.4: Risk of death by smoking habit relative to risk in non-smokers: circulatory disease. (Source: Doll *et al.*, 1990.)

explanation for this is not clear, although it could be that smoking habit at entry in this study did not truly reflect previous smoking habits.

Although the introduction of filtered low-tar and low-nicotine cigarettes and the progessive reduction in tar and nicotine yields over the last 30 years or so have (along with the decline in smoking prevalence) contributed to a fall in the death rate of smokers, there is little evidence that these changes have reduced CHD mortality rates in smokers (Castelli *et al.*, 1981).

It is now clear that smoking is a major risk factor for strokes as well as for CHD. In the British Doctors Study, the increase in risk was by about a third but in the British Regional Heart Study there was a twofold increase in risk (Shaper *et al.*, 1991). A recent meta-analysis of all published studies suggests an overall relative risk of about 1.5, with this relative risk, as with CHD, being greater at a younger age and a dose response effect being apparent in some studies (Shinton and Beavers 1989). However, there are considerable differences in relative risk amongst stroke subtypes (2.9 for subarachnoid haemorrhage, 1.9 for cerebral infarction, and 0.7 for cerebral haemorrhage).

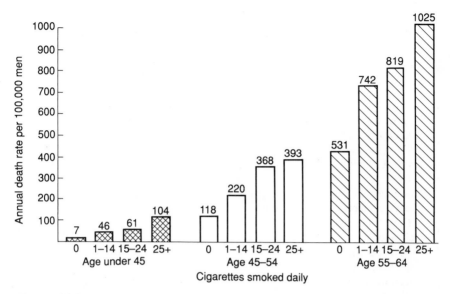

Figure 18.2: Mortality from coronary heart disease in male non-smokers and current smokers by age and smoking category (numbers above columns are numbers of deaths). (Source: Doll and Peto, 1976; Royal College of Physicians, 1977.)

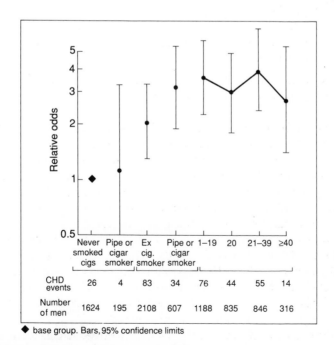

Figure 18.3: Age-adjusted relative odds of a major CHD event by smoking status at screening. (Source: Cook *et al.*, 1986.)

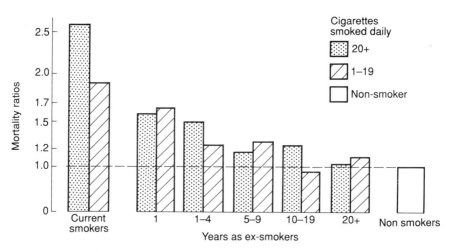

Figure 18.4: Diminished risk of death from coronary heart disease in former light and heavy smokers. (Source: Hammond and Garfinkel, 1969.)

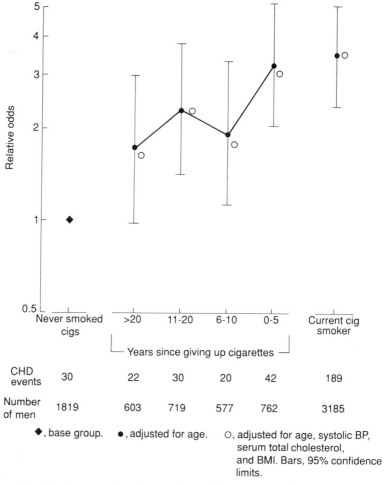

Figure 18.5: Relative odds of a major CHD event in relation to years since stopping smoking cigarettes. (Source: Cook *et al.*, 1986.)

Are there benefits from stopping smoking and, if so, how quickly are they achieved?

An important question is whether stopping smoking reduces excess risk. The observational studies provide evidence of reduction in excess risk of heart attack or death from CHD in those who stop smoking compared with those who continue (Figure 18.4) (Hammond and Garfinkel, 1969; Rosenberg *et al.*, 1990). Evidence from controlled trials of smoking cessation is not substantial, but is consistent with the observational studies. The Oslo Study (Hjermann *et al.*, 1981) involved both dietary change and advice to stop smoking, and the analysis suggested that the major determinant of the reduction in fatal and non-fatal MI was reduction in total cholesterol and to a lesser extent reduction in smoking. The randomized trial of smoking cessation advice in the Whitehall Study (Rose and Colwill, 1992) showed a small reduction in CHD and all causes of mortality at the 20-year follow-up. So there is little dispute that stopping smoking reduces risk, although debate revolves around the issue of the rapidity with which this excess risk attenuates. The British Doctors Study and many other observational studies suggest that the excess risk declines fairly rapidly, especially in younger smokers. However in the British Regional Heart Study (Cook *et al.*, 1986) there was no decline within five years of stopping smoking, and only a slow decline after that (Figure 18.5).

Stopping smoking after MI is associated with a substantial reduction in risk of non-fatal recurrences and of cardiovascular death, both short-term and long-term (Figure 18.6) (Wilhelmsson *et al.*, 1975; Daly *et al.*, 1983).

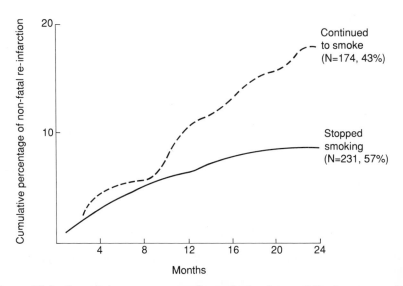

Figure 18.6: Cumulative percentage of non-fatal relapses following myocardial infarction (N = 405). (Source: Wilhelmsson *et al.*, 1975.)

Passive smoking is now a significant public health issue. While the evidence of an association between passive smoking and increased risk of lung cancer is now clear, a similar association with cardiovascular risk from prolonged exposure to environmental tobacco smoke is less firmly established; but a recent overview of ten epidemiological studies suggests passive smoking may increase the risk CHD death by as much as 25% (Beaglehole, 1990).

References

Beaglehole R (1990). Does passive smoking cause heart disease? (Editiorial). *British Medical Journal.* **301**:1343–4.

Castelli WP *et al.* (1981) The filter cigarette and coronary heart disease. *The Lancet.* **ii**:109.

Cook DG *et al.* (1986) Giving up smoking and the risk of heart attacks: a report from the British Regional Heart Study. *The Lancet.* **ii**:1376–9.

Daly LE *et al.* (1983) Long term effect on mortality of stopping smoking after unstable angina and myocardial infarction. *British Medical Journal.* **287**:324–6.

Doll R and Hill AB (1950) Smoking and carcinoma of the lung. *British Medical Journal.* **2**:739.

Doll R and Hill AB (1956). Lung cancer and other causes of death in relation to smoking. *British Medical Journal.* **2**:1071–81.

Doll R and Peto R (1976). Mortality in relation to smoking: 20 years observation of British doctors. *British Medical Journal.* **4**:1525.

Doll R *et al* (1980) Mortality in relation to smoking: 22 years observation of female British doctors. *British Medical Journal.* **1**:967.

Doll R *et al.* (1990) Tobacco related diseases. *Journal of Smoking Related Diseases.* **1**:3–13.

Hammond EC and Garfinkel (1969) Coronary heart disease, stroke and aortic aneurysm: factors in aetiology. *Archives of Environmental Health.* **19**:167.

Hjermann T *et al.* (1981) Effect of diet and smoking intervention on incidence of coronary heart disease. The Oslo Study. *The Lancet.* **ii**:1303–10.

Keys A (1970) Coronary heart disease in seven countries. *Circulation.* **41** (Suppl. 1).

Marmot MG (1986) Epidemiology and the art of the soluble. *The Lancet.* **i**:897–900.

Martin MJ *et al.* (1986) Serum cholesterol, blood pressure, and mortality: implications from a cohort of 361 662 men. *The Lancet.* **ii**:933–6.

OPCS (1990) Cigarette smoking 1972–88. *OPCS Monitor.* 5590/2.

Reid DD *et al.* (1976). Smoking and other risk factors for coronary heart disease in British civil servants. *The Lancet.* **ii**:979–83.

Rose G and Colwill L (1992) Randomised controlled trial of anti-smoking advice: final (20 year) results. *Journal of Epidemiology and Community Health.* **42**:75–7.

Rosenberg L *et al.* (1990) Decline in risk of myocardial infarction among women who stop smoking. *New England Journal of Medicine.* **322**:213–17.

Royal College of Physicians (1977) *Smoking or health?* Pitman Medical, London.

Shaper AG *et al.* (1985) Risk factors for ischaemic heart disease: the prospective phase of the British Regional Heart Study. *Journal of Epidemiology and Community Health.* **35**:197–209.

Shaper AG *et al.* (1991) Risk factors for stroke in middle aged British men. *British Medical Journal.* **302**:1111–15.

Shinton R and Beavers G (1989) Meta-analysis of relation between cigarette smoking and stroke. *British Medical Journal.* **298**:789.

Wilhelmsson C *et al.* (1975) Smoking and myocardial infarction. *The Lancet.* **i**:415.

Wynder EL and Graham EA (1950) Tobacco smoking as a possible etiological factor in bronchogenic carcinoma. *Journal of the American Medical Association.* **143**:329.

19

Cigarette Smoking and Atherosclerosis

N WOOLF, RM PITTILO, PM ROWLES, AA NORONHA-DUTRA AND
MM EPPERLEIN

A recent article in *The Lancet* states that, on current smoking patterns, just over 20% of those now living in developed countries will owe their deaths to cigarette smoking (Peto *et al.*, 1992). A large proportion of these will be due to atherosclerosis-related diseases, and there can be little or no doubt that there is a very strong epidemiological association between such disorders and cigarette smoking (Doll *et al.*, 1990). Doll (1983) estimated that cigarette smoking accounted for about 25% of the mortality from ischaemic heart disease. It is clear that this baneful effect of cigarette smoking might be mediated via a number of different pathways, which include changes in clotting indices and in the behaviour of platelets, and this view gains some support from the steady decline in risk of a major ischaemic event which results from stopping smoking. In addition, data from the long-running Framingham study show that the increment of clinical risk in cigarette smokers finds its chief expression in myocardial infarction and sudden death rather than in stable angina pectoris (Doyle *et al.*, 1964).

Is there increased atherogenesis in cigarette smokers?

Nevertheless it would be wrong to conclude that cigarette smoke has no effect on the extent and severity of atherosclerosis. Retrospective studies of material derived from necropsies on smokers and non-smokers have consistently shown more extensive and severe atherosclerosis in the former (Pittilo and Woolf, 1993). A prospective study carried out by Rhoads *et al.* (1976) in a group of Japanese-American men showed that there was a statistically independent association between the daily consumption of cigarettes and the degree of aortic and coronary atherosclerosis.

The mechanisms which operate in the genesis and natural history of atherosclerotic plaques are complex and it is virtually certain that many different cell types take part (Ross, 1986).

Despite the convincing epidemiological data which have been alluded to above, the mechanisms by which cigarette smoke produces its effects are still largely unknown. Cigarette smoke is an immensely complex mixture, with more than 3000 components already identified; so ascribing these effects to one or other component will certainly not be easy. Even the targets related to artery wall structure and function are multiple and heterogeneous. Cigarette smoke produces changes in the ability of platelets and endothelial cells to produce prostanoids (Jeremy and Mikhailidis, 1990); it produces alterations in platelet function (Kutti, 1990; Murray *et al.*, 1990; Schmidt *et al.*, 1990); it alters plasma lipoprotein profiles (Olsson and Molgaard, 1990) and produces changes in the pattern of aortic proteoglycans and glycosoaminoglycans (Latha *et al.*, 1991). In addition, cigarette smoking changes have been recorded in relation to blood flow and to artery wall mechanics (Caro, 1990).

Endothelium and cigarette smoke

If potentially cytotoxic components of cigarette smoke do indeed gain access to the blood stream, the first component of the circulatory system with which they are likely to interact is the endothelium. The day is long past when endothelium could be regarded as a more or less passive barrier between the elements of flowing blood and the sub-endothelial tissues. It is now appreciated that endothelial cells have a very wide repertoire in respect of synthesis and secretion and that endothelial products include surface molecules important in blood cell/endothelium adhesion, growth factors which can affect arterial smooth muscle cells and components which take part in the activation and regulation of coagulation and fibrinolytic pathways (Petty and Pearson, 1989). In the same way, our ideas as to what constitutes endothelial injury have undergone a change. Where once this concept was restricted to instances when endothelial cell denudation could be recognized on ultrastructural examination, we now know that endothelial cell loss can occur with no morphological evidence of denudation. As in the case of any other cell, the meaning of the term 'injury' should be extended to include a variety of alterations in cell function some of which may (although some may not) be associated with morphological changes (Reidy, 1985).

Cigarette smoke-related morphological changes in endothelium

From the morphological point of view, human arteries are the most relevant for studying the effects of cigarette smoking. For obvious reasons, opportunities for this are restricted. Asmussen and her colleagues have studied umbilical artery endothelium from cords of infants born to smoking or to non-smoking mothers. Arteries from the former showed sub-endothelial oedema and the endothelial cells were swollen and appeared contracted. In addition the luminal plasma membranes showed the presence of irregular, bleb-like projections. Basement membranes were thickened and there was widening of the intercellular junctions (Asmussen and Kjeldsen, 1975; Asmussen, 1978, 1982*a,b,c*, 1984). Changes in the pattern of endothelial nuclear chromatin have also been described in the endothelial cells of infants born to smoking mothers (Asmussen 1982*a*), and endothelial cells from such infants contain more mitochondria than those of 'controls' (Asmussen, 1984). Morphological changes have also been reported in endothelial cells in uterine arteries from smokers (Bylock *et al.*, 1979). Not everyone accepts that these sites are suitable for the study of the effects of cigarette smoke, and at least one study (Staubesand *et al.*, 1984) suggests that changes similar to those alluded to above can be seen in the umbilical arteries of infants born to non-smoking mothers as well. Perhaps a more important reservation concerns the ease with which artefactual changes can be produced in endothelium, emphasizing the importance of employing standardized, precise and comparable methodology in preparing specimens for ultrastructural examination (Buss and Hollweg, 1977; Pittilo, 1988).

Morphological changes in endothelium associated with exposure of animals to cigarette smoke

Examination of arterial specimens from animals exposed to cigarette smoke has a number of potential advantages. First, the dosimetry of the smoke exposure can be accurately controlled. This is important since, quite apart from standardizing the amount of smoke exposure, variations (eg in the burning temperature of the cigarette) are associated with variations in smoke chemistry, as is the degree of freshness of the smoke. Secondly, the treatment of the specimens can reduce the chances of artefact. In small animals, the whole circulatory bed can be perfused with oxygenated and buffered solutions and then fixed under pressure before undertaking any dissection, which may cause artefactual changes.

Cigarette smoke exposure has been shown to result regularly in morphological changes in the aortic endothelium of rats and rabbits, the nature of these changes being basically similar in both species (Pittilo, 1990) (*see* Figures 19.1–19.4). On scanning electron microscopy many of the endothelial cells appear swollen and irregular. Their plasma membranes show some striking abnormalities which include the presence of projections, some of which are bleb-like and some microvillus in appearance. In addition there are large numbers of small, rounded and well demarcated defects which, it has been suggested, represent the stomata of plasmalemmal vesicles. Transmission electron microscopy confirms the presence of these plasma membrane abnormalities (Pittilo *et al.*, 1990), which bear a close resemblance to those seen in cells which have been subjected to oxidant stress with consequent peroxidation of unsaturated lipids in their plasma membranes (Noronha-Dutra and Steen, 1982).

Platelet/vessel wall interactions

Both in rats and in rabbits, exposure to cigarette smoke is associated with the presence of groups of platelets adhering to an apparently intact endothelial surface. These platelet aggregates, which were present in the vast majority of the animals studied, were found mostly in relation to ostia of intercostal arteries. At these branches, the platelets were found in the proximal portion of

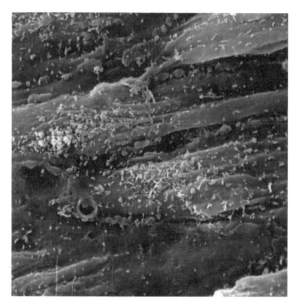

Figure 19.1: Scanning electron micrograph of rat aorta following exposure to cigarette smoke. The normally smooth lumenal plasma membrane is covered with small blebs and microvillous processes. × 8000

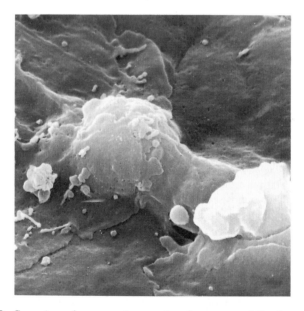

Figure 19.2: Scanning electron micrograph of rat aorta following exposure to cigarette smoke. The endothelial cell in the centre of the field shows swelling and contraction, and at its right extremity a leucocyte can be seen penetrating between endothelial cells to reach the sub-endothelial space. × 15 600

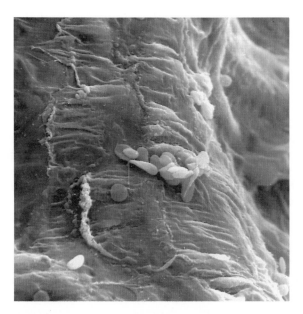

Figure 19.3: Scanning electron micrograph of rat aorta following exposure to cigarette smoke. The field chosen shows the proximal part of the ostium of a branch on which a small group of aggregated platelets can be seen adhering to the underlying endothelial surface. × 4800

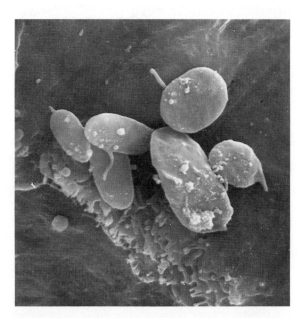

Figure 19.4: Scanning electron micrograph of rat aorta following exposure to cigarette smoke, showing a small number of platelets adhering to an intact but morphologically abnormal endothelial surface. × 13 200

the ostia, where the wall shear rates are low and the 'dwell time' of cells is longest.

In the *ex vivo* situation, exposure of cultured mesothelial cells to plasma samples derived from human volunteer smokers has also been shown to be associated with morphological changes (Pittilo *et al.*, 1985). Mesothelial cells were chosen since they are not only very easy to culture, but also constitute a non-thrombogenic surface, perhaps because of their ability to produce prostacyclin (Blow, 1988). Compared with pre-smoking samples of plasma, those obtained after the volunteers had smoked two cigarettes, produced—after 30 minutes' exposure, following by removal of the plasma and replacement with culture medium—some striking morphological changes in which blebbing of the plasma membranes was again a prominent feature.

In another *ex vivo* model, smoking has been shown to alter platelet/vessel wall interactions. Non-abraded aorta from rabbits was exposed in a Baumgartner flow chamber to pre- and post-smoking samples of whole blood from human volunteers who had smoked two medium-tar cigarettes. Passage of the post-smoking samples of blood was associated with the adherence of very numerous platelets to the endothelial surfaces of the rabbit aortae. It is not clear whether this was due to an alteration in the expression of platelet surface adhesion molecules or whether the endothelium played a major role. However, while smoking produces no significant degree of change in adenosine diphosphate (ADP) or collagen-induced platelet aggregation, a rise in the plasma concentrations of Factor VIII related antigen was reported in six of eight volunteers after smoking two cigarettes (Pittilo *et al.*, 1984).

The effects of cigarette smoke on prostacyclin production by endothelial cells

The finding of activated platelets on apparently intact endothelial surfaces, in the arteries of animals exposed to cigarette smoke, raises a number of questions, including whether cigarette smoke influences platelet/vessel wall interactions by depressing endothelial prostacyclin production.

Aortic rings obtained from anaesthetized rats which had been exposed to fresh smoke showed a decrease in their ablity to produce prostacyclin, when compared with tissue taken from 'sham-smoked' animals (Pittilo *et al.*, 1982; Lubawy *et al.*, 1986); and umbilical arteries from the cords of infants born to mothers who were smokers produce less prostacyclin than those derived from the cords of infants of mothers who were non-smokers (Dadak *et al.*, 1981).

In humans, the data relating to the effects of cigarette smoking on PGI_2 production are somewhat conflicting, although the majority of studies indicate that a cigarette smoke-related depression of prostacyclin production does indeed exist (Nadler *et al.*, 1983; Jeremy *et al.*, 1985; Reinders *et al.*, 1986). Apart from a putative role in modulating platelet/vessel wall interaction, prostacyclin may also exert some cytoprotective effect on endothelium. Infusion of prostacyclin into patients with peripheral vascular disease has been followed by a fall in the number of circulating endothelial cells (Sinzinger *et al.*, 1988) and an increase in circulating endothelial cells has been reported in patients with sickle cell disease following cigarette smoking (Sowemimo-Coker *et al.*, 1989).

As stated above, cigarette smoke is so complex a mixture that it is not possible to examine the effects of all its individual constituents. However, data on nicotine do exist.

The effect of nicotine on endothelial morphology and function

Giving nicotine orally to rabbits has been associated with changes in aortic arch endothelium which include what has been described as 'ruffling' and microvillus formation (Booyse *et al.*, 1981*a*). Acute administration of nicotine in quite large doses (10 mg/kg) has failed to produce any of the morphological changes described as occurring after exposure to cigarette smoke (Pittilo and Bull, 1988), although a subacute regime—in which nicotine was administered to rats via a subcutaneous infusion pump for a period of seven days—was associated with morphological changes in endothelium which were characterized by microvillus projections from the plasma membranes, platelet adhesion and some separation of adjacent endothelial cells (Pittilo *et al.*, 1990). No morphological changes were detected in dog arterial endothelium after intravenous administration of nicotine (Allen *et al.*, 1988). In the rat, however, intravenous injections of nicotine have been associated with a rise in the number of circulating endothelial cells (Hladovec, 1978).

In endothelial cell cultures, very high concentrations of nicotine outside the usual range encountered in human smokers are required before any morphological abnormalities can be detected (Booyse *et al.*, 1981*b*; Bull *et al.*, 1985). Blaes *et al.* (1986) found that treatment of cultured human umbilical vein endothelial cells with nicotine led to an increased secretion of Factor VIII/Vwf and a decrease both of fibronectin secretion and the intracellular content of fibronectin. High concentrations of nicotine did succeed in decreasing prostacyclin production by cultured human endothelial cells (Bull *et al.*, 1985), but the concentrations used were greater than those which occur in the plasma of human smokers.

Free radicals: a possible role in cigarette smoke-mediated endothelial change

The presence of free radicals in cigarette smoke has been known for almost 35 years (Lyons *et al.*, 1958), and it has been shown that there is an association between lipid peroxidation and endothelial cell injury (Hennig and Chow, 1988). As already pointed out, the morphological changes seen in aortic endothelium of animals exposed to cigarette smoke, and those seen in cultured cells treated with plasma from volunteer smokers, closely resemble what is seen in cardiac myocytes and other cell types following free radical mediated lipid peroxidation in their plasma membranes (Woolf and Wilson-Holt, 1981; Noronha-Dutra and Steen, 1982; Noronha-Dutra et al., 1984; Pittilo et al., 1985).

Cigarette smoke radicals fall into two classes (Pryor et al., 1990). The first are long-lived radicals which are associated with the particulate or tar phase of the smoke. These are semiquinone radicals which are associated with the redox shuttling which can occur between quinones and hydroquinones in the tar. The quinones and hydroquinones in smoke include catechol and other quinoid compounds which may be present in smoke or generated by oxidation of polycyclic hydrocarbons.

The second category of radical is associated with the vapour phase of smoke which contains carbon and oxygen-centred radicals. These have structures which predict a very short lifespan, but spin trap experiments have shown that these radicals have apparent stability in excess of five minutes. This suggests that there is a dynamic equilibrium in which there is both continuous formation and continuous destruction of these radicals (Church and Pryor, 1985). One possible chain of events which might account for the observed data starts with the rather slow oxidation of nitric oxide to nitrogen dioxide. Nitrogen dioxide could then react with such constituents of smoke as isoprene, butadiene and acrolein leading to the formation of carbon-centred radicals. These then react with the oxygen in smoke to give peroxyl radicals, which are deoxygenated by nitric oxide to potentially cytotoxic alkoxyl radicals.

Noronha-Dutra et al. (1993) have studied some of the biochemical events which occur after cultured human umbilical vein endothelium is treated with plasma samples derived from volunteer smokers, or with plasma samples to which standard doses of fresh cigarette smoke had been added. In both circumstances there was evidence of activation of the hexose–monophosphate shunt and a sharp increase in the total glutathione content of the culture medium, which are suggestive of oxidant stress. There was also evidence of some degree of cell injury as manifested by a decrease in the ability of the cells to produce ATP.

Red blood cells from smokers contain more glutathione than those of non-smokers, and when these cells are added to endothelial cell cultures they exert a greater degree of protection against hydrogen peroxide-mediated damage than do red cells from non-smokers (Toth et al., 1986). This suggests that repetitive oxidant stress, such as might occur in smokers, might lead to an adaptive up-regulation of scavenging mechanisms in the red cell. Another piece of circumstantial evidence has been the finding that cigarette smoking is followed by an increased output of pentane in the breath, which is regarded by some as evidence of lipid peroxidation. High doses of Vitamin E have been reported as suppressing this effect (Hoshino et al., 1990).

These data, although clearly incomplete, suggest that the generation of free radicals within cigarette smoke may be an important pathogenetic pathway in cigarette smoke-related cell injury, both within and without the circulatory system.

Acknowledgement

These studies were supported by a grant from the Tobacco Products Research Trust.

References

Allen DR *et al.* (1988) The effect of cigarette smoke, nicotine and carbon monoxide on the permeability of the arterial wall. *Journal of Vascular Surgery.* 7:139–52.

Asmussen I (1978) Arterial changes in infants of smoking mothers. *Postgraduate Medical Journal.* 54:200–4.

Asmussen I (1982*a*) Chromatin changes of endothelial cells in umbilical arteries in smokers. *Clinical Cardiology.* 5:653–6.

Asmussen I (1982*b*) Ultrastructure of the umbilical arteries from new-born children of smoking and non-smoking mothers. *Acta Pathologica Scandinavica.* 90:375–83.

Asmussen I (1982*c*) Ultrastructure of the umbilical artery from a newborn delivered at term by a mother who smoked 80 cigarettes per day. *Acta Pathologica Scandinavica.* 90:397–404.

Asmussen I (1984) Mitochondrial proliferation in endothelium. Observations on umbilical arteries from newborn children of smoking mothers. *Atherosclerosis.* 50:203–8.

Asmussen I and Kjeldsen K (1975) Intimal ultrastructure from newborn children of smoking and non-smoking mothers. *Circulation Research.* 36:577–89.

Blaes N *et al.* (1986) Nicotine alters fibronectin and factor VIII/vWF in human vascular endothelial cells. *British Journal of Haematology.* 64:675–8.

Blow CM (1988) Mesothelium as a non-thrombogenic surface. In: Pittilo RM and Machin SJ (ed) *Platelet-vessel wall interactions, the Bloomsbury series in clinical science.* Springer, London. pp. 103–19.

Booyse FM *et al.* (1981*a*) Effects of chronic oral consumption of nicotine on the rabbit aortic endothelium. *American Journal of Pathology.* 102:93–102.

Booyse FM *et al.* (1981*b*) Effects of nicotine on cultured bovine aortic endothelial cells. *Thrombosis Research.* 23:169–85.

Bull HA *et al.* (1985) The effects of nicotine on PGI_2 production by rat aortic endothelium. *Thrombosis and Haemostasis.* **54**:472–4.

Buss H and Hollweg HG (1977) Scanning electron microscopy of blood vessels. A review. In: Pittilo RM and Machin SJ (ed) *Scanning electron microscopy II.* IITRI, Chicago. pp. 467–75.

Bylock A *et al.* (1979) Surface ultrastructure of human arteries with special reference to the effects of smoking. *Acta Pathologica et Microbiologica Scandinavica.* **87**:201–9.

Caro CG (1990) Cigarette smoking causes acute changes in arterial wall mechanics and the pattern of arterial blood flow in healthy subjects: possible insight into mechanisms of atherosclerosis. *Advances in Experimental Medicine and Biology.* **273**:273–80.

Church DF and Pryor WA (1985) Free radical chemistry of cigarette smoke and its toxicological implications. *Environmental Health Perspectives.* **64**:111–26.

Dadak CH *et al.* (1981) Diminished prostacyclin formation in umbilical arteries of babies born to women who smoke. *The Lancet.* **i**:94.

Doll R (1983) Prospects for prevention. *British Medical Journal.* **80**:445–53.

Doll R (1990) Tobacco related diseases. *Journal of Smoking Related Disorders.* **1**:3–13.

Doyle JT *et al.* (1964) The relationship of cigarette smoking to coronary heart disease; the second report of the combined experience of the Albany, N.Y. and Framingham, Mass. studies. *Journal of the American Medical Association.* **190**:886–90.

Henning B and Chow C (1988) Lipid peroxidation and endothelial cell injury: implications in atherosclerosis. *Free Radicals in Biology and Medicine.* **4**:99–106.

Hladovec J (1978) Endothelial injury by nicotine and its prevention. *Experientia.* **34**:1585–6.

Hoshino E *et al.* (1990) Vitamin E suppresses increased lipid peroxidation in cigarette smokers. *Journal of Parenteral and Enteral Nutrition.* **14**:300–5.

Jeremy JY *et al.* (1985) Cigarette smoke extracts, but not nicotine, inhibit prosta-cyclin (PGI_2) synthesis in human, rabbit and rat vascular tissue. *Prostaglandins and Leukotrienes in Medicine.* **19**:261–70.

Jeremy JY and Mikhailidis DP (1990) Smoking and vascular prostanoids: the relevance to the pathogenesis of atheroma. *Journal of Smoking Related Disorders.* **1**:59–69.

Kutti J (1990) Smoking, platelet reactivity and fibrinogen. *Advances in Experimental Medicine and Biology*. **273**:129–45.

Latha MS *et al.* (1991) Changes in the glycosaminoglycans and glycoproteins in the tissues of rats exposed to cigarette smoke. *Atherosclerosis*. **86**:49–54.

Lubawy WC *et al.* (1986) Alterations in prostacyclin and thromboxane formation by chronic cigarette smoke exposure: temporal relationships and whole smoke vs. gas phase. *Journal of Applied Toxicology*. **6**:77–80.

Lyons MJ *et al.* (1958) Free radicals produced in cigarette smoke. *Nature*. **181**:1003–4.

Murray JJ *et al.* (1990) Platelet-vessel wall interactions in individuals who smoke cigarettes. *Advances in Experimental Medicine and Biology*. **273**:189–98.

Nadler JL *et al.* (1983) Cigarette smoking inhibits prostacyclin production. *The Lancet*. i:1248–50.

Noronha-Dutra AA and Steen EM (1982) Lipid peroxidation as a mechanism of injury in cardiac myocytes. *Laboratory Investigation*. **47**:346–53.

Noronha-Dutra AA *et al.* (1984) The early changes induced by isoproterenol in the endocardium and adjacent myocardium. *American Journal of Pathology*. **114**:231–9.

Noronha-Dutra AA *et al.* (In press) The effect of cigarette smoking on cultured human umbilical vein endothelial cells. *Cardiovascular Research*.

Olsson AG and Molgaard J (1990) Relations between smoking, food intake and plasma lipoproteins. *Advances in Experimental Medicine and Biology*. **273**:237–43.

Petty RG and Pearson JD (1989) Endothelium—the axis of vascular health and disease. *Journal of the Royal College of Physicians of London*. **23**:92–102.

Peto R *et al.* (1992) Mortality from tobacco in developed countries: indirect estimation from national vital statistics. *The Lancet*. i:1268–78.

Pittilo RM (1988) Endothelium and the vessel wall. In: Pittilo RM and Machin SJ (ed) *Platelet–vessel wall interactions, the Bloomsbury series in clinical science*. Springer, London. pp. 33–59.

Pittilo RM (1990) Cigarette smoking and endothelial injury: a review. *Advances in experimental medicine and biology*. **273**:61–78.

Pittilo RM *et al.* (1982) Effects of cigarette smoking on the ultrastructure of rat thoracic aorta and its ability to produce prostacyclin. *Thrombosis and Haemostasis*. **48**:173–6.

Pittilo RM *et al.* (1984) Cigarette smoking and platelet adhesion. *British Journal of Haematology.* **58**:627–32.

Pittilo RM *et al.* (1985) Cigarette smoke-induced injury of peritoneal mesothelial cells. *British Journal of Experimental Pathology.* **65**:365–70.

Pittilo RM *et al.* (1990) Nicotine and cigarette smoking: effects on the ultrastructure of aortic endothelium. *International Journal of Experimental Pathology.* **71**:573–86.

Pittilo RM and Bull HA (1988) The effects of nicotine on endothelial morphology and prostacyclin production. In: Rand M and Tharau K (eds) *The pharmacology of nicotine.* pp. 176–7. IRL Press, Oxford.

Pittilo RM and Woolf N (1993) Cigarette smoking, endothelial cell injury and atherosclerosis. *Journal of Smoking Related Disorders.* **4**:17–25.

Pryor WA *et al.* (1990) A comparison of the free radical chemistry of tobacco burning cigarettes and cigarettes that only heat tobacco. *Free Radicals in Biology and Medicine.* **8**:275–9.

Reidy MA (1985) Biology of disease. A reassessment of endothelial injury and arterial lesion formation. *Laboratory Investigation.* **53**:513–20.

Reinders JH *et al.* (1986) Cigarette smoke impairs endothelial cell prostacyclin production. *Arteriosclerosis.* **6**:15–23.

Rhoads GG, Gulbrandsen GL and Kagan A (1976) Serum lipoproteins and coronary heart disease in a population study of Hawaiian-Japanese men. *New England Journal of Medicine.* **294**:293–8.

Ross R (1986) The pathogenesis of atherosclerosis–an update. *New England Journal of Medicine.* **314**:488–96.

Schmidt KG *et al.* (1990) Acute platelet activation induced by smoking cigarettes: *in vivo* and *ex vivo* studies in humans. *Advances in Experimental Medicine and Biology.* **273**:199–209.

Sinzinger H *et al.* (1988) Beneficial effect of PGI_2 on circulating endothelial cells. *Basic Research in Cardiology.* **83**:597–601.

Sowemimo-Coker SO *et al.* (1989) Increased circulating endothelial cells in sickle cell crisis. *American Journal of Hematology.* **31**:263–5.

Staubesand J *et al.* (1984) Intimal ultrastructural morphology of umbilical cord vasculature in babies born to smoking mothers. *Vasa.* **13**:138–46.

Toth KM *et al.* (1986) Erythrocytes from cigarette smokers contain more glutathione and catalase and protect endothelial cells from hydrogen peroxide better than erythrocytes from non-smokers. *American Review of Respiratory Diseases.* 134:281–4.

Woolf N and Wilson-Holt RMC (1981) Cigarette smoking and atherosclerosis. In: *Smoking and arterial disease.* Pitman Medical, London. pp. 46–59.

20

Fibrinogen and other Clotting Factors in Cardiovascular Disease, with Particular Reference to Smoking

TW MEADE

It was not until the early 1980s that a thrombotic component in ischaemic heart disease (IHD) was generally recognized (Meade *et al.*, 1992). However, Morris had drawn attention to the involvement of a major process other than atherogenesis as early as 1951 through his analysis of post-mortem findings at the London Hospital (Morris, 1951). There was no increase—if anything there was a decrease—in the prevalence of advanced atheroma over a period during which mortality from IHD had increased many times. Morris pointed out that the main epidemic had started just after the First World War and that some environmental change that had occurred about then might provide at least a partial explanation. One such possibility was the widespread adoption of smoking by men. The findings suggested a relatively short-term, acute effect of smoking rather than a longer-term influence. This is also indicated by the much closer relationship of smoking with clinically manifest IHD, which is nearly always preceded by thrombosis, than with coronary atheroma (Meade *et al.*, 1992). The plasma fibrinogen concentration is raised by smoking and is strongly associated with the later risk of IHD. This review summarizes the determinants, pathogenetic effects and clinical consequences of high fibrinogen levels.

Prevalence studies

Prevalence or cross-sectional studies may give a useful preliminary indication of relationships with cardiovascular disease (CVD) although interpretation of the associations so demonstrated is difficult. Table 20.1 summarizes the fibrinogen results of the Northwick Park Heart Study (NPHS) (Meade, 1987*a*), a whole population (as distinct from a case-control) study in which cases and those so far affected or unaffected by clinically manifest IHD are drawn from the same groups. Other studies have also reported higher levels of fibrinogen or its products in those with a past history of MI (Yarnell *et al.*, 1985) and in patients with unstable angina (Kruskal *et al.*, 1987).

	MI	Angina	All IHD	No IHD
	N = 38	N = 33	N = 71	N = 1350
Fibrinogen g/l	3.24*	3.21*	3.22*	2.91

Compared with no IHD: * $P < 0.01$

Table 20.1: Mean values by presence or absence of IHD at entry to NPHS. Numbers of cases (all IHD) by low, middle and high thirds of fibrinogen distribution are 12, 23 and 35 (one missing value). (Source: Meade, 1987*a*.)

Prospective studies

Northwick Park Heart Study (NPHS)

In 1980, Meade *et al.* (1980) showed preliminary results suggesting that high levels of factor VII activity, VII_c, and of plasma fibrinogen, and possibly also of factor VIII activity, were associated with mortality from CVD, principally IHD. The findings on VII_c and fibrinogen were confirmed and amplified in the main NPHS results in 1986 (Meade *et al.*, 1986). The relationships of VII_c and fibrinogen with the incidence of IHD itself within five years of recruitment were if anything stronger than for cholesterol although the latter relationship —as expected—was also demonstrated. There were no clear relationships between VII_c or fibrinogen and the incidence of cancer, the commonest non-vascular cause of illness and death, so that the findings appear to be specific for vascular disease.

Göteborg Study

Wilhelmsen *et al.* (1984) showed a relationship in a study of 792 men born in 1913 between high fibrinogen levels and the incidence of both IHD and, in particular, stroke. The data on stroke suggested a possible interaction between fibrinogen and systolic blood pressure, men with high levels of both being at considerably greater risk than might have been expected from the sum of the two effects separately, although the small number of events on which this analysis is based needs to be taken into account.

Leigh Study

In 1985, Stone and Thorp (1985) reported an association between high fibrinogen levels and IHD incidence in a group of 297 men aged between 40 and 69 who were followed for up to 20 years. The relationship was stronger than for cholesterol, blood pressure or smoking. In this study, too, there was suggestive evidence of an interaction between fibrinogen and blood pressure. Thus, men whose systolic blood pressure and plasma fibrinogen levels fell in the top third of the respective distributions experienced 12 times the incidence of IHD compared with those both of whose levels fell in the low third.

	Normotensive		Mild hypertension		Definite hypertension	
Fibrinogen g/l	Men	Women	Men	Women	Men	Women
<2.65	2.27	1.53	4.21	1.92	5.39	3.78
2.65–3.11	2.61	1.54	5.19	2.40	4.10	2.82
>3.12	4.67	2.18	5.38	3.78	7.08	5.43

Table 20.2: CVD by fibrinogen and hypertensive status: Framingham Study subjects 45–79 years of age, 12-year rate per 1000. (Source: Kannel, 1987.)

Framingham Study

In 1985, Kannel *et al.* (1985) reported an association between high fibrinogen levels and the incidence of CVD in 554 men and 761 women aged between 45 and 79 who had not previously experienced a cardiovascular event, CVD being defined as the sum of IHD, stroke, heart failure and peripheral arterial disease. Subsequent publications (Kannel, 1987; Kannel *et al.*, 1987) established a clear relationship between fibrinogen and the incidence of IHD in both men and women and between fibrinogen and stroke in men but not in women (perhaps because of small numbers) and, again, also suggested that the effects of simultaneously high levels of fibrinogen and blood pressure may be of particular importance (Table 20.2).

Caerphilly Study

Most recently, the Caerphilly Study (Yarnell *et al.*, 1991) has also shown a strong relationship between fibrinogen and IHD incidence that remained significant after adjusting for a variety of characteristics, including smoking habit. Viscosity was also associated with IHD.

The relationship of fibrinogen to the patency of femoropopliteal vein grafts has also been established (Wiseman *et al.*, 1989). In those with plasma fibrinogen concentrations below the median value, 90% of grafts were patent at one year compared with 57% in those with values above the median. The plasma fibrinogen level, followed by thiocyanate concentration as a measure of smoking, were the two most powerful predictors of graft status in this study. Other work also indicates the involvement of fibrinogen in the progression of peripheral arterial disease (Dormandy *et al.*, 1973; Banerjee *et al.*, 1992) and probably in its onset, too (Kannel and D'Agostino 1990).

Thus, prospective studies are very consistent in suggesting a strong relationship between the plasma fibrinogen level and the subsequent onset of clinically manifest IHD, of stroke (at least in men) and of progression in established peripheral arterial disease. The relationship between fibrinogen and stroke contrasts with the less certain association between cholesterol and stroke, thus indicating the potential value of fibrinogen as a particularly useful index of the risk of major CVD defined as the sum of IHD and stroke.

Other clotting factors

As already indicated, NPHS also established a strong relationship between the level of factor VII activity, VII_c, and the subsequent onset of IHD (Meade *et al.*, 1986).

Although considerably weaker than for VII_c and fibrinogen, there were also suggestive associations in NPHS of high factor VIII levels and poor fibrinolytic activity with incidence (Meade *et al.*, 1980, 1986). Impaired fibrinolytic activity may also influence the recurrence of myocardial infarction (MI) (Hamsten *et al.*, 1987*a*). In the case of factor VIII, supporting evidence comes from studies showing a lower than expected incidence of IHD in haemophiliacs (Rosendaal *et al.*, 1989) and from other results (Egeberg, 1962).

However, association does not automatically prove causation. Besides prospective studies, other types of evidence also have to be considered in establishing whether high fibrinogen and other clotting factor levels are associated with the subsequent incidence of CVD because they are causally involved or simply because they are markers of another process—a question of particular relevance in the case of fibrinogen in view of its response to a variety of stimuli. The results of randomized controlled trials are particularly valuable in this context providing, as they do, unbiased evidence on the consequences of altering clotting factor levels.

Clinical trials

The WHO clofibrate trial (Committee of Principal Investigators, 1978, 1980, 1984) was actually based on the relationship between cholesterol (not fibrinogen) and IHD and was carried out in men with hyperlipidaemia, using the cholesterol-lowering property of clofibrate. There was a significant reduction, of about 20%, in the incidence of IHD attributable to clofibrate but there was also an increase in deaths from a variety of causes for reasons which are still unclear but which preclude the general use of clofibrate. However, it is known that clofibrate also lowers fibrinogen levels (Dormandy *et al.*, 1974; Green *et al.*, 1989). Furthermore, the beneficial effect of clofibrate against infarction appears to have been confined, as Table 20.3 shows, to heavy smokers who were also hypertensive (Green *et al.*, 1989). The heavy smokers will have had high fibrinogen levels. Besides suggesting that the effect of clofibrate may have been to reduce the risk of MI through its effect on fibrinogen (as well as on cholesterol), this analysis is interesting in further supporting the possibility of an interaction between blood pressure and fibrinogen, already referred to, since it was in those at risk on both accounts that the benefit of treatment was mostly seen. The other source of evidence from trials is a series of studies (Becker, 1988) in both man and animals showing that ancrod, a defibrinating agent, reduces thrombosis and improves clinical function in immune kidney disease.

	Non-smokers		Smokers			
			<20/d		20+/d	
	Active	Placebo	Active	Placebo	Active	Placebo
Normotensive	3.4	3.5	6.2	9.6	9.6	9.1
Hypertensive	3.9	6.0	12.1	14.3	8.7	*18.3

*$P < 0.01$

Table 20.3: Heart attacks per 1000 per annum in WHO clofibrate trial. (Source: Green *1l.*, 1989.)

Thus evidence from trials is compatible with a causal role for high fibrinogen levels although it is certainly not yet conclusive.

General epidemiological characteristics

Another approach to clarifying the nature of the relationship between high clotting factor levels and the incidence of IHD is to establish how far these levels vary according to personal and environmental characteristics associated with IHD. With a high degree of consistency, fibrinogen levels tend to be high or low in association with characteristics which respectively raise or lower the risk of IHD (Figure 20.1). Considering smoking in more detail, all the large-scale prospective studies already referred to (and several cross-sectional studies) have found the highest fibrinogen levels in smokers, intermediate levels in ex-smokers and the lowest levels in non-smokers (Meade, 1987*b*). There is a dose-response relationship between the number of cigarettes smoked and the fibrinogen level (Wilkes *et al*, 1988). Figure 20.2, from data at entry to NPHS, shows a rapid initial decline in fibrinogen on stopping but levels remain above those for non-smokers for up to five and perhaps 10 years after discontinuation (Meade *et al.*, 1987*a*), also observed in Welsh and Scottish studies (Yarnell *et al.*, 1987; Lee *et al.*, 1990). This time course mirrors the decline in the risk of IHD itself after smoking cessation (Cook *et al.*, 1986; Dobson *et al.*, 1991). The effect has also been shown prospectively (Meade *et al.*, 1987*a*). Thus, over the six-year follow-up period in NPHS, fibrinogen levels rose (over and above the increase with age) in those who started or resumed smoking while they fell in those who discontinued. The rapid initial fall in fibrinogen after discontinuation (Meade *et al.*, 1987*a*; Yarnell *et al.*, 1987; Lee *et al.*, 1990; Dobson *et al.*, 1991; Rothwell *et al.*, 1991) is one of the reasons for questioning the frequent assertion that high fibrinogen levels associated with the incidence of IHD only reflect the extent of underlying atheroma. Bearing in mind the difficulty of achieving the regression of atheroma other than by fairly intensive methods not ordinarily used by those who are giving up smoking, it is most unlikely that the fall in fibrinogen soon after discontinuation is due to a reduction in atheroma.

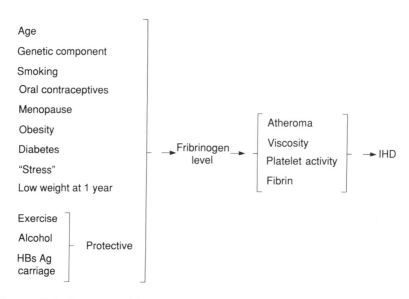

Figure 20.1: Summary of determinants and thrombogenic pathways of fibrinogen in pathogenesis of IHD.

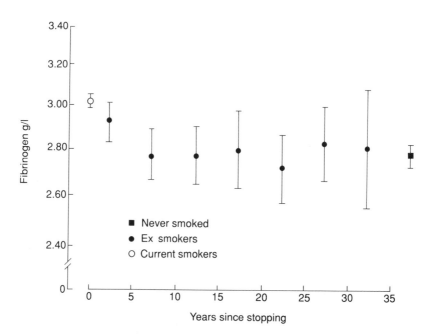

Figure 20.2: Plasma fibrinogen (age-adjusted) by time since stopping smoking in 518 ex-smokers, in current smokers and in non-smokers. Log scale. Bars show 95% confidence intervals. (Source: Meade *et al.*, 1987*a*.)

The extent to which fibrinogen levels are genetically determined (see below) also represents a component of high fibrinogen levels that cannot be explained as a response to atheroma. Given the strong relationship between fibrinogen levels and the risk of IHD or stroke, the fall in fibrinogen in ex-smokers is enough to account for a large part of the decline in their risk of IHD and strengthens the conclusion that much of the relationship between smoking and IHD is mediated through the fibrinogen level. It is, however, important to remember that high levels are associated with an increased risk of IHD in non-smokers (Meade *et al.*, 1986; Yarnell *et al.*, 1991) as well as in smokers.

There are quite strong although poorly appreciated indications of an increased risk of vascular disease following infection. For example, patients admitted for acute MI had significantly higher serological indices of chronic chlamydial infection than a control group (Saikku *et al.*, 1988). In a case-control study in patients under the age of 50, there was a relative risk of no less than 9.0 for brain infarction associated with a febrile infection during the previous month (Syrjanen *et al.*, 1988). There would of course have been changes in many acute and chronic phase proteins but one of these would almost have certainly been an increase in fibrinogen. In another study, dental health was significantly worse in patients with acute MI than in controls (Mattila *et al.*, 1989). Again, a rise in fibrinogen levels is only one of several possible explanations but there is a strong case for further work to confirm or exclude it. Other studies linking virus infection to development of atheroma might also be explained through effects on fibrinogen levels, at least in part (The Lancet, 1978). The apparently high cardiovascular mortality in patients with rheumatoid arthritis (Mutru *et al.*, 1985) and the possible involvement of fibrin deposition in Crohn's disease (Wakefield, 1989) could also perhaps be partly explained through the effects of these diseases on fibrinogen levels. If raised fibrinogen levels do to some extent explain the fairly clear increase in risk associated with these conditions—and it it must be emphasized that this is at present speculative—they illustrate the importance of not dismissing elevations in fibrinogen that may be due to relatively non-specific stimuli as uninteresting or biologically insignificant. It is also worth bearing in mind that high fibrinogen levels are also found in neoplastic disease and in pregnancy, both of which are also associated with an increased risk of thromboembolism. There appears to be a striking seasonal variation in plasma fibrinogen concentrations in older individuals (Stout and Crawford, 1991). Levels are highest during the coldest months when mortality from both MI and stroke are also at their highest levels. It might be that the high fibrinogen and thus mortality levels during the colder months are partly explained by respiratory and other infections which are, of course, also commonest during colder weather. However, there was no seasonal variation in white cell count in the study under consideration, which argues against this particular explanation although white cell counts may not rise as much in older as in younger patients in response to infection. The origin of high fibrinogen levels is certainly a question of considerable interest, but whatever they are—genetic, environmental or non-specific—they may lead to an increased risk of thrombosis.

Some characteristics protective against IHD are associated with below-average fibrinogen levels. Thus there is little doubt that moderate alcohol consumption leads to a lowering of fibrinogen levels. This conclusion is based not only on cross-sectional studies (Meade *et al.*, 1979; Lee *et al.*, 1990; Folsom *et al.*, 1991) but also on the fall in fibrinogen observed prospectively in NPHS with increased alcohol consumption (Meade *et al.*, 1987*a*). A German cross-sectional study (Balleisen *et al.*, 1985), however, has reported no association between alcohol consumption and fibrinogen. While the magnitude of the effect of alcohol consumption on fibrinogen levels may not be large and may suggest only a modest degree of protection against IHD, it is nevertheless compatible with the evidence from studies on the relationship between alcohol consumption and IHD incidence (Marmot and Brunner, 1991). Thus the apparent effect of alcohol consumption on fibrinogen levels and direct studies of the relationship between alcohol consumption and IHD complement each other in suggesting that there is, indeed, some protection against IHD from moderate consumption.

Several studies are consistent in suggesting or quite firmly establishing an inverse relationship between exercise and the fibrinogen level, ie lower levels in those taking most exercise or in those who are physically 'fittest' (Davey-Smith *et al.*, 1989; Moller and Kirstensen, 1991; Connelly *et al.*, 1992).

It is also likely that carriers of hepatitis B surface antigen, who seem to experience considerably less IHD than non-carriers, have lower fibrinogen levels than the latter (Hall *et al.*, 1985; Meade *et al.*, 1987*b*).

Genetic contribution

Encouraging early progress has been made in characterizing the genetic contribution to fibrinogen levels. Two restriction fragment length polymorphisms (RFLPs) associated with variation in fibrinogen levels have been identified (Humphries *et al.*, 1987; Thomas *et al.*, 1991), although the finding on one of them (Humphries *et al.*, 1987) has not been confirmed in a Scandinavian study (Berg and Kierulf, 1989). Methodological differences or true variations in the association of this RFLP with fibrinogen in different populations are possible explanations. At the same time, the RFLP in question is associated with the risk of peripheral vascular disease (Fowkes *et al.*, 1992). The variations at the fibrinogen locus suggested by RFLPs account for between 3% and 15% of the variance in fibrinogen levels although because the studies in question were based on single fibrinogen measurements, these proportions are likely to be underestimates. Using path analysis, another study (Hamsten *et al.*, 1987*b*) accounted for 51% of the variance in fibrinogen in genetic terms. As the authors of this study themselves concluded, a substantial genetic determination weakens the explanation that high fibrinogen levels are only or mainly due to non-specific influences such as atheroma.

Fibrinogen and thrombogenic pathways

As Figure 20.1 shows, there are at least four ways in which high fibrinogen levels may predispose to thrombosis.

Atheroma

Several studies have now established a relationship between the fibrinogen level and the extent of atheroma, both in the coronary and carotid circulations (Schneidau *et al.*, 1989; Broadhurst *et al.*, 1990). The contribution of fibrinogen and fibrin to the atheromatous plaque throughout its evolution and development is increasingly recognized and supported by other biochemical and pathological observations (Smith *et al.*, 1990).

Viscosity

Large, asymmetrical molecules such as fibrinogen have a marked effect on blood viscosity and there is little doubt that increasing viscosity increases the risk of thrombosis (Lowe, 1986; Yarnell *et al.*, 1991).

Fibrin formation

In the rabbit, the fibrinogen concentration when coagulation is initiated influences the amount of fibrin deposited (Gurewich *et al.*, 1976; Chooi and Gallus, 1989). Kinetic experiments support the same conclusion (Naski and Shafer, 1991). Thus, the claim on theoretical grounds that high fibrinogen levels will not influence thrombogenesis because they are in excess of those needed for haemostasis is not borne out.

Platelet aggregation

Plasma fibrinogen is a cofactor for platelet aggregation. But it also affects aggregability throughout its physiological range (Meade *et al.*, 1985*a*). Experimental studies show either by defibrination with ancrod (Lowe *et al.*, 1979) or through the addition of further fibrinogen (Meade *et al.*, 1985*b*) that it is indeed high fibrinogen levels that influence aggregability, not *vice versa*.

Summary and implications

The pathways summarized in Figure 20.1, and the fact that lowering fibrinogen levels probably reduces the incidence of thrombotic episodes, now leave little doubt that high fibrinogen levels are of causal significance. It is thus clear that the plasma fibrinogen level occupies a central place in the pathogenesis of IHD (and almost certainly of stroke). What, therefore, are the practical implications? As with other approaches to the prevention of IHD, lifestyle modifications and pharmacological intervention should both be considered. Much the most important lifestyle change is the discontinuation or avoidance of smoking (although the relationship between high fibrinogen levels and IHD in non-smokers as well as smokers should not be overlooked). Although fibrinogen levels in ex-smokers do begin to fall quite soon after discontinuation, they remain above non-smoking levels for several years, as does the risk of IHD itself. The apparently beneficial effect of strenuous exercise on fibrinogen now provides both doctors and patients with a valuable and practical incentive towards prevention, particularly where IHD risk is substantially due to raised fibrinogen levels. Since the independent relationship between fibrinogen and IHD is about as strong as the relationship between cholesterol and IHD, it is reasonable to suggest the inclusion of fibrinogen in the IHD risk profile and to use the information in making general decisions about prophylactic measures. However, the strong relationship between fibrinogen and IHD does raise the question of pharmacological intervention in some circumstances. The case for clofibrate has already been considered and it may yet prove that its general abandonment after the WHO trial was premature. Bezafibrate also probably lowers fibrinogen levels (Cook and Ubben, 1990). While gemfibrozil reduces the incidence of IHD, it raises rather than lowers fibrinogen levels (Wilkes *et al.*, 1992), but it reduces thrombin production: the benefit of which, along with its lipid-lowering properties, outweighs the fibrinogen rise. Indeed, the numerous effects of gemfibrozil illustrate the importance of clinical rather than surrogate end-points in prophylactic trials. Pentoxifylline has benefical effects on blood flow (Cook and Ubben, 1990) and may be particularly useful in peripheral vascular disease. Stanozolol produces a marked reduction in fibrinogen (Cook and Ubben, 1990) but may adversely effect high-density lipoprotein (HDL) cholesterol levels as well as having androgenic properties. Ancrod markedly lowers fibrinogen levels through its defibrinating effect but is given by infusion and is only used in rather extreme circumstances. Recently, the calcium channel blocking agent nisoldipine has been reported to lower fibrinogen levels substantially and significantly (Salmasi *et al.*, 1991). Ticlopidine may also do so (Finelli *et al.*, 1991).

In conclusion, fibrinogen can and should be increasingly used as part of the IHD risk profile. The avoidance of smoking and the encouragement of physical exertion are lifestyle modifications further supported by the evidence on fibrinogen and IHD risk. Finally, fibrinogen-lowering agents should be increasingly considered in those who have already experienced thrombotic episodes while the evaluation of agents such as the fibrates in primary prevention may soon be indicated.

References

Balleisen L *et al.* (1985) Epidemiological study on factor VII, factor VIII and fibrinogen in an industrial population I: baseline data on the relation to age, gender, body-weight, smoking, alcohol, pill-using, and menopause. *Thrombosis and Haemostasis*. 54:475–9.

Banerjee AK *et al.* (1992) A six year prospective study of fibrinogen and other risk factors associated with mortality in stable claudicants. *Thrombosis and Haemostasis*. 68:261–3.

Berg K and Kierulf P (1989) DNA polymorphisms at fibrinogen loci and plasma fibrinogen concentration. *Clinical Genetics*. 36:229–35.

Broadhurst P *et al.* (1990) Fibrinogen, factor VII clotting activity and coronary artery disease severity. *Atherosclerosis*, 85:169–73.

Chooi CC and Gallus AS (1989) Acute phase reaction, fibrinogen level and thrombus size. *Thrombosis Research*. 53:493–501.

Committee of Principal Investigators (1978) Co-operative trial in the primary prevention of ischaemic heart disease using clofibrate. *British Heart Journal*. **40**: 1069–118.

Committee of Principal Investigators (1980) WHO co-operative trial on primary prevention of ischaemic heart disease using clofibrate to lower serum cholesterol: mortality follow-up. *The Lancet*. ii:379–85.

Committee of Principal Investigators (1984) WHO co-operative trial on primary prevention of ischaemic heart disease using clofibrate to lower serum cholesterol: final mortality follow-up. *The Lancet*, ii:600–4.

Connelly JB *et al.* (1992) Strenuous exercise and plasma fibrinogen. *British Heart Journal*. 67:351–4.

Cook DG *et al.* (1986) Giving up smoking and the risk of heart attacks. *The Lancet*. ii:1376–80.

Cook NS and Ubben D (1990) Fibrinogen as a major risk factor in cardiovascular disease. *Trends in Pharmacological Sciences*. 11:444–51.

Davey-Smith G *et al.* (1989) *A work stress-fibrinogen pathway as a potential mechanism for employment grade differences in coronary heart disease rates*. Abstracts, 2nd international conference on preventive cardiology, Washington DC.

Dobson AJ *et al.* (1991) How soon after quitting smoking does risk of heart attack decline? *Journal of Clinical Epidemiology*. 44:1247–53.

Dormandy JA *et al.* (1973) Prognostic significance of rheological and biochemical findings in patients with intermittent claudication. *British Medical Journal.* 4:581–3.

Dormandy JA *et al.* (1974) Effect of clofibrate on blood viscosity in intermittent claudication. *British Medical Journal.* 4:259–62.

Egeberg O (1962) Clotting factor levels in patients with coronary atherosclerosis. *Scandinavian Journal of Clinical and Laboratory Investigations.* 14:253–8.

Finelli C *et al.* (1991) Ticlopidine lowers plasma fibrinogen in patients with polycythaemic rubra vera and additional thrombotic risk factors. *Acta Haematologica.* 85:113–18.

Folsom AR *et al.* (1991) Population correlates of plasma fibrinogen and factor VII, putative cardiovascular risk factors. *Atherosclerosis.* 91:191–205.

Fowkes FGR *et al.* (1992) Fibrinogen genotype and risk of peripheral atherosclerosis. *The Lancet.* 339:693–6.

Green KG *et al.* (1989) Blood pressure, cigarette smoking and heart attack in the WHO co-operative trial of clofibrate. *International Journal of Epidemiology.* 18: 355–60.

Gurewich V *et al.* (1976) The effect of the fibrinogen concentration and the leukocyte count on intravascular fibrin deposition from soluble fibrin monomer complexes. *Thrombosis and Haemostasis.* 36:605–14.

Hall AJ *et al.* (1985) Mortality of hepatitis B positive blood donors in England and Wales. *The Lancet.* i:91–3.

Hamsten A *et al.* (1987*a*) Plasminogen activator inhibitor in plasma: risk factor for recurrent myocardial infarction. *The Lancet.* ii:3–9.

Hamsten A *et al.* (1987*b*) Genetic and cultural inheritance of plasma fibrinogen concentration. *The Lancet.* ii:988–91.

Humphries SE *et al.* (1987) Role of genetic variation at the fibrinogen locus in determination of plasma fibrinogen concentrations. *The Lancet.* i:1452–5.

Kannel WB *et al.* (1985) *Fibrinogen and cardiovascular disease.* Abstract of paper for 34th Annual Scientific Session of the American College of Cardiology, March 1985, Anaheim, California.

Kannel WB (1987) Hypertension and other risk factors in coronary heart disease. *American Heart Journal.* 114:918–25.

Kannel WB *et al.* (1987) Fibrinogen and risk of cardiovascular disease. *Journal of the American Medical Association.* 258:1183–6.

Kannel WB and D'Agostino RB (1990) Update of fibrinogen as a major cardiovascular risk factor: the Framingham Study. *Journal of the American College of Cardiology.* **15**:156A.

Kruskal JB *et al.* (1987) Fibrin and fibrinogen-related antigens in patients with stable and unstable coronary artery disease. *New England Journal of Medicine.* 317:1361–5.

The Lancet (1978) Virus infections and atherosclerosis. (Editorial.) *The Lancet.* ii:821–2.

Lee AJ *et al.* (1990) Plasma fibrinogen and coronary risk factors: the Scottish heart health study. *Journal of Clinical Epidemiology.* **43**:913–19.

Lowe GDO *et al.* (1979) Increased platelet aggregates in vascular and non-vascular illness: correlation with plasma fibrinogen and effect of ancrod. *Thrombosis Research.* 14:377–86.

Lowe GDO (1986) Blood rheology in arterial disease. *Clinical Science.* **71**:137–46.

Marmot M and Brunner E (1991) Alcohol and cardiovascular disease: the status of the U shaped curve. *British Medical Journal.* **303**:565–8.

Mattila KJ *et al.* (1989) Association between dental health and acute myocardial infarction. *British Medical Journal.* **298**:779–81.

Meade TW *et al.* (1979) Characteristics affecting fibrinolytic activity and plasma fibrinogen concentrations. *British Medical Journal.* **1**:153–6.

Meade TW *et al.* (1980) Haemostatic function and cardiovascular death: early results of a prospective study. *The Lancet.* i:1050–4.

Meade TW *et al.* (1985*a*) Epidemiological characteristics of platelet aggregability. *British Medical Journal.* **290**:428–32.

Meade TW *et al.* (1985*b*) The effect of physiological levels of fibrinogen on platelet aggregation. *Thrombosis Research.* **38**:527–34.

Meade TW *et al.* (1986) Haemostatic function and ischaemic heart disease: principal results of the Northwick Park Heart Study. *The Lancet.* ii:533–7.

Meade TW (1987*a*) Epidemiology of atheroma, thrombosis and ischaemic heart disease. In: Bloom AM and Thomas DP (eds) *Haemostasis and thrombosis, 2nd edn.* Churchill Livingstone, Edinburgh. pp. 597–720.

Meade TW (1987*b*) The epidemiology of haemostatic and other variables in coronary artery disease. In: Verstraete M *et al. Thrombosis and haemostasis 1987.* Leuven University Press, Leuven. pp 37–60.

Meade TW *et al.* (1987*a*) Effects of changes in smoking and other characteristics on clotting factors and the risk of ischaemic heart disease. *The Lancet.* ii:986–8.

Meade TW *et al.* (1987*b*) Carriers of hepatitis B surface antigen: possible association between low levels of clotting factors and protection against ischaemic heart disease. *Thrombosis Research.* **45**:709–13.

Meade TW, *et al.*(1992) Characteristics associated with the risk of arterial thrombosis and the prethrombotic state. In: Fuster V and Verstraete M (eds) *Thrombosis in cardiovascular disorders.* W.B. Saunders, Philadelphia. pp. 79–97.

Moller L and Kirstensen TS (1991) Plasma fibrinogen and ischaemic heart disease risk factors. *Arteriosclerosis and Thrombosis.* **11**:344–50.

Morris JN (1951) Recent history of coronary disease. *The Lancet.* i:1–7, 69–73.

Mutru O *et al.* (1985) Ten year mortality and causes of death in patients with rheumatoid arthritis. *British Medical Journal.* **290**:1797–9.

Naski MC and Shafer JA (1991) A kinetic model for the α-thrombin-catalysed conversion of plasma levels of fibrinogen to fibrin in the presence of antithrombin III. *Journal of Biological Chemistry.* **266**:13003–10.

Rosendaal FR *et al.* (1989) Mortality and causes of death in Dutch haemophiliacs, 1973–86. *British Journal of Haematology.* **71**:71–6.

Rothwell M *et al.* (1991) Haemorheological changes in the very short term after abstention from tobacco by cigarette smokers. *British Journal of Haematology.* **79**: 500–3.

Saikku P *et al.* (1988) Serological evidence of an association of a novel chlamydia, twar, with chronic coronary heart disease and acute myocardial infarction. *The Lancet.* ii:983–6.

Salmasi A–M, *et al.* (1991) Improvement of silent myocardial ischaemia and reduction of plasma fibrinogen during nisoldipine therapy in occult coronary arterial disease. *International Journal of Cardiology.* **31**:71–80.

Schneidau A *et al.* (1989) Arterial disease risk factors and angiographic evidence of atheroma of the carotid artery. *Stroke.* **20**:1466–71.

Smith EB *et al.* (1990) Fate of fibrinogen in human intima. *Arteriosclerosis.* **10**: 263 –75.

Stone MC and Thorp JM (1985) Plasma fibrinogen—a major coronary risk factor. *Journal of the Royal College of General Practitioners.* **35**:565–9.

Stout RW and Crawford V (1991) Seasonal variations in fibrinogen concentrations among elderly people. *The Lancet.* **338**:9–13.

Syrjanen J *et al.* (1988) Preceding infection as an important risk factor for ischaemic brain infarction in young and middle aged patients. *British Medical Journal.* **296**:1156–60.

Thomas AE *et al.* (1991) Variation in the promoter region of the *B* fibrinogen gene is associated with plasma fibrinogen levels in smokers and non-smokers. *Thrombosis and Haemostasis.* **65**:487–90.

Wakefield AJ *et al.* (1989) Pathogenesis of Crohn's disease: multifocal gastrointestinal infarction. *The Lancet.* **ii**:1057–62.

Wilhelmsen L *et al.* (1984) Fibrinogen as a risk factor for stroke and myocardial infarction. *New England Journal of Medicine.* **311**:501–5.

Wilkes HC *et al.* (1988) Smoking and plasma fibrinogen. *The Lancet.* **i**:307–8.

Wilkes HC *et al.* (1992) Gemfibrozil reduces plasma prothrombin fragment F1+2 concentration, a marker of coagulability, in patients with coronary heart disease. *Thrombosis and Haemostatis.* **67**:503–6.

Wiseman S *et al.* (1989) Influence of smoking and plasma factors on patency of femoropopliteal vein grafts. *British Medical Journal.* **299**:643–6.

Yarnell JWG *et al.* (1985) Haemostatic factors and ischaemic heart disease. The Caerphilly study. *British Heart Journal.* **53**:483–7.

Yarnell JWG *et al.* (1987) Some long term effects of smoking on the haemostatic system: a report from the Caerphilly and Speedwell collaborative surveys. *Journal of Clinical Pathology.* **40**:909–13.

Yarnell JWG *et al.* (1991) Fibrinogen, viscosity, and white blood cell count are major risk factors for ischemic heart disease. The Caerphilly and Speedwell Collabortive Heart Disease Studies. *Circulation.* **83**:836–44.

21

Clotting Factors and Rheology: Mechanisms of Damage and Intervention

MW RAMPLING

Introduction

It is well established that smoking is an important risk factor for cardiovascular disease (Reid *et al.*, 1976; Abbott *et al.*, 1986; Gotto, 1986) While the precise causative mechanisms are not clear, there is little doubt that they relate, at least in part, to smoking-induced alterations in other risk factors such as haematocrit (Galea and Davidson, 1985; Ernst *et al.*, 1987), concentrations of plasma proteins and haemostatic factors (Belch *et al.*, 1984), especially fibrinogen (Meade *et al.*, 1987), and leucocyte count (Ernst *et al.*, 1987). An indication of the dose dependence of some of these is given in Table 21.1.

The potential importance of these risk factors is not always clear. Even where it seems obvious—for instance the relationship between clotting and thrombosis—there may be hidden factors. This chapter discusses the possible role of haemorheology, ie the flow properties of the blood, and the way in which it is affected by disturbances in other risk factors. However, in view of the specialist nature of haemorheology, a brief summary will first be given of its general relevance to the vascular system.

The determinants of the flow rate of simple liquids (those that have constant viscosity, such as water) through a cylindrical tube are related by Poiseuille's equation:

$$\frac{Q}{t} = \frac{\pi}{8} \frac{(P_{in} - P_{out})}{v} \frac{r^4}{l} \qquad \text{(equation 1)}$$

where Q/t is the volume flow rate, P_{in} and P_{out} are the entrance and exit pressures, r and l are the vessel radius and length and v is the viscosity of the liquid. This equation can be rewritten

$$\frac{Q}{t} = \frac{\pi}{8} \frac{(P_{in} - P_{out})}{v \quad (l/r^4)} \qquad \text{(equation 2)}$$

which can be reduced to

$$\frac{Q}{t} = \frac{\pi}{8} \frac{(P_{in} - P_{out})}{\underset{\substack{\text{(viscous} \\ \text{resistance)}}}{} \quad \underset{\substack{\text{(geometric} \\ \text{resistance)}}}{}} \qquad \text{(equation 3).}$$

	Fibrinogen (g/l)	Thrombin clotting time (s)	White cell count (10^9/l)	Haematocrit (%)
Non-smoker	3.5	36	5.9	46.3
	(0.8)	(13)	(1.2)	(3.1)
Smoker (1–14)	3.9	28	7.7	46.7
	(0.9)	(11)	(2.0)	(3.8)
Smoker (15–24)	4.0	29	8.1	47.2
	(0.8)	(12)	(2.0)	(3.7)
Smoker (>24)	4.05	27	8.25	48.2
	(0.8)	(10)	(2.2)	(3.4)

Table 21.1: Comparison of a number of risk factors in male smokers (cigarettes per day) and non-smokers. Approximately 300 subjects per group. Mean (SD). (Source: Yarnell *et al.*, 1987.)

Blood, as will be seen, is not a simple liquid in the above sense since it has complex viscous properties. Nevertheless the principles of equation 3 still apply to it, so blood viscosity is an important determinant of flow rate or flow resistance in the circulation. However, a variety of factors affect it and most are influenced by smoking.

Factors affecting blood viscosity

The principal factors affecting the viscous properties of blood are plasma viscosity, shear rate and haematocrit. The viscosity of plasma is significant because its magnitude depends on the concentration of plasma proteins: particularly the large asymmetric proteins such as the immunoglobulins, and most especially fibrinogen (Lowe and Barbenel, 1988). It has been shown above (*see* Table 21.1) that fibrinogen concentration increases with smoking and hence it is to be expected that plasma viscosity will also increase. This is relevant because, to a reasonable approximation, the viscosity of whole blood increases in proportion to the increase in the viscosity of the plasma, at least at high shear rates (Lowe, 1988).

The two factors with the greatest influence on blood viscosity are the shear rate and the haematocrit.

Shear rate

When a liquid flows through a tube, the velocity varies across the tube. It is lowest at the walls and highest in the centre of flow (Figure 21.1), the velocity profile being curved. Hence the planes of liquid flow past one another at

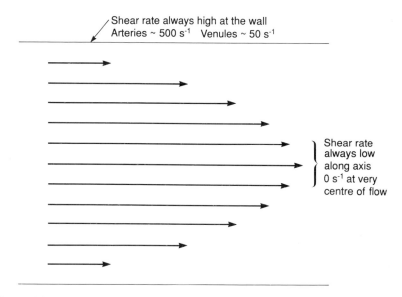

Shear rate always high at the wall
Arteries ~ 500 s^{-1} Venules ~ 50 s^{-1}

Shear rate
always low
along axis
0 s^{-1} at very
centre of flow

Figure 21.1: Variation of the velocity of a liquid across the bore of a cylindrical tube and the range of shear rates present.

varying rates. The rate of separation of these planes is the shear rate. It is defined as the difference in velocity between adjacent planes divided by the distance between them, and the units are inverse seconds or s^{-1}.

In the context of blood, low shear rates are usually taken as less than about 10s^{-1} and vice versa. The shear rate at the wall of a blood vessel is always high, ranging from about 500s^{-1} in arteries to about 50s^{-1} in venules and small veins (Chien, 1987). In the centre of flow it is always low, however, irrespective of the size or type of vessel; indeed in the very centre of flow it is zero. For simple viscous liquids, such as water, this is of no consequence because their viscosity is constant with shear rate. However, blood is different: its viscosity is very variable with shear rate (Figure 21.2). At high shear rate the viscosity changes relatively little, but in the low shear region the rate of change is very significant. Over the whole shear-rate range shown in Figure 21.2, the change in viscosity is about ten fold.

The causes of this somewhat unusual rheological behaviour are two properties of the erythrocytes (Lowe and Barbenel, 1988), their deformability and their propensity to form rouleaux (ie loose aggregates). At low shear rates, the large rouleaux lead to the high viscosity. As the shear rate rises the weak forces holding the aggregates together are overcome by the shear, the aggregates are progressively broken down and the viscosity falls rapidly until, at about 10s^{-1} in normal blood, the cells are monodispersed. After this the small continuing fall is due to progressive deformation of the cells by the increasing shear forces in the flowing system.

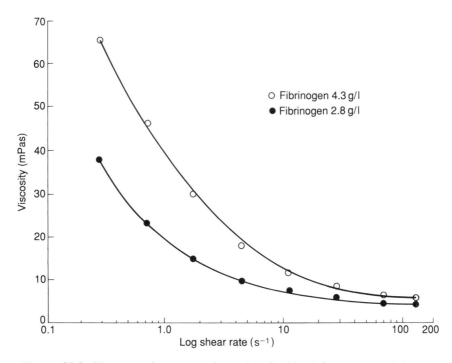

Figure 21.2: Viscosity: shear rate relationship for blood from a normal (●--●) and a diabetic subject (○--○).

The deformability of the red cell is reputed to be changed in association with a number of pathologies, but in very few is the change enough to affect blood viscosity significantly. The alteration that has been reported in smokers (Norton and Rand, 1981; Ernst and Matrai, 1987) is also not enough to be relevant in this respect. However, the low shear-rate effect of rouleaux formation is increased very significantly in many pathologies, and this is illustrated for a typical diabetic patient in Figure 21.2. In this case, as in most, it is due largely to the increased fibrinogen concentration which is a common concomitant of many pathologies and the fact that fibrinogen is the most potent rouleaux-inducing plasma protein (Rampling, 1988). As has been shown earlier, fibrinogen concentration is raised in smokers and hence can be expected to lead to an increase in low shear-rate blood viscosity.

Haematocrit

Haematocrit is the most potent of all the factors that affect blood viscosity, and the approximate relationship between them is semi-logarithmic, ie:

$$\log(\text{viscosity}) = C + K.H \qquad \text{(equation 4)}$$

where C and K are shear-rate-dependent constants and H is the haematocrit.

This is illustrated for a normal individual in Figure 21.3 where the haematocrit has been manipulated by adding or removing autologous plasma. It can be seen that the viscosity increases rapidly as the haematocrit rises, but this is particularly so at low shear rate. Again, because haematocrit is increased in smokers (*see* Table 21.1), their blood viscosity should be raised.

These effects that increase blood viscosity also increase viscous resistance in the circulation. However, the influence is exaggerated in regions where the flow is sluggish and thus where the shear rates are low, for example where driving pressure is reduced, typically distal to vascular obstructions such as atheroma.

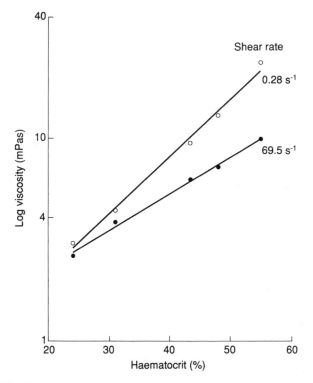

Figure 21.3: Blood viscosity: haematocrit relationship for a normal individual.

The same effects are to be found behind valve pockets in the veins. It is of interest that these are the regions where thrombotic events are particularly common and it is thought that there is a cause-and-effect relationship between the sluggish flow and thrombosis (Lowe, 1984). It is also of relevance that there is a strong correlation between elevated blood viscosity, particularly at low shear rate, and vascular occlusive disease in general (Dintenfass, 1971), and hypertension (Letcher *et al.*, 1981) and stroke (Lechner *et al.*, 1986) in particular.

Microvascular flow

So far this chapter has concentrated on blood viscosity as the prime rheological parameter, and in large vessels—where the red cell is small in comparison with the vessel bore—this is correct. In the microvasculature, however, where the relative dimensions are similar, blood viscosity loses its usefulness as a parameter. Instead the other rheological factors must be considered separately, ie plasma viscosity, red cell rigidity and rouleaux formation, increases in any of which are thought to limit flow or affect flow resistance. Furthermore at this level the white cell is important because, even though it is present in relatively small numbers, its deformability is down by some three orders of magnitude on that of the erythrocyte (Chien, 1987). This is relevant because smokers have raised white cell counts (*see* Table 21.1). Unfortunately the theory of microvascular flow has not been worked out fully so it is not clear what the relative influences of these various parameters are at this level.

Smoking and rheology

It has been shown above that a variety of haematological variables are disturbed in the smoker, and that several of these are influential on haemorheology in general, so it can be expected to disturb haemorheology in the smoker as well. A number of studies have shown this to be the case (Belch *et al.*, 1984; Galea and Davidson, 1985; Ernst *et al.*, 1987), and data from one of these are shown in Table 21.2 to illustrate the important haematological disturbances. There were about 30 healthy males in each group. It can be seen that haematocrit,

	Haematocrit (%)	Plasma oncotic pressure (mmHg)	Fibrinogen (g/l)
Non-smoker	44.1 (3.4)	26.4 (1.3)	2.7 (0.4)
Smoker (10–20)	45.7 (3.8)	28.1* (1.6)	3.0 (0.3)
Smoker (21–40)	46.6* (3.2)	28.9* (2.2)	3.2 (0.4)
Smoker (>40)	48.2* (3.5)	28.7* (2.0)	3.4* (0.5)

*$P = < 0.01$ cf non-smoker

Table 21.2: Disturbances in haematological factors in smokers (cigarettes per day) compared with non-smokers. Mean (SD). (Source: Ernst *et al.*, 1987.)

	Plasma viscosity (mPas)	Blood viscosity, low shear rate $0.7s^{-1}$ (mPas)	Blood viscosity, high shear rate $94.5s^{-1}$ (mPas)
Non-smoker	1.20 (0.06)	23.3 (8.0)	4.4 (0.6)
Smoker (10–20)	1.24* (0.06)	27.4* (8.1)	4.8 (0.9)
Smoker (21–40)	1.26* (0.07)	29.8* (10.2)	5.1* (0.8)
Smoker (>40)	1.26* (0.06)	31.2* (9.7)	5.2* (0.9)

$*P = {} < 0.01$ cf non-smoker

Table 21.3: Differences in viscometric properties of blood from smokers (cigarettes per day) and non-smokers. Mean (SD). (Source: Ernst *et al.*, 1987.)

plasma oncotic pressure (and therefore plasma protein concentration) and fibrinogen are raised, and that the disturbances are dose-dependent.

Since all of these are influential on haemorheological factors, they too are disturbed (as shown in Table 21.3, using data from the same study). Blood viscosity is raised at high and low shear rates in response to the raised haematocrit, but especially so at low shear rate due to the elevated fibrinogen concentration (and enhanced rouleaux formation). The plasma viscosity is also raised in response to the increase in plasma protein concentration. The ultimate causes of all these changes are probably smoking-induced fluid movement to the extravascular space leading to haemoconcentration, coupled with a low-grade inflammatory response. Incidentally, Ernst *et al.* (1987) also found a decrease in erythrocyte deformability (as did Norton and Rand, 1981) and an increase in white cell count (as did Yarnell *et al.*, 1987), both of which should affect microvascular flow.

Effects of stopping smoking

The only reasonable way to try to reverse these changes in smokers is to get them to abstain, and the Surgeon General has been quoted as saying that cigarette smoking is the single most preventable cause of death from heart disease in the United States (Gotto, 1986). What, then, are the effects of stopping?

Ernst *et al.* (1987) compared the haemorheological profile of 30 healthy male non-smokers with that of 30 matched ex-smokers who had given up the habit one or two years previously. A synopsis of their results is shown in Table 21.4. It can be seen that after long-term abstention all values are normalized.

However, there is evidence elsewhere for much more rapid changes in the haematological parameters that normally affect haemorheology (Isager and

	Haematocrit	White cell count (10^9/l)	PV (mPas)	BV 1s 0.7s^{-1} (mPas)	BV hs 94.5s^{-1} (mPas)	Fib (g/l)
Non-smoker	44.1 (3.4)	5.9 (2.1)	1.20 (0.06)	23 (8)	4.4 (0.6)	2.7 (0.4)
Ex-smoker	44.9 (3.5)	6.4 (1.9)	1.21 (0.07)	24 (9)	4.5 (0.7)	2.7 (0.5)

PV, plasma viscosity; BV, blood viscosity at ls (low shear rate) and hs (high shear rate); Fib, fibrinogen concentration.

Table 21.4: Haemorheological profiles of non-smokers compared to ex-smokers of 1–2 years' duration. Mean (SD). (Source: Ernst *et al.*, 1987.)

Haglerup, 1971). Rapid haemorheological changes have been looked for by others (Galea and Davidson, 1985) but the data of Ernst and Matrai (1987) are shown in Table 21.5. It is clear that normalization has occured after only eight weeks. However, neither of these studies was adequately controlled because there was no objective test of abstention, it being checked only by questionnaire. Again only males were used by Ernst and Matrai (1985), and

	Smoker base-line (N = 14)	4 weeks (N = 14)	8 weeks (N = 10)	Non Smoker (N = 24)
BV 1s 0.7s^{-1} (mPas)	30.2 (9.1)	26.0* (8.2)	24.1* (7.5)	22.4* (8.2)
BV hs 94.5s^{-1} (mPas)	5.2 (0.9)	4.9* (0.8)	4.6* (0.7)	4.4* (0.7)
PV (mPas)	1.26 (0.04)	1.24* (0.04)	1.22* (0.06)	1.19* (0.06)
Haematocrit (%)	49.1 (4.0)	46.3 (3.6)	45.7* (3.5)	44.3* (3.8)
Fib (g/l)	3.8 (1.2)	2.9 (0.9)	2.4* (1.0)	2.4* (1.2)
WBC (10^9/l)	7.4 (2.0)	7.2* (2.0)	6.2* (1.7)	5.7* (2.4)

*$P < 0.01$ cf base-line. (See Table 21.4 for abbreviations.)

Table 21.5: Changes in viscometric parameters of smokers in the first 8 weeks following abstention from tobacco. Mean (SD). (Source: Ernst and Matrai, 1987.)

the two sexes were not separated in the other study (Galea and Davidson, 1985).

In a very recent study (Rampling *et al.*, 1991) the two sexes were separated, but the crucial difference from other studies was that compliance with the abstention protocol was checked by testing the urine of the subjects for nicotine and cotenene levels. Only if these were negligible were a subject's data included. Base-line readings were taken while the subjects were smoking normally; they stopped smoking two weeks later and were retested two weeks after that. This time-scale was chosen because of the effects of menstruation on haemorheo-logy (Buchan and Macdonald, 1980); by retesting after four weeks they could be expected to be insignificant. The result was a group of 14 healthy females and eight males (aged 30–58 years) (Table 21.6). Although all parameters decreased by similar amounts for both sexes after two weeks of abstention, the female data were more significant than those of the males— probably due to the small number of the latter subjects. Thus this study showed that, on complete abstention, a considerable degree of normalization takes place within two weeks in females as well as in males.

These investigators then looked at even shorter time-scales. A group of young subjects (aged 19–30 years), all healthy, who smoked 10–35 cigarettes per day were persuaded to abstain. Again the urine was tested to confirm compliance. The females all entered the study on the day their periods started to synchronize menstrual effects and blood was processed on a daily basis for two weeks. A synopsis of the data is given in Figure 21.4 (Rothwell *et al.*, 1991). The changes were seen to be very rapid. The viscosity of the blood at both high and low shear rates reached a new base-line within two days, and reflected the drop in haematocrit. The associated factors all behaved similarly in the males, ie the plasma viscosity, plasma protein and fibrinogen levels, reaching new lower plateaux in the same time. The females also showed rapid falls within two days, but a rebound followed in some parameters: probably because they had started the study on the first day of their periods. The rebound was probably related to the fact that smoking leads to a reduction in oestrogen level which is acutely raised on abstention from smoking, and this in turn leads to an acute increase in protein production (Jensen *et al.*, 1985).

Conclusion

It has been shown that significant disturbances are present in the haemorheological profile of smokers. These can be explained as resulting from smoking-induced haemoconcentration coupled with a low-grade inflammatory response. The disturbances are largely removed by abstention from smoking and there is evidence that these changes are very rapid: indeed within two days a very considerable degree of normalization occurs.

Unfortunately, however, the area is complicated. There appear to be differences in the responses of males and females, they are dose-dependent (ie they

	Before	Female After	Non-smoker	Before	Male After	Non-smoker
	(N = 14)		(N = 6)	(N = 8)		(N = 19)
BV 1s 0.277s^{-1} (mPas)	38.9 (4.3)	33.2* (7.2)	32.6 (9.4)	52.1 (5.7)	47.6 (6.2)	41.9† (7.1)
BV hs 128.5s^{-1} (mPas)	4.28 (0.21)	4.16 (0.42)	4.1 (0.6)	5.0 (0.4)	4.75 (0.23)	4.60 (0.3)
Haematocrit (%)	44.0 (2.3)	42.2* (2.5)	40.5† (1.9)	48.6 (2.3)	46.4* (2.8)	44.1† (2.5)
PV (mPas)	1.37 (0.04)	1.33 (0.05)	1.34 (0.08)	1.50 (0.20)	1.40 (0.10)	1.34 (0.08)
Fib (g/l)	3.4 (0.6)	2.8* (0.6)	3.2 (0.6)	4.0 (0.7)	3.7 (1.41)	3.2 (0.6)
PP (g/l)	72.4 (4.0)	71.3 (8.0)		78.7 (6.2)	72.2 (8.5)	

*$P < 5\%$ before vs after, †$P < 5\%$ after vs non-smoker.

PP, plasma protein concentration. (See Table 21.4 for other abbreviations.)

Table 21.6: Comparison of the haemorheological profiles of non-smokers and smokers before and two weeks after abstention from tobacco. Mean (SD). (Source: Rampling et al., 1991.)

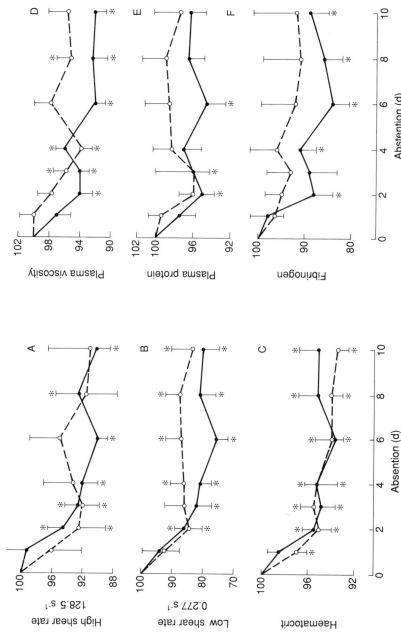

Figure 21.4: Percentage change from base-line in (A) high and (B) low shear rate blood viscosity, (C) haematocrit, (D) plasma viscosity, (E) plasma protein and (F) fibrinogen concentrations after abstention from smoking (m+/−sem). Closed circles for males, open circles for females; asterisks indicate significant change from baseline ($P<0.05$)

depend on numbers and strengh of cigarettes smoked, inhalation patterns etc), and will probably depend of the duration of the habit and on any underlying pathology. More data are needed in this area.

However, the principal conclusion is that within a very short time (two days or so) a considerable degree of normalization in haemorheological factors occurs with abstention from cigarettes. In view of the association of these factors with cardiovascular risk the benefits of abstention from smoking may be much more rapidly felt than was hitherto thought.

References

Abbott RD *et al.* (1986) Risk of stroke in male cigarette smokers. *New England Journal of Medicine.* **315**:718–20.

Belch JTF *et al.* (1984) The effects of acute smoking on platelet behaviour, fibrinolysis and haemorheology in habitual smokers. *Thrombosis and Haemostasis.* **51**:6–8.

Buchan PC and Macdonald HN (1980) Rheological studies in obstetrics and gynaecology. In: Lowe GDO *et al.* (eds) *Aspects of blood viscosity and cell deformability.* Springer, Berlin. pp. 175–92.

Chien S (1987) Physiological and pathophysiological significance of hemorheology. In: Chien S *et al.* (eds) *Clinical haemorheology.* Martinus Nijhoff, Dordrecht. pp. 123–64.

Dintenfass L (1971) *Blood-microrheology-viscosity factors in blood flow, ischaemia and thrombosis.* Butterworth, London.

Ernst E *et al.* (1987) Dose-effect relationship between smoking and blood rheology. *British Journal of Haematology.* **65**:485–7.

Ernst E *et al.*, (1987) Dose-effect relationship between smoking and blood rheology. *British Journal of Haematology.* **65**:485–7.

Galea G and Davidson RJL (1985) Haematological and haemorheological changes associated with cigarette smoking. *Journal of Clinical Pathology.* **38**:978–84.

Gotto AM (1986) Interactions of the major risk factors for coronary heart disease. *American Journal of Medicine.* **80** (Suppl. 2A):48–55.

Isager H and Hagelrup L (1971) Relationship between smoking and high packed cell volume and haemoglobin levels. *Scandinavian Journal of Haematology.* **8**:241–4.

Jensen J *et al.* (1985) Cigarette smoking, serum estrogens and bone loss during hormone replacement therapy early after menopause. *New England Journal of Medicine.* **16**:973–5.

Lechner H *et al*. (1986) Follow up studies of the haemorheological profile in acute ischaemic stroke. *Clinical Hemorheology*. **6**:3–9.

Letcher RL *et al*. (1981) Direct relationship between blood pressure and blood viscosity in normal and hypertensive subjects. Role of fibrinogen and concentration. *American Journal of Medicine*. **70**:1195–202.

Lowe GDO (1984) Blood rheology and venous thrombosis. *Clinical Hemorheology*. **4**:571–88.

Lowe GDO (1988) Rheology of paraproteinaemias and leukemias. In: Lowe GDO (ed.) *Clinical blood rheology*, Volume II. CRC Press, Boca Raton. pp. 67–85.

Lowe GDO and Barbenel JC (1988) Plasma and blood viscosity. In: Lowe GDO (ed.) *Clinical blood rheology*, Volume I. CRC Press, Boca Raton. pp. 11–44.

Meade TW *et al*. (1987) Effects of changes in smoking and other characteristics on clotting factors and the risk of ischaemic heart disease. *The Lancet*. **i**:986–8.

Norton JM and Rand PW (1981) Decreased deformability of erythrocytes from smokers. *Blood*. **5**:671–4.

Rampling MW (1988) Red cell aggregation and yield stress. In: Lowe GDO (ed.) *Clinical blood rheology*, Volume I. CRC Press, Boca Raton. pp. 45–64.

Rampling MW *et al*. (1991) The short term effects of abstention from tobacco by cigarette smokers on blood viscosity and related parameters. *Clinical Hemorheology*. **11**:441–6.

Reid DD *et al*., (1976) Smoking and other risk factors for coronary heart disease in British civil servants. *The Lancet*. **i**:979–83.

Rothwell M *et al*., (1991) Haemorheological changes in the very short term after abstention from tobacco by cigarette smokers. *British Journal of Haematology*. **79**: 500–3.

Yarnell JWG *et al*. (1987) Some long term effects of smoking on the haemostatic system: a report from the Caerphilly and Speedwell collaborative surveys. *Journal of Clinical Pathology*. **40**:909–13.

22

Coffee and Lack of Dietary Fibre as Risk Factors for Cardiovascular Disease

TAB SANDERS

It has been claimed for some years that coffee consumption (Jick *et al.*, 1973) and a lack of dietary fibre (Trowell, 1975) may increase the risk of cardiovascular disease (CVD). This chapter reviews the evidence and discusses possible mechanisms of action.

Evidence for the relationship between dietary fibre intake and CVD is drawn mainly from ecological studies of rural communities in Africa compared with Western countries. However, many Far Eastern countries have low rates of coronary heart disease (CHD) but intakes of fibre that are similar to those of Western countries. Moreover, it is now recognized that the term 'dietary fibre' may be inappropriate (British Nutrition Foundation, 1990) to describe the myriad of substances such as gums, lignans and cellulose of which it is comprised. The term 'non-starch polysaccharide' (NSP) is used to describe indigestible complex carbohydrates consisting of more than 18 monosaccharide units, and this can be divided into a water-soluble fraction and an insoluble fraction. Some forms of starch are poorly digested and may behave like NSP and act as a substrate for the colonic microflora. It has been argued that when fermentable carbohydrate reaches the large bowel it is converted to short-chain fatty acids which are absorbed into the portal system and may have effects on plasma lipids. Diets high in NSP also tend to be high in starch and to contain less fat. A high intake of NSP may decrease the digestibility of fat and retard the absorption of glucose and decrease postprandial insulin effects. Thus the intake of NSP may indirectly affect risk of CHD.

High intakes of dietary fibre derived from cereals emerged as a protective factor in a prospective study in the UK (Morris *et al.*, 1977) but these findings were not confirmed by Burr and Sweetnam (1982). Thus the role of dietary fibre in the primary prevention of CVD is uncertain, but countries with high intakes of complex carbohydrates generally have low intakes of saturated fatty acids and low rates of CHD. A secondary prevention trial in patients who had previously suffered from a myocardial infarction (MI) was carried out by Burr *et al.* (1989a): patients were advised to increase their intake of cereal fibre, and the incidence of CHD and death were followed over the next two years. Total mortality rates were non-significantly greater in the group advised about fibre than in the group which did not receive the advice.

Proponents of the fibre hypothesis argue that other types of fibre, such as the soluble forms found in oat-bran and some legumes, may have different effects from wheat fibre. Much publicity has been given to oats and their potential to reduce plasma cholesterol and thus CHD. However, countries where oats are widely consumed (Scotland, Finland) have some of the highest rates of CHD in the world. A high intake of oat fibre can compromise the absorption of certain minerals from the diet, particularly calcium and zinc.

In contrast, the epidemiological evidence for the relationship between coffee consumption and CHD has been derived almost entirely from prospective and cross-sectional studies (Thelle et al., 1991). Strong relationships between coffee consumption and CHD have been found in Nordic countries and in some, but not all, North American studies (Kovar et al., 1983). The interaction between lifestyle habits such as smoking does not make interpretation easy. Coffee consumption and smoking habits are often strongly related. However, a study of American physicians—who comprise a predominantly non-smoking population—found a strong relationship between coffee consumption and risk of CHD (La Croix et al., 1986) after adjusting for other risk factors. Heavy coffee consumption was associated with a twofold or threefold risk of CHD. The association was strongest with the most recent assessment of intake, and a dose response relationship was demonstrated. These studies, however, can never entirely control for lifestyle or personality factors that might be related to risk.

Several cross-sectional as well as prospective studies show a positive relationship between serum cholesterol concentrations and coffee consumption (Thelle et al., 1983, 1987; Williams et al., 1985; Solvoll et al., 1989; Tverdal et al., 1990; Kohlmeier et al., 1991; Salvaggio et al., 1991). This effect appears to be independent of other known dietary factors, and the association is strongest where heated unfiltered coffee or boiled coffee is consumed. However, the increased risk of CHD with coffee consumption cannot be explained solely by the increased risk posed by raised cholesterol (La Croix et al., 1986; Tverdal et al., 1990). This implies that coffee—or the life-style associated with coffee consumption—exerts other effects on CHD.

Influence of fibre and coffee on plasma lipoprotein

Various types of dietary fibre have been shown to influence plasma total cholesterol and low-density lipoprotein (LDL) cholesterol (Miettenen, 1987; British Nutrition Foundation, 1990). Wheat bran and rice bran have no significant effect (Kestin et al., 1990) on plasma cholesterol or LDL concentrations in man (Sanders and Reddy, 1992). Barley (McIntosh et al., 1991) and oats (Judd and Truswell, 1981; Kestin et al., 1990) have a modest cholesterol-lowering effect in subjects with mild hypercholesterolaemia. Both oats and barley contain significant amounts of soluble fibre. Other foods containing soluble fibre such as pectin and guar gum lower plasma cholesterol at doses between 8 and 30 g/d in both normal and hypercholesterolaemic subjects. Such doses are not readily provided by diets and so should be regarded as pharmacological rather than nutritional. Guar gum has been the most extensively studied material; it is used therapeutically in doses of 15–30 g/d and can lead to reductions in LDL cholesterol in the order of 15% (Tuomilehto et al., 1988, 1989). It is, however, poorly tolerated because of gastrointestinal side-effects. Soluble fibre increases the excretion of bile acids and neutral sterols and thus decreases the hepatic intracellular cholesterol concentration, leading to up-regulation of LDL receptors (Topping et al., 1990). Human kinetic studies have found that guar gum increases the fractional catabolic rate of LDL, similar to cholestyramine (Turner et al., 1990).

It has also been argued that the fermentation of NSP to short-chain fatty acids may inhibit the action of HMGCoA reductase, the rate limiting step in the synthesis of cholesterol. However, subjects given lactulose, a carbohydrate that is fermented in the large bowel, show a paradoxical increase in LDL cholesterol concentrations (Jenkins et al., 1991). It was been suggested that acetate resulting from the fermentation acted as a substrate for hepatic cholesterol synthesis.

The putative beneficial effects of high-fibre diets in the management of hypercholesterolaemia have been seized on with alacrity by the food industry who have used heart-shaped breakfast cereals in heart-shaped bowls to assert their claims for cholesterol-lowering properties. Consequently the role of dietary fibre in the management of hyperlipidaemia is often exaggerated by dietitians and other health professionals, whereas the impact that high-fibre diets have on plasma cholesterol concentrations is relatively small. For example, oat bran products do lead to a small (5%) reduction in plasma cholesterol when 60–100 g are consumed daily (Swain et al., 1990). Yet an average portion of oat bran containing breakfast cereal weighs only 30–40 g, an insufficient amount to influence plasma cholesterol concentrations.

Thelle et al. (1983) showed a difference in total cholesterol concentration of 0.79 and 0.72 mmol/l in men and women respectively, from the lowest to the highest coffee consumption category. It was then demonstrated that abstinence from coffee led to a fall in plasma cholesterol concentration and that reintroduction of coffee led to a prompt rise in serum cholesterol (Arnesen et al., 1984; Førde et al., 1985).

Later studies showed that the method of brewing was a crucial factor, and that instant and filtered coffee were not as potent in raising serum cholesterol as boiled coffee (Aro et al., 1990). The cholesterol-elevating substance is largely removed by the filtration of boiled coffee (Aro et al., 1990; van Dusseldorp et al., 1991); it is retained by the filter paper (Ahola et al., 1991) and is present in the fat fraction of coffee. Using volunteers, Zock et al. (1990) showed that a lipid fraction derived from boiled coffee led to a 29% rise in plasma cholesterol concentration. The exact nature of the substance has yet to be identified.

Bak and Grobbee (1989) suggested that more moderate heating of coffee led to this undesirable effect. They compared the effect of coffee prepared using a filter with that using the same coffee prepared by adding boiling water to coffee grounds in a Thermos flask which was left for at least 10 minutes before consumption. The latter was referred to as boiled coffee, although the temperature of the coffee was below 100°C. The filtered coffee had no effect, but the boiled coffee increased cholesterol concentrations by about 10%. Measurement of blood and salivary caffeine revealed no differences between the two types of coffee preparations, demonstrating that no more caffeine was extracted in the boiled coffee. The same workers (Bak and Grobbee, 1991) conducted a double-blind trial of caffeine versus placebo in subjects given filtered decaffeinated coffee. Neither treatment influenced plasma cholesterol or LDL concentrations, thus exonerating caffeine as the cholesterol-elevating factor.

While the LDL cholesterol-raising effect of boiled coffee is clearly established, the effects of other types of coffee on blood cholesterol are less clear-cut. In Italy, where filter or expresso coffee is consumed, there is also a relationship between coffee intake and plasma cholesterol concentration (Salvaggio *et al*., 1991). However, the difference between light and heavy consumers is much smaller (0.25 mmol/d) than in Nordic countries. Burr *et al*. (1989*b*), in a cross-over trial in the UK, found only a weak non-statistically significant effect of coffee consumption on plasma cholesterol level. However, in this study coffee intakes were relatively low.

An early study by Naismith *et al*. (1970) suggested that instant decaffeinated coffee slightly raised plasma cholesterol more than regular instant coffee. We repeated these studies and were unable to demonstrate any difference between instant decaffeinated and regular instant coffee on apoprotein B levels. However, both types of instant coffee led to a 4–5 mg/d increase in apoprotein B concentration (unpublished data). Superko *et al*. (1991) reported that filtered coffee prepared from decaffeinated beans slightly increased (9 mg/dl) apoprotein B and LDL cholesterol (0.23 mmol/l) concentrations compared with filtered coffee, and increased the activity of hepatic lipase while reducing that of lipoprotein lipase. They attributed the difference between the decaffeinated and caffeinated coffee brands to the coffee varieties used to make them. The more expensive Arabica variety is more commonly used to make regular caffeinated filter coffee, whereas the cheaper Robusta variety, which has a higher content of caffeine and other pharmacologically active materials, is used to make decaffeinated and instant brands.

Fried *et al*. (1992) showed that 720 ml of filtered caffeinated coffee raised LDL cholesterol by about 0.25 mmol/l compared with no coffee, or 300 ml of filtered or decaffeinated coffee, thus demonstrating that even filtered coffee has a cholesterol-raising effect, if consumed in sufficient quantity.

Coffee is an extremely complex mixture and undergoes several chemical changes during processing. For example, nicotinic acid is present in relatively high concentrations in instant coffee but is relatively low in green coffee beans.

Varying procedures are used for the production of coffee and some involve heating the coffee liquor prior to drying. It is not possible to increase plasma cholesterol concentration in hamsters by incorporating coffee into their basal diet (Mensink *et al.* 1992; Sanders and Sandaradura, 1992). However, if they are given a diet containing lard and cholesterol to down-regulate their LDL receptors, they show an increase in LDL cholesterol (Sanders and Sandaradura, 1992). Thus the mechanism for the increase in cholesterol is likely to be due to an increased rate of synthesis of LDL rather than an effect on the expression of LDL receptors.

References

Ahola I *et al.* (1991) The hypercholesterolaemic factor in boiled coffee is retained by a paper filter. *Journal of Internal Medicine.* **230**:293–7.

Arnesen E *et al.* (1984) Coffee and serum cholesterol. *British Medical Journal.* **228**:1960.

Aro A *et al.* (1990) Dose-dependent effect on serum cholesterol and apoprotein B concentrations by consumption of boiled, non-filtered coffee. *Atherosclerosis.* **83**: 257–61.

Bak AA and Grobbee DE (1989) The effect on serum cholesterol levels of coffee brewed by filtering or boiling. *New England Journal of Medicine.* **321**:1432–7.

Bak AA and Grobbee DE (1991) Caffeine, blood pressure, and serum lipids. *American Journal of Clinical Nutrition.* **53**:971–5.

British Nutrition Foundation (1990) *Complex carbohydrates in foods.* Chapman and Hall, London.

Burr ML and Sweetnam PM (1982) Vegetarianism, dietary fiber, and mortality. *American Journal of Clinical Nutrition.* **36**:873–7.

Burr ML *et al.* (1989*a*) Effects of change in fat, fish and fibre intakes on death and myocardial infarction: Death and Reinfarction Trial (DART). *The Lancet.* **ii**:757– 60.

Burr ML *et al.* (1989*b*) Coffee, blood pressure and plasma lipids. A randomized controlled trial. *European Journal of Clinical Nutrition.* **43**:477–83.

Førde OH *et al.* (1985) The Tromsø Heart Study: coffee consumption and serum lipid concentration in men with hypercholesterolaemia: a randomised intervention study. *British Medical Journal.* **290**:893.

Fried RE *et al.* (1992) The effect of filtered-coffee consumption on plasma lipid levels. Results of a randomized clinical trial. *Journal of the American Medical Association.* **267**:811–15.

Jenkins DJA *et al.* (1991) Specific types of colonic fermentation may raise low-density-lipoprotein cholesterol concentrations. *Annals of the Journal of Clinical Nutrition.* **54**:141–7.

Jick H *et al.* (1973) Coffee and myocardial infarction. *New England Journal of Medicine.* **289**:63–4.

Judd PA and Truswell AS (1981) The effect of rolled oats on blood lipids and fecal steroid excretion in man. *American Journal of Clinical Nutrition.* **34**:2061–7.

Kestin M *et al.* (1990) Comparative effect of three cereal brans on plasma lipids, blood pressure, and glucose metabolism in mildly hypercholesterolemic men. *American Journal of Clinical Nutrition.* **52**:661–6.

Kohlmeier L *et al.* (1991) The relationship between coffee consumption and lipid levels in young and older people in the Heidelberg-Michelstadt-Berlin study. *European Heart Journal.* **12**:869–74.

Kovar MG *et al.* (1983) Coffee and cholesterol. (Letter.) *New England Journal of Medicine.* **309**:1249.

La Croix AZ *et al.* (1986) Coffee consumption and the incidence of coronary heart disease. *New England Journal of Medicine.* **315**:976.

McIntosh GH *et al.* (1991) Barley and wheat foods: influence on plasma cholesterol concentrations in hypercholesterolemic men. *American Journal of Clinical Nutrition.* **53**:1205–9.

Mensink RP *et al.* (1992) Boiled coffee does not increase serum cholesterol in gerbils and hamsters. *Zeitschrift Ernahrungswiss.* **31**:82–5.

Miettenen TA (1987) Dietary fiber and lipids. *American Journal of Clinical Nutrition.* **45**:1237–42.

Morris JN *et al.* (1977) Diet and heart: a postscript. *British Medical Journal.* **2**:1307–14.

Naismith DJ *et al.* (1970) The effect in volunteers of coffee and decaffeinated coffee on blood glucose, insulin, plasma lipids and some factors involved in blood clotting. *Nutrition and Metabolism.* **12**:144–51.

Salvaggio A *et al.* (1991) Coffee and cholesterol, an Italian study. *American Journal of Epidemiology.* **134**:149–56.

Sanders TAB and Reddy S (1992) The influence of rice bran on plasma lipids and lipoproteins in human volunteers. *European Journal of Clinical Nutrition.* **46**:167–72.

Sanders TAB and Sandaradura S (1992) The cholesterol-raising effect of coffee in the Syrian hamster. *British Journal of Nutrition.* **68**:431–4.

Solvoll K *et al.* (1989) Coffee, dietary habits, and serum cholesterol among men and women 35–49 years of age. *American Journal of Epidemiology.* **129**:1277–88.

Superko HR *et al.* (1991) Caffeinated and decaffeinated coffee effects on plasma lipoprotein cholesterol, apolipoproteins, and lipase activity: a controlled, randomized trial. *American Journal of Clinical Nutrition.* **54**:599–605.

Swain JF *et al.* (1990) Comparison of the effects of oat bran and low-fiber wheat on serum lipoprotein levels and blood pressure. *New England Journal of Medicine.* **322**:147–52.

Thelle DS *et al.* (1983) The Tromsø Heart Study. Does coffee raise serum cholesterol? *New England Journal of Medicine.* **308**:1250.

Thelle DS *et al.* (1987) Coffee and cholesterol in epidemiological and experimental studies. *Atherosclerosis.* **67**:97–103.

Thelle DS (1991) Coffee and cholesterol: what is brewing? (Editorial.) *Journal of Internal Medicine.* **230**:289–91.

Topping DL *et al.* (1990) Modulation of the hypolipidemic effect of fish oils by dietary fiber in rats: studies with rice and wheat bran. *Journal of Nutrition.* **120**: 325–30.

Trowell H (1975) Ischaemic heart disease, atheroma and fibrinolysis. In: Burkitt DP and Trowell HC (eds) *Refined carbohydrate foods and disease.* Academic Press, London. pp. 195–226.

Tuomilehto J *et al.* (1988) Long term treatment of severe hypercholesterolaemia with guar gum. *Atherosclerosis.* **72**:157–62.

Tuomilehto J *et al.* (1989) Guar gum and gemfibrozil—an effective combination in the treatment of hypercholesterolaemia. *Atherosclerosis.* **76**:71–7.

Turner PR *et al.* (1990) Metabolic studies on the hypolipidaemic effect of guar gum. *Atherosclerosis.* **81**:145–50.

Tverdal A *et al.* (1990) Coffee consumption and death from coronary heart disease in middle aged Norwegian men and women. *British Medical Journal.* **300**:566–9.

van Dusseldorp M *et al.* (1991) Cholesterol-raising factor from boiled coffee does not pass a paper filter. *Arteriosclerosis and Thrombosis.* **11**:586–93.

Williams PT *et al*. (1985) Coffee intake and elevated cholesterol and apoprotein B levels in men. *Journal of the American Medical Association*. **253**:1407–11.

Zock PL *et al*. (1990) Effect of a lipid-rich fraction from boiled coffee on serum cholesterol. *The Lancet*. **8700**:1235–7.

23

Microalbuminuria

PETER H WINOCOUR

Procedures for the measurement of urinary albumin in small concentrations were first developed in the early 1960s (Berggard and Risinger, 1961; Keen and Chlouverakis, 1963). The term 'microalbuminuria', coined in the 1980s to describe this, is defined as persistent elevation of urinary albumin excretion which is above reference values but undetectable using conventional semiquantitative test strips.

It reflects glomerular, or less commonly tubulointerstitial dysfunction, and it is usually deemed present only after renal tract structural pathology or infection has been excluded. Semiquantitative test strips have also recently been validated for detection of microalbuminuria. At present they remain expensive (Marshall *et al.*, 1991, 1992), and their role is still uncertain.

Classification of microalbuminuria has been hampered by (1) a lack of consensus on the most appropriate type of urine collection and quantitative expression of albuminuria (Marshall, 1991), (2) considerable intra-individual postural and diurnal variation (Marshall, 1991), and (3) a suggestion of ethnic differences in its prevalence (Allawi *et al.*, 1988; Haffner *et al.*, 1990; Winocour *et al.*, 1992). An early morning urine sample with an albumin:creatinine ratio >3.0 has been said to be the most suitable preliminary screening method, predicting an overnight excretion rate >30 μg/min with 97% sensitivity and >90% specificity (Marshall *et al.*, 1991). This negates the need for precise timing of urine collections, which are only then necessary to confirm those with positive screening values. According to a recent international consensus meeting (Mogensen *et al.*, 1985), microalbuminuria is best categorized as albumin excretion rates of 20–200 μg/min in at least two out of three timed overnight collections within a period of six months.

Microalbuminuria of this degree is an independent predictor of impending nephropathy and of predominantly cardiovascular morbidity and mortality in both insulin-dependent diabetes mellitus (IDDM) and non-insulin-dependent diabetes mellitus (NIDDM) (Messent *et al.*, 1992; Viberti *et al.*, 1982; Jarrett *et al.*, 1984; Mogensen, 1984). It also predicts mortality from cardiovascular disease (CVD) and cancer in the elderly (Damsgaard *et al.*, 1990), and perhaps also coronary and peripheral vascular disease in the general population (Yudkin *et al.*, 1988).

The mechanism whereby microalbuminuria identifies people at risk of CVD is not fully understood, but two broad mechanisms have been proposed, predominantly in the area of diabetes: first that microalbuminuria is associated with an excess of known and potential cardiovascular risk factors, and secondly that it is a marker of established CVD. These mechanisms are not mutually exclusive.

The prevalence of microalbuminuria in the general population has been reported to be 2.2% in white Caucasian adults aged 20–65 (Winocour *et al.*, 1992), but 13–20% in those aged 60–74 (Damsgaard and Mogensen, 1986) or in Mexican Americans aged 25–64 (Haffner *et al.*, 1990). In NIDDM and IDDM the true prevalence is respectively 7–10% (Gatling *et al.*, 1988; Marshall and Alberti, 1989) and 3.7–6.7% (Marshall and Alberti, 1989; Microalbuminuria Collaborative Study Group, 1992). Blood glucose control may be an important determinant of microalbuminuria (Wiseman *et al.*, 1984), and this—together with variable classification criteria and patient selection—may account for a reported prevalence of microalbuminuria in IDDM as high as 22% (Parving *et al.*, 1988).

Microalbuminuria is closely associated with hypertension, not only in diabetes (Jones *et al.*, 1989; Allawi *et al.*, 1990; Marshall and Alberti, 1989), but also in benign essential hypertension (Parving *et al.*, 1974), the general and elderly populations (Gosling and Beevers, 1989; Damsgaard *et al.*, 1990; Haffner *et al.*, 1990; Winocour *et al.*, 1992), and those with established CVD (Yudkin *et al.*, 1988). In diabetes and the elderly it has been shown to exert a synergistic effect with blood pressure in predicting CVD morbidity and mortality (Jarrett *et al.*, 1984; Mogensen, 1984; Damsgaard *et al.*, 1990).

Microalbuminuria may also be a marker of dyslipoproteinaemia in diabetes. The most consistent abnormality is a reduction in concentrations of high-density lipoprotein (HDL) (predominantly HDL_2) cholesterol and apoA1 (Vannini *et al.*, 1984; Jones *et al.*, 1989; Watts *et al.*, 1989; Niskanen *et al.*, 1990; Winocour *et al.*, 1991*a,b*), although increases in total serum and very low-density lipoprotein (VLDL) triglycerides and low-density lipoprotein (LDL) cholesterol have been noted (Vannini *et al.*, 1984; Watts *et al.*, 1989; Seghieri *et al.*, 1990). Alterations in the composition of triglyceride-rich lipoproteins (Winocour *et al.*, 1991*a*) and increased Lp(a) concentrations (Kapelrud *et al.*, 1991; Winocour *et al.*, 1991*b*) have also been recorded. In non-diabetic subjects, increases in serum triglycerides and reductions in HDL cholesterol may accompany microalbuminuria (Haffner et al., 1990; Winocour *et al.*, 1992). It has been suggested in both diabetes and in non-diabetic individuals that microalbuminuria and the combination of high serum triglycerides and low HDL cholesterol may be characterized by insulin resistance (Reaven, 1988; Haffner *et al.*, 1990; Winocour *et al.*, 1992), which itself may play a role in CVD (Reaven, 1988).

More recently, insulin insensitivity has been recorded in IDDM complicated by hypertension and microalbuminuria, in association with increased red cell sodium lithium counter-transport activity (Lopes de Faria *et al.*, 1992; Trevisan *et al.*, 1992). This constellation of factors may particularly mark out those at greatest risk of CVD.

Reports of significant increases in platelet aggregability and turnover and increases in other haemostatic measures in association with microalbuminuria have been confined to IDDM (Jensen *et al.*, 1988; O'Donnell *et al.*, 1991), while no clear differences have been reported in NIDDM or the general population (Schmitz and Ingerslev, 1990; Winocour *et al.*, 1992). Similarly, the suggestion that microalbuminuria is a marker of widespread endothelial dysfunction is based mainly on reports of increased circulating endothelial constituents in IDDM, such as thrombomodulin and von Willebrand factor (Deckert *et al.*, 1989; Iwashima *et al.*, 1990) although an increased transcapillary escape of protein has been noted in both IDDM and essential hypertension (Deckert *et al.*, 1989 Parving *et al.*, 1977). The hypothesis that microalbuminuria and generalized endothelial damage is due to genetic polymorphism in enzymes involved in the metabolism of glycosaminoglycan components of the extracellular matrix (Deckert *et al.*, 1989) has yet to be substantiated, and may only be applicable to diabetes.

Autonomic neuropathy, which is also associated with microalbuminuria (Winocour *et al.*, 1986), is a particularly poor prognostic marker for CVD death (often sudden) in diabetes (Ewing *et al.*, 1980). Its prevalence in non-diabetic subjects is not known.

An increased frequency of both symptomatic and asymptomatic electrocardiographic evidence of coronary heart disease (CHD) has been associated with diabetic and non-diabetic microalbuminuria (Yudkin *et al.*, 1988; Haffner *et al.*, 1990; Gall *et al.*, 1991; Winocour *et al.*, 1992), although the link is by no means inevitable. The prevalence of abnormal electrocardiograms in microalbuminuric subjects may be no more than 30% (Yudkin *et al.*, 1988; Gall *et al.*, 1991; Winocour *et al.*, 1992), whilst microalbuminuria has been recorded in 20% of those with documented CHD (Yudkin *et al.*, 1988).

In IDDM there are reports that microalbuminuria may be associated with functional cardiac abnormalities prior to the development of clinical features of CHD. Intraventricular septal hypertrophy and reduced left ventricular filling in diastole have been documented in the absence of significant hypertension (Sampson *et al.*, 1990*a,b*), and it has been hypothesized these are the consequence of marginal increases in blood pressure and a specific diabetic microvascular cardiomyopathy.

Many of the previously noted associations with microalbuminuria are even more evident in diabetic and non-diabetic subjects with overt proteinuria (Vannini *et al.*, 1984; Winocour *et al.*, 1987, 1991*a, b*; Jensen *et al.*, 1988), which is a clear predictor of a greatly enhanced risk of CHD mortality in diabetic, hypertensive and general populations (Bulpitt *et al.*, 1979; Kannel *et al.*, 1984; Borch-Johnsen *et al.*, 1985; Nelson *et al.*, 1988). It should be stressed that even in IDDM, overt proteinuria may be recorded in less than 50% of those with established CHD (Orchard *et al.*, 1990).

Microalbuminuria may also be a non-specific marker of acute illness (Gosling and Shearman, 1988) (including myocardial infarction), where it may be operating as an acute-phase reactant, and of malignancy, where it probably reflects a microvacular response to tumour-related antigens (Sawyer *et al.*, 1988). The presence of microalbuminuria in these situations may also be of prognostic value.

In conclusion, microalbuminuria is uncommon in the absence of established CVD or other cardiovascular risk factors. Screening for microalbuminuria appears justified at present in diabetic and hypertensive populations, and possibly in the elderly, since it appears to identify those at greatest risk of early mortality. There is some evidence, at least in diabetes, that both microalbuminuria and the subsequent excess risk of nephropathy and CVD could be amenable to correction (Feldt-Rasmussen *et al.*, 1986; Mathiesen *et al.*, 1991).

It remains to be seen whether similar dividends will be evident in elderly or essential hypertensive patients with microalbuminuria, but in such cases consideration might at least be given to more active management of hypertension, and possibly also of malignancy.

References

Allawi J *et al.* (1988) Microalbuminuria in non-insulin-dependent diabetes: its prevalence in Indian compared with Europid subjects. *British Medical Journal.* **296**:462–4.

Allawi J and Jarrett RJ (1990) Microalbuminuria and cardiovascular risk factors in type 2 diabetes mellitus. *Diabetic Medicine.* **7**:115–18.

Berggard I and Risinger C (1961) Quantitative immunochemical determination of albumin in normal human urine. *Acta Societodis Medicorum Upsaliensis.* **66**:217–29.

Borch-Johnsen K *et al.* (1985) The effect of proteinuria on relative mortality in type 1 (insulin dependent) diabetes mellitus. *Diabetologia.* **28**:590–6.

Bulpitt CJ *et al.* (1979) Risk factors for death in treated hypertensive patients. Report from the DHSS hypertension care computing project. *The Lancet.* **ii**:134–7.

Damsgaard EM and Mogensen CE (1986) Microalbuminuria in elderly hyperglycaemic patients and controls. *Diabetic Medicine.* **3**:430–5.

Damsgaard EM *et al.* (1990) Microalbuminuria as predictor of increased mortality in elderly people. *British Medical Journal.* **300**:297–300.

Deckert T *et al.* (1989) Albuminuria reflects widespread vascular damage. The Steno hypothesis. *Diabetologia.* **32**:219–26.

Ewing DJ *et al.* (1980) The natural history of diabetic autonomic neuropathy. *Quarterly Journal of Medicine.* **49**:95–108.

Feldt-Rasmussen B *et al.* (1986) Effect of two years of strict metabolic control on progression in incipient nephropathy in insulin dependent diabetes. *The Lancet.* ii:1300–4.

Gall MA *et al.* (1991) Prevalence of micro- and macroalbuminuria, arterial hypertension, retinopathy, and large vessel disease in European Type 2 (non-insulin-dependent) diabetic patients. *Diabetologia.* 34:655–61.

Gatling W *et al.* (1988) Microalbuminuria in diabetes: a population study of the prevalence and an assessment of three screening tests. *Diabetic Medicine.* 5:343–7.

Gosling P and Shearman CP (1988) Increased levels of urinary proteins: markers of vascular permeability? *Annals of Clinical Biochemistry.* 25 (Suppl):150–1s.

Gosling P and Beevers DG (1989) Urinary albumin excretion and blood pressure in the general population. *Clinical Science.* 76:39–42.

Haffner SM *et al.* (1990) Microalbuminuria. Potential marker for increased cardiovascular risk factors in nondiabetic subjects? *Arteriosclerosis.* 10:727–31.

Iwashima Y *et al.* (1990) Elevation of plasma thrombomodulin level in diabetic patients with early diabetic nephropathy. *Diabetes.* 39:983–8.

Jarrett RJ *et al.* (1984) Microalbuminuria predicts mortality in non-insulin-dependent diabetes. *Diabetic Medicine.* 1:17–20.

Jensen T *et al.* (1988) Abnormalities in plasma concentrations of lipoproteins and fibrinogen in type 1 (insulin-dependent) diabetic patients with increased urinary albumin excretion. *Diabetologia* 31:142–5.

Jones SL *et al.* (1989) Plasma lipid and coagulation factor concentrations in insulin dependent diabetics with microalbuminuria. *British Medical Journal.* 298:487–90.

Kannel WB *et al.* (1984) The prognostic significance of proteinuria. The Framingham study. *American Heart Journal.* 108:1347–52.

Kapelrud H *et al.* (1991) Serum Lp(a) lipoprotein concentrations in insulin dependent diabetic patients with microalbuminuria. *British Medical Journal.* 303:675–8.

Keen H and Chlouverakis C (1963) An immunoassay method for urinary albumin at low concentrations. *The Lancet.* ii:913–14.

Lopes de Faria J *et al.* (1992) Sodium-lithium countertransport activity and insulin resistance in normotensive IDDM patients. *Diabetes.* 41:610–15.

Marshall SM and Alberti KGMM (1989) Comparison of the prevalence and associated features of abnormal albumin excretion in insulin-dependent and non-insulin-dependent diabetes. *Quarterly Journal of Medicine.* 70:61–71.

Marshall SM (1991) Screening for microalbuminuria: which measurement? *Diabetic Medicine*. 8:706–11.

Marshall SM *et al.* (1992) Evaluation of Micral-test strips for screening for microalbuminuria. *Clinical Chemistry*. 38:588–91.

Mathiesen ER *et al.* (1991) Efficacy of captopril in postponing nephropathy in normotensive insulin dependent diabetic patients with microalbuminuria. *British Medical Journal*. 303:81–7.

Messent JWC *et al.* (1992) Prognostic significance of microalbuminuria in insulin-dependent diabetes mellitus: a twenty-three year follow-up study. *Kidney International*. 41:836–9.

Microalbuminuria Collaborative Study Group (1992) Microalbuminuria in type 1 diabetic patients. Prevalence and clinical characteristics. *Diabetes Care*. 15:495–501.

Mogensen CE (1984) Microalbuminuria predicts clinical proteinuria and early mortality in maturity-onset diabetes. *New England Journal of Medicine*. 310:356–60.

Mogensen CE *et al.* (1985) *Uremia Investigations*. 9:85–95.

Nelson RG *et al.* (1988) The effect of proteinuria on mortality in NIDDM. *Diabetes*. 37:1499–504.

Niskanen L *et al.* (1990) Microalbuminuria predicts the development of serum lipoprotein abnormalities favouring atherogenesis in newly diagnosed type 2 (non-insulin-dependent) diabetic patients. *Diabetologia*. 33:237–43.

O'Donnell MJ *et al.* (1991) Platelet behaviour and haemostatic behaviour in type 1 (insulin-dependent) diabetic patients with and without albuminuria. *Diabetic Medicine*. 8:624–8.

Orchard TJ *et al.* (1990) Prevalence of complications in IDDM by sex and duration. Pittsburgh epidemiology of diabetes complications study II. *Diabetes*. 39:1116–24.

Parving HH *et al.* (1974) Increased urinary albumin excretion rate in benign essential hypertension. *The Lancet*. i:1190–2.

Parving HH *et al.* (1977) Increased transcapillary escape rate of albumin and IgG in essential hypertension. *Scandinavian Journal of Clinical and Laboratory Investigations*. 37:223–7.

Parving HH *et al.* (1988) Prevalance of microalbuminuria, arterial hypertension, retinopathy and neuropathy in patients with IDD. *British Medical Journal*. 296: 156–60.

Reaven GM (1988) The role of insulin resistance in human disease. *Diabetes.* **37**:1595–607.

Sampson MJ *et al.* (1990*a*) Intraventricular septal hypertrophy in type 1 diabetic patients with microalbuminuria or early proteinuria. *Diabetic Medicine.* **7**:126–31.

Sampson MJ *et al.* (1990*b*) Abnormal diastolic function in patients with type 1 diabetes and early nephropathy. *British Heart Journal.* **64**:266–71.

Sawyer N *et al.* (1988) Prevalence, concentration, and prognostic importance of proteinuria in patients with malignancies. *British Medical Journal.* **296**:1295–8.

Schmitz A and Ingerslev J (1990) Haemostatic measures in type 2 diabetic patients with microalbuminuria. *Diabetic Medicine.* **7**:521–5.

Seghieri G *et al.* (1990) Serum lipids and lipoproteins in type 2 diabetic patients with persistent microalbuminuria. *Diabetic Medicine.* **7**:810–14.

Trevisan R *et al.* (1992) Clustering of risk factors in hypertensive insulin-dependent diabetics with high sodium-lithium countertransport. *Kidney International.* **41**: 855–61.

Vannini P *et al.* (1984) Lipid abnormalities in insulin-dependent diabetic patients with albuminuria. *Diabetes Care.* **7**:151–4.

Viberti GC *et al.* (1982) Microalbuminuria as a predictor of clinical nephropathy in insulin-dependent diabetes mellitus. *The Lancet.* **i**:1430–2.

Watts GF *et al.* (1989) Serum lipids and lipoproteins in insulin-dependent diabetic patients with persistent microalbuminuria. *Diabetic Medicine.* **6**:25–30.

Winocour PH *et al.* (1986) The relationship between autonomic neuropathy and urinary sodium and albumin excretion in insulin-treated diabetics. *Diabetic Medicine.* **3**:436–40.

Winocour PH *et al.* (1987) Influence of proteinuria on vascular disease, blood pressure and lipoproteins in insulin dependent diabetes mellitus. *British Medical Journal.* **294**:1648–51.

Winocour PH *et al.* (1991*a*) The influence of early diabetic nephropathy on very low density lipoprotein (VLDL), intermediate density lipoprotein (IDL), and low density lipoprotein (LDL) composition. *Atherosclerosis.* **89**:49–57.

Winocour PH *et al.* (1991*b*) Lipoprotein (a) and microvascular disease in type 1 (insulin dependent) diabetes mellitus. *Diabetic Medicine.* **8**:922–7.

Winocour PH *et al.* (1992) Microalbuminuria and associated risk factors in the community. *Atherosclerosis.* **93**:71–81.

Wiseman M *et al.* (1984) Glycaemia, arterial pressure and microalbuminuria in type 1 (insulin-dependent) diabetes mellitus. *Diabetologia.* **26**:401–5.

Yudkin JS *et al.* (1988) Microalbuminuria as a predictor of vascular disease in non-diabetic subjects. Islington Diabetes Survey. *The Lancet.* **ii**:530–3.

24

Psychosocial Factors in Perspective

M KORNITZER, I BERIOT, F KITTEL AND M DRAMAIX

Whereas the concepts of atherosclerosis and thrombosis were laid down by two 19th century pathologists, Virchow and Rokitanski, myocardial infarction was not described clinically until the beginning of the 20th century by Straschesko in 1910 and Herrick in 1912 (Leibowitz, 1970). Epidemiological evidence for the aetiological determinants of coronary heart disease (CHD) was delayed for another 40 years until the first results of the Framingham Study were published. This prospective study was followed by numerous European and American studies concerning coronary as well as other cardiovascular diseases (CVD) due to atherosclerosis. A multifactorial concept emerged from these prospective studies, whereby 'risk' factors having both environmental and genetic determinants were related to atherogenesis and thrombogenesis which, with imbalance of the autonomic nervous system (increasing the risk of arrhythmia), would lead to clinical CHD.

Both short-term and long-term studies have shown that a predictive model where age, total serum cholesterol, systolic blood pressure, smoking behaviour, obesity and physical activity are introduced in a multiple logistic equation can detect population groups with large differences in risk of CHD. Ten studies with 23–30 years' follow-up have shown consistency in the long-term independent prediction of CHD for high serum cholesterol, high blood pressure and cigarette smoking (Kornitzer and Goldberg, 1993). Nevertheless, not all of the differences in the risk of CHD are explained by these major coronary risk factors (even in the Framingham model, where high-density lipoprotein (HDL) cholesterol, diabetes and left ventricular hypertrophy are added to the model).

Marmot et al. (1984) showed that, in the Whitehall Civil Servant Study, the major coronary risk factors could only partly explain the large differences in coronary mortality or all-cause mortality between employment grades. Cassel (1976) raised the possibility of social factors contributing to host resistance or host susceptibility to disease, and claimed that social environment could have a non-specific negative influence on both disease occurrence and disease evolution, leading to premature mortality.

If these psychosocial factors play a role in the occurrence of CHD in a normal population, they could be influenced by primary prevention, or influence the natural history and lethality of CHD; and at this point, secondary prevention could play a beneficial role.

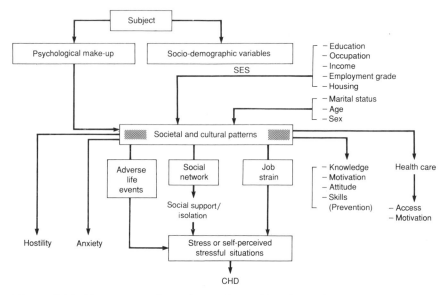

Figure 24.1: Emergence of psychosocial variables from the interaction of the individual with societal patterns. Most of these variables by way of stress (self-perceived or not) increase the risk of CHD.

Figure 24.1 proposes a broad concept in which each subject is defined according to psychological make-up and sociodemographic variables such as socio-economic and marital status, age and sex. We are all shaped by the particular cultural patterns and norms of our own society. The resulting psychosocial factors could help to explain the differences in risk or evolution of CHD.

Socio-economic status and CHD

We would like to propose the level of education as a good marker for socio-economic status. When looking at the relationship between level of education and CHD mortality in the USA, Feldman *et al.* (1989) observed that there were almost no differences in CHD mortality in 1960 according to level of education, but that 10 to 15 years later differences emerged as the decline of CHD mortality was steeper in the most compared to the least educated people, both for males and females. Taking into account the evolution of CHD mortality trends in Great Britain (Marmot *et al.*, 1978) as well as in America, it seems that about 60 years ago, there was a direct correlation between the level of education and risk of CHD, that this disappeared somewhere between 1950 and 1960 and thereafter an inverse association appeared (Marmot *et al.*, 1991; Woodward *et al.*, 1992). Indeed a steep inverse relationship between employment grade and both CHD and total mortality was observed at the 10-year follow-up of the Whitehall I study (Marmot *et al.* 1984), whereby men in the lowest grade had three times the mortality rate of CHD compared to those with the highest grade. Differences in major CHD factors could only explain part of these differences. A Finnish study (Salonen, 1982) and the Chicago Heart Association Detection Project in Industry (Liu *et al.*, 1982) also demonstrated an inverse relationship between level of education and age-adjusted mortality for CVD and all causes. Similarly amongst Oslo males aged 40–49; the lowest social class exhibited a much higher rate of lung cancer, accidents, homicides and CHD than the other classes (Holme *et al.*, 1980).

In summary, it seems clear that both in Europe and in the United States there was an inverse relationship between socio-economic markers and risk of CHD mortality during the 1970s and 1980s.

Socio-economic status (SES) and coronary risk factors

The major coronary risk factors do not seem to explain the whole of the gradient between SES and CHD mortality. It is nevertheless important to look at these risk factors in relation to level of education. In the Belgian Interuniversity Research on Nutrition and Health (BIRNH), 5567 males aged 25–74 were screened between 1980 and 1985 (Kornitzer and Bara, 1989). No significant differences were observed between level of education and total serum cholesterol, HDL cholesterol and non-HDL cholesterol. There was a significant positive association for systolic blood pressure with level of education. Body mass index (weight/height^2) was inversely related to level of education. Height, a marker of early environmental influences, was directly and significantly related to level of education (Table 24.1).

Cigarette smoking shows a significant trend, with the highest prevalence in those with least education. Stopping smoking is least common in this group.

Nutrition seems to play a key role in the processes of atherogenesis and thrombogenesis. Table 24.2 shows the relation in the BIRNH Study between some nutrients derived from 24-hour record and level of education. We observed a slightly higher saturated fat and cholesterol intake in the lower educated, who also tended to have a lower fibre intake ($P < 0.097$).

The Belgian Physical Fitness Study was initiated at the end of the 1970s in 2329 middle-aged males (Sobolski *et al.*, 1981). There was an increased odds ratio for low level of total leisure time physical activity and for absence of any heavy leisure time activity during the previous 12 months amongst the less educated (Table 24.3).

In the Tromso Heart Study of 12 368 males and females (Jacobsen and Thelle, 1988), the same patterns emerged with the highest educated tending to be less overweight, to smoke less, to be more active in leisure time and have food habits thought to be less atherogenic (eg lower coffee consumption, greater intakes of soft margarines, low-fat milk, fruits and vegetables). In the

	Primary	Secondary	Tertiary	P
Serum cholesterol, mg/dl (mmol/l)	233 (6.0)	233 (6.0)	234 (6.03)	NS
HDL cholesterol, mg/dl (mmol/l)	48.4 (1.25)	49.2 (1.29)	48.7 (1.25)	NS
Non-HDL cholesterol, mg/dl (mmol/l)	185 (4.77)	184 (4.74)	185 (4.77)	NS
Systolic blood pressure mmHg	135.0	137.1	137.0	<0.003
BMI W/H^2	26.5	25.2	24.4	<0.001
Height, cm	171.0	172.6	173.9	<0.001
Cigarette smokers	48%	39%	32%	<0.001
Ex-smokers	26%	31%	30%	<0.001

Table 24.1: Level of education and risk factors (age adjusted) in the BIRNH Study of males aged 25–74 years.

	Primary	Secondary	Tertiary	P
Saturated fats, % cal	17.5	17.5	16.9	0.028
Polyunsaturated fats, % cal	7.5	7.7	7.8	NS
Poly unsaturated/saturated ratio	0.50	0.52	0.53	NS
Cholesterol intake, mg	448	423	411	0.002
Fibre intake, g/1000 cal	8.2	8.4	8.7	0.097

Table 24.2: Level of education and nutritional patterns (age-adjusted) of males aged 25–74 years in the BIRNH Study.

	Low level of total leisure-time physical activity			No heavy activity during leisure time		
	OR (age-adjusted)	Confidence interval (95%)	P	OR (age-adjusted)	Confidence interval (95%)	P
Tertiary	1			1		
Secondary	1.29	(0.93;1.77)	0.123	1.64	(1.21;2.21)	<0.001
Primary	1.40	(0.99;1.97)	0.059	2.69	(1.95;3.72)	<0.001

Table 24.3: Level of education and leisure-time physical activity among males aged 40–55 years in the Physical Fitness Study.

same study, mean serum total cholesterol and systolic blood pressure were negatively associated with education level, whereas in women education and high-density lipoprotein were positively associated. In the Dutch Nutrition Surveillance System (Hulshof *et al.*, 1991), an SES index combining education level, occupation and occupational position showed that those with the highest status consumed more alcohol-based drinks, drank less coffee, were less obese and smoked less. The P/S ratio was higher in the low SES group compared to the high group, but no differences in cholesterol intake or dietary fibre were observed in that study. Butter accounted for about 25% of total fat intake in the higher SES class and for only 10% in the lowest class. In the Chicago Heart Association Detection Project in Industry, an inverse association was observed at baseline between education and blood pressure, independently of age and relative weight. For three Chicago cohorts, a significant graded and inverse association was also recorded between education and cigarette use at entry (Liu *et al.*, 1982). In 18 000 males from Oslo aged 20–49, screened for CHD and other atherosclerotic disease, a social index combining income and education was computed. Again the authors observed a substantial decrease in the frequency of cigarette smoking with increasing social status and a sharp increase in the percentage of ex-smokers. Serum cholesterol and triglycerides

	Primary	Secondary	Tertiary	P
Theoretical knowledge of CHD prevention	17.5	18.6	19.3	<0.0001
Practical knowledge of CHD prevention	15.2	16.6	17.5	<0.0001
Attitude towards prevention of CHD	24.7	25.4	26.0	<0.001

Table 24.4: Level of education (age-adjusted) of males aged 25–74 years in the BIRNH Study.

concentrations decreased with increasing SES, just as an index of obesity increased with higher status; the degree of physical activity during leisure time was higher among high-status men than among those with low status, and blood pressure showed a slight downward trend in relation to higher SES (Holme *et al.*, 1976). Low education was positively correlated with a lack of a social network in a Finnish study (Salonen, 1988). Finally, independent of smoking habit, fibrinogen levels were higher in lower SES subjects (Markowe *et al.*, 1985).

In summary, the major coronary risk factors as well as atherogenic nutritional patterns are more prevalent in the less-educated and would account for part of the differences in CHD between poorly and well educated middle-aged males.

The lower CHD rates in the well educated may be mediated partly by greater knowledge of and a more favourable attitude towards primary and secondary prevention of CHD. This was supported by the results of a questionnaire on theoretical knowledge, practical knowledge on CHD risk factors and attitude towards CHD prevention completed in the BIRNH Study (Table 24.4).

The general practitioner may be able to narrow the gap between social classes by increasing knowledge, motivation and skills in the prevention of CHD in the less educated: modifying nutritional patterns, decreasing prevalence of overweight and smoking, and increasing physical activity in the less educated could achieve that goal.

Social network and disease

Following Cassel (1976), the concept of the contribution of social environment to disease occurrence and mortality was tested empirically by Berkman and Syme (1979). This concept concerns the relation between a quantitative social network index and disease and proposes that a low social network could be a non-specific harbinger for different diseases including CHD. Table 24.5 summarizes eight studies published between 1979 and 1988 which address this question. They substantiate the concept of a low social network as a risk factor

Authors	Study	Follow-up	End points	Association
Berkman and Syme (1979)	Alameda County (M+F)	9 years	All causes	M:S RR:2.3
				F:S RR:2.8
House et al. (1982)	Tecumseh (M+F)	12 years	All causes	(SRR)M:S F:NS
Reed et al. (1983)	Hawaii (Japanese) (M)	7 years	Prevalence CHD	S
			Incidence CHD	S FOR NF MI
Reed et al. (1984)	Hawaii (Japanese) (M)	7 years	All cause mortality	NS
			Cancer incidence	NS
			Stroke incidence	NS
Welin et al. (1985)	Gothenburg (M)	9 years	All causes	S
Schoenbach et al. (1986)	Evans County (M+F)	13 years	All causes	S (SHR:1.5)
Orth-Gomer and Johnson (1987)	Sweden (M+F)	6 years	All causes	S (RR:1.46)
			Cardiovascular	M:S (RR:1.37)
Kaplan et al. (1988)	Finland (M+F)	5 years	All causes	M:S RR:1.54
			Cardiovascular	M:S RR:1.54
			CHD mortality	M:S RR:1.34

Table 24.5: Social network and disease. (S significant; NS non-significant.)

for incidence and/or mortality of different diseases including CHD, but we need more longitudinal data on morbidity and mortality in males and females, blacks and whites. Regarding the risk of low social support in subjects with CHD, Case *et al.* (1992) have shown that in males who have had a myocardial infarction, living alone was an independent risk factor with a hazard ratio of 1.54 for recurrent cardiac events. In a Swedish Study of 150 middle-aged men, including healthy men and subjects with clinical manifest CHD or coronary risk factors, followed for 10 years, non-survivors were discriminated from survivors by several factors including relative social isolation, indicated by a low social activity level which emerged as one of the three predictive factors in a multivariate analysis (Orth-Gomer *et al.*, 1988). Orth-Gomer and Undén (1990) also observed that in socially isolated type A cardiac patients (*see* below), the 10-year mortality experience was 69% versus only 17% in socially integrated type A men. Looking at 159 males and females after coronary angiography, Seeman and Syme (1987) observed that a network providing instrumental support and feelings of being loved were more important in predicting coronary atherosclerosis than the size of the network, this being independent of other coronary risk factors, with a relative risk of critical atherosclerosis for low versus high social support of 1.74. Blumenthal *et al.* (1987) observed a higher degree of atherosclerosis in type A subjects with little social support compared to type A subjects with much social support. Williams *et al.* (1992) showed, amongst subjects who had undergone coronary angiography and in those with CHD, that married patients had a better survival than unmarried patients. However there was a significant interaction between marital status and confidant availability, which may be considered as markers of social network or social isolation. In fact, unmarried patients without a confidant had a more than threefold increase in risk of death within five years compared with patients who were either married or had a close confidant.

In the search for pathogenetic pathways, Rosengren *et al.* (1990) observed a higher plasma fibrinogen in those with a low social network and a higher 24-hour average blood pressure was observed in those with low social network by Undén *et al.* (1991).

Behavioural variables: type A behaviour and hostility

In the 1970s, a type of behaviour characterized by high activity, speed and impatience, job-involvement, self-imposed deadlines, facial tics and overt hostility was labelled type A behaviour. The first publications showed that subjects with type A behaviour pattern had at least a twofold increase of a risk of CHD than type B subjects (Rosenman *et al.*, 1975). A review of subsequent papers (Kornitzer, 1992) revealed that out of 12 incidence studies (11 in males), seven did not find a significant relationship between type A behaviour and CHD. Part of the inconsistency in the results may be explained by the difference in instruments used to assess type A behaviour. On the other hand,

Authors	Study	Follow-up	Technique	End point	Association
Theorell et al. (1975)	Sweden (M)	2 years	Swedish	MI incidence	Yes
Haynes et al. (1980)	Framingham (F)	8 years	Framingham	CHD incidence	Yes
Shekelle et al. (1983)	Chicago (M)	10 years	MMPI	CHD incidence	No
		20 years	MMPI	All cause mortality	Yes
Barefoot et al. (1983)	USA (M)	25 years	MMPI	CHD incidence	Yes
				All cause mortality	Yes
Mc Cranie et al. (1986)	US physicians (M)	25 years	MMPI	CHD incidence	No
				All cause mortality	No
Koskenvuo et al. (1988)	Finland (M)	3 years	Finnish	CHD incidence	No
Leon et al. (1988)	USA (M)	30 years	MMPI	CHD incidence	No
Hearn et al. (1989)	USA (M)	33 years	MMPI	CHD incidence	No
				CHD mortality	No
				All causes	No
Barefoot et al. (1989)	USA (M)	25 years	MMPI	All causes	Yes
Almada et al. (1991)	USA (M)	25 years	MMPI (cynicism)	All causes	Yes
Carmelli et al. (1991)	WCGS (M)	27 years	Type A Hostility Score	CHD mortality	Yes
				CHD mortality	Yes

Table 24.6: Hostility and CHD.

the majority of the studies looking for a biological plausibility did not observe a higher degree of coronary atherosclerosis in type A subjects compared to type B subjects, nor was there a relation of type A behaviour with catecholamine urinary excretion.

Whilst the concept of type A behaviour was fading away, another related concept has emerged during the last 10 years: that of a pattern of repressed or overt hostility in relation to an increased risk of CHD. Table 24.6, summarizes 11 studies investigating this area, published between 1977 and 1991. Of these studies, five observed a significant relationship between hostility levels with CHD and one with all causes of mortality. Regarding pathological plausibility, two studies observed a higher degree of coronary atherosclerosis in subjects with high levels of hostility (Williams et al., 1980; Dembroski et al., 1985), but Helmer et al. (1991) did not.

We would like to emphasize that in an American study of 5115 young adults (Scherwitz et al., 1991), a hostility scale was negatively related to level of education and social support, and positively related to adverse life events. In this cross-sectional study it is impossible to know the temporal relationships: is it high hostility that leads to low social support or the reverse, and do both increase the risk of adverse life events? In summary, a high degree of hostility assessed by the Cook and Medley scale of the MMPI (Barefoot et al., 1989) may be related to an increased risk of CHD although the reviewed literature is not consistent. Large incidence studies which are under way in both Europe and the USA should help to clarify this situation.

From stress to job strain

The concept of stress as a non-specific response of the human body to any threat was first described by Hans Selye about 60 years ago. He described a normal biological reaction mediated both through the adrenal medulla and cortex. This concept received little attention in epidemiological studies in CHD until the beginning of the 1980s, when the concept of stress reappeared in cardiovascular epidemiology through a model by the American sociologist Robert Karasek (Figure 24.2). Based on stress at the work site, each working subject is categorized by low or high demand and high or low decision latitude or control (which has since been extended to low intellectual discretion or a monotonous job). According to the author of the model, job-strain occurs when high demand is associated with low decision latitude (Karasek et al., 1982).

Table 24.7 summarizes 10 studies, published between 1975 and 1990, which investigated this area. All except Theorell's study were based on the Karasek model and all reported a significant association of job strain with CHD prevalence, incidence or mortality.

The Karasek concept has recently been enlarged by adding a measure of social support at the work site, so that we have a three-dimensional model wherein the high risk of CHD would be expected in those with high job

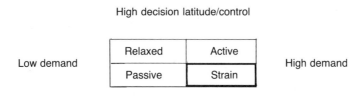

Figure 24.2: Concept of job-strain within the Karasek model.

demands, low work control, and low work support (Johnson and Hall, 1988). Johnson published one prevalence and one prospective study (Johnson and Hall, 1988; Johnson et al., 1989), both showing an association of high demand, low control and low support with increased prevalence of CHD and CVD mortality.

The relation between job strain and the classic coronary risk factors was reported in a meta-analysis of five US databases, (Pieper et al., 1989); low decision latitude was related to cholesterol level and smoking in the predicted directions. Psychological demands, however, were not related to any of the risk factors, although the tendency was in the predicted direction. Concerning the relation of job stress to blood pressure, Matthews et al. (1987) observed a significant independent positive correlation between stressful work conditions as well as overall job dissatisfaction with diastolic blood pressure. Furthermore, in an American case control study, comparing 87 cases of hypertension to a random sample of 128 controls, job strain was significantly related to hypertension with an estimated odds ratio of 3.1 after adjusting for age, race, BMI, type A behaviour, alcohol consumption, smoking, 24-hour urine sodium excretion, education and physical demand of the job. The same authors observed that those with high job strain had a left ventricular mass which was on average significantly higher than those without job strain (Schnall et al., 1990). Similarly, using the Karasek job content survey, Pickering (1990) observed that men in high-strain jobs had a higher prevalence of hypertension and of left ventricular hypertrophy than men in less stressful jobs. However Aro et al. (1984) and Chapman et al. (1990), did not observe any relation between incidence of hypertension and perceived work stress. In search for biological plausibility, Frankenhaeuser and Gardell (1976) compared males working under stress with those in low-demand jobs and found that the sympathetic adrenal medullary activity, as assessed by the urinary excretion of adrenalin and noradrenalin, was significantly higher in the 'high-risk' than in the control group. (High-risk men carried out machine-paced work characterized by short work cycles and a lack of control over the work process.) The authors hypothesized that the common origin of the high urinary catecholamine output and high frequency of psychosomatic symptoms of which they complained was the monotonous coercive machine-paced nature of their work. More recently, Theorell et al. (1990) have

Job strain and CHD

Authors	Type of study	Association with CHD
Theorell *et al.* (1975) Sweden	Prospective	Incidence of MI

Karasek *et al.* (1981) Sweden	Prospective	CHD mortality
		  Hectic work OR : 4
		  Low-control OR : 6.6

Alfredsson *et al.* (1982) Sweden	Prospective (Job strain: indirect)	Incidence of MI
Alfredsson *et al.* (1983) Sweden	Case-control (Job strain: indirect)	MI RR : 2
Alfredsson *et al.* (1985) Sweden	Prospective (Job strain: indirect)	Hospitalization for MI RR : 1.6

Theorell *et al.* (1987) Sweden	Case-control
	(< 45 years)
		MI survival
		  (Hectic work + low level
		  of intellectual discretion)
		  SOR* 1.5–1.6

Karasek *et al.* (1988) USA	Prevalence of MI (Job strain: indirect)	Incidence of MI SOR* 4.9
Haan (1988) Finland	Prospective	No association with CHD
Reed *et al.* (1989) US (Japanese ancestry)	Prospective	CHD incidence
Siegrist *et al.* (1990) Germany (blue collars)	Prospective	Work pressure SOR* 3.4 Need for control SOR* 4.5

*SOR : standardized odds ratio.

Table 24.7: Job strain and CHD.

	Low Social Network Index			Job strain			High Hostility		
	OR*	CI(95%)†	P	OR*	CI(95%)†	P	OR*	CI(95%)†	P
Tertiary	1			1			1		
Secondary	0.96	(0.60;1.5)	NS	2.73	(1.78;4.18)	0.001	2.27	(1.53;3.36)	<0.001
Primary	1.75	(1.11;2.77)	0.03	4.28	(2.75;6.68)	0.001	1.44	(0.98;2.1)	<0.059

Table 24.8: Level of education and psychosocial variables among males aged 25–64 years in the MONICA Ghent-Charleroi Study. (*Age-adjusted odds ratio; †confidence interval.)

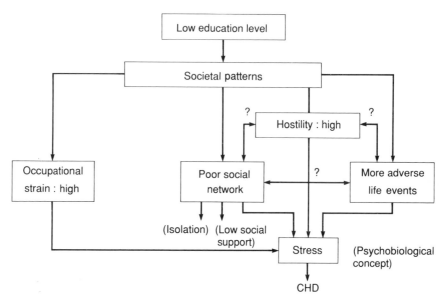

Figure 24.3: Concept of the key-role of low education level in the occurrence of high prevalence rates of psychosocial factors related to CHD.

shown that in working subjects aged 35–60 years, rated by amount of job strain, the serum level of immunoglobulin G was observed to rise progressively with rising job strain. The reported adequacy of social support was negatively associated with that of the serum level of immunoglobulin and, when job strain increased, the serum level of immunoglobulin increased mainly among those with poor levels of social support. Rosengren *et al.* (1991) followed up 6935 men aged 47–55 years questioned at base-line for self-perceived stress. After a mean follow-up of 11.8 years, 6% of the men with the four lowest stress ratings had either developed a non-fatal myocardial infarction or died from CHD, whereas the corresponding figures among the men with the highest two stress ratings was 10%, (the odds ratio was 1.5 after controlling for age and other risk factors). This is comparable with earlier data from Devereux *et al.* (1983), who demonstrated a relationship between left ventricular hypertrophy and higher blood pressure during self-perceived stressful occupations. Finally, Kaplan *et al.* (1983) showed that stress among adult male monkeys fed a low-fat choles-terol diet developed more extensive coronary atherosclerosis than unstressed controls and this group did not differ in serum lipids, blood pressure, serum glucose or ponderosity at the start. This would suggest that even in the absence of elevated serum lipids, psychosocial factors could increase the risk of athero-sclerosis.

In summary, psychosocial or behavioural variables such as low social net-work, job strain and high hostility may be independent risk factors for CHD. They seem to be related to low level of education, as suggested by data from a population survey of males aged 25–64 in the MONICA Ghent-Charleroi project (Table 24.8).

The inter-relationships of the variables discussed above are outlined in Figure 24.2, and in Figure 24.3, the mechanism whereby low education level could play a pivotal role is proposed.

References

Alfredsson L *et al.* (1982) Myocardial infarction risk and psychosocial work environment: an analysis of the male Swedish working force. *Social Science of Medicine.* **16**:463–7.

Alfredsson L *et al.* (1983) Job characteristics of occupations and myocardial infarction risk: effect of possible confounding factors. *Social Science of Medicine.* **17**:1497–503.

Alfredsson L *et al.* (1985) Type of occupation and near-future hospitalization for myocardial infarction and some other diagnoses. *International Journal of Epidemiology.* **14**:378–88.

Almada SJ *et al.* (1991) Neuroticism and cynicism and risk of death in middle-aged men: the Western Electric Study. *Psychosomatic Medicine.* **53**:165–75.

Aro S *et al.* (1984) Occupational stress, health-related behavior, and blood pressure: a 5-year follow-up. *Preventive Medicine.* **13**:333–48.

Barefoot JC *et al.* (1983) Hostility, CHD incidence, and total mortality: a 25-year follow-up study of 255 physicians. *Psychosomatic Medicine.* **45**:59–63.

Barefoot JC *et al.* (1989) The Cook-Medley hostility scale: item content and ability to predict survival. *Psychosomatic Medicine.* **51**:46–57.

Berkman LF and Syme SL (1979) Social networks, host resistance and mortality: a nine-year follow-up study of Alameda county residents. *American Journal of Epidemiology.* **109**:186–204.

Blumenthal JA *et al.* (1987) Social support, type A behavior and coronary artery disease. *Psychosomatic Medicine.* **49**:331–40.

Carmelli D *et al.* (1991) 27-year mortality in the western collaborative group study: construction of risk groups by recursive partitioning. *Journal of Clinical Epidemiology.* **44**:1341–51.

Case RB *et al.* (1992) Living alone after myocardial infarction. Impact on prognosis. *Journal of the American Medical Association.* **267**:515–19.

Cassel J (1976) The contribution of the social environment to host resistance. *American Journal of Epidemiology.* **104**:107–23.

Chapman A *et al.* (1990) Chronic perceived work stress and blood pressure among Australian government employees. *Scandinavian Journal of Work and Environmental Health.* **16**:258–69.

Dembroski TM *et al.* (1985) Components of type A, hostility and anger in relationship to angiographic findings. *Psychosomatic Medicine.* **47**:219–33.

Devereux RB *et al.* (1983) Left ventricular hypertrophy in patients with hypertension: importance of blood pressure response to regularly recurring stress. *Circulation.* **68**:470–6.

Feldman JJ *et al.* (1989) National trends in educational differentials in mortality. *American Journal of Epidemiology.* **129**:919–33.

Frankenhaeuser M and Gardell B (1976) Underload and overload in working life: outline of a multidisciplinary approach. *Journal of Human Stress.* **2**:35–46.

Haan MN (1988) Job strain and ischaemic heart disease: an epidemiologic study of metal workers. *Annals of Clinical Research.* **20**:143–5.

Haynes SG *et al.* (1980) The relationship of psychosocial factors to coronary heart disease in the Framingham study: eight-year incidence of coronary heart disease. *American Journal of Epidemiology.* **111**:37–58.

Hearn MD *et al.* (1989) Hostility, coronary heart disease, and total mortality: a 33-year follow-up study of university students. *Journal of Behavioral Medicine.* **12**:105–21.

Helmer DC *et al.* (1991) Hostility and coronary artery disease. *American Journal of Epidemiology.* **133**:112–22.

Holme I *et al.* (1976) Coronary risk factors and socioeconomic status. The Olso Study. *The Lancet.* **ii**:1396–8.

Holme I *et al.* (1980) Four-year mortality by some socioeconomic indicators: the Olso Study. *Journal of Epidemiology and Community Health.* **34**:48–52.

House JS *et al.* (1982) The association of social relationships and activities with mortality: prospective evidence from the Tecumseh community health study. *American Journal of Epidemiology.* **116**:123–40.

Hulshof KAFM *et al.* (1991) Diet and other life-style factors in high and low socio-economic groups (Dutch Nutrition Surveillance System). *European Journal of Clinical Nutrition.* **45**:441–50.

Jacobsen BK and Thelle DS (1988) Risk factors for coronary heart disease and level of education, the Tromso Heart Study. *American Journal of Epidemiology.* **127**:923–32.

Johnson JV and Hall EM (1988) Job strain, work place social support, and cardiovascular disease: a cross-sectional study of a random sample of the Swedish working population. *American Journal of Public Health*. **78**:1336–42.

Johnson JV *et al*. (1989) Combined effects of job strain and social isolation on cardiovascular disease morbidity and mortality in a random sample of the Swedish male working population. *Scandinavian Journal of Work and Environmental Health*. **15**:271–9.

Kaplan GA *et al*. (1988) Social connections and mortality from cardiovascular disease: prospective evidence from eastern Finland. *American Journal of Epidemiology*. **128**:370–80.

Kaplan JR *et al*. (1983) Social stress and atherosclerosis in normocholesterolaemic monkeys. *Science*. **220**:733–5.

Karasek R *et al*. (1981) Job decision latitude, job demands, and cardiovascular disease: a prospective study of Swedish men. *American Journal of Public Health*. **71**:694–705.

Karasek RA *et al*. (1982) Job, psychological factors and coronary heart disease. Swedish prospective findings and US prevalence findings using a new occupational inference method. *Advance in Cardiology*. **29**:62–7.

Karasek RA *et al*. (1988) Job characteristics in relation to the prevalence of myocardial infarction in the US health examination survey (HES) and the health and nutrition examination survey (HANES). *American Journal of Public Health*. **78**:910–18.

Kornitzer M and Bara L (1989) Clinical and anthropometric data, blood chemistry and nutritional patterns in the Belgian population according to age and sex. *Acta Cardiologica*. **44**:101–44.

Kornitzer M and Goldberg R (1993) Editorial: The contribution of long-term follow-up to the prediction of coronary heart disease. *Cardiology*. (In press.)

Kornitzer M (1992) Type A behavior and coronary heart disease: an update. *Nutrition, Metabolism and Cardiovascular Disease*. **2**:86–93.

Koskenvuo M *et al*. (1988) Hostility as a risk factor for mortality and ischaemic heart disease in men. *Psychosomatic Medicine*. **50**:330–40.

Leibowitz JO (1970) *The history of coronary heart disease*. University of California Press, Berkeley and Los Angeles. pp. 1–214.

Leon GR *et al*. (1988) Inability to predict cardiovascular disease from hostility scores or MMPI items related to type A behavior. *Journal of Consulting and Clinical Psychology*. **56**:597–600.

Liu K *et al.* (1982) Relationship of education to major risk factors and death from coronary heart disease, cardiovascular diseases and all causes: findings of Three Chicago Epidemiologic Studies. *Circulation.* 66:1308–14.

Markowe HJL *et al.* (1985) Fibrinogen: a possible link between social class and coronary heart disease. *British Medical Journal.* 291:1312–14.

Marmot MG *et al.* (1978) Changing social-class distribution of heart disease. *British Medical Journal.* 2:1109–12.

Marmot MG *et al.* (1984) Inequalities in death-specific explanations of general patterns? *The Lancet.* i:1003–6.

Marmot MG *et al.* (1991) Health inequalities among British civil servants: the Whitehall II Study. *The Lancet.* 338:1387–93.

Matthews KA *et al.* (1987) Stressful work conditions and diastolic blood pressure among blue collar factory workers. *American Journal of Epidemiology.* 126:280–91.

McCranie EW *et al.* (1986) Hostility, coronary heart disease (CHD) incidence, and total mortality: lack of association in a 25-year follow-up study of 478 physicians. *Journal of Behavioral Medicine.* 9:119–25.

Orth-Gomer K and Johnson JV (1987) Social network interaction and mortality. A six year follow-up study of a random sample of the Swedish population. *Journal of Chronic Disease.* 40:949–57.

Orth-Gomer K *et al.* (1988) Social isolation and mortality in ischemic heart disease. A 10-year follow-up study of 150 middle-aged men. *Acta Medica Scandinavia.* 224:205–15.

Orth-Gomer K and Undén AL (1990) Type A behavior, social support, and coronary risk: interaction and significance for mortality in cardiac patients. *Psychosomatic Medicine.* 52:59–72.

Pickering TG *et al.* (1990) Does psychological stress contribute to the development of hypertension and coronary heart disease? *European Journal of Clinical Pharmacology.* 39:S1–S7.

Pieper C *et al.* (1989) The relation of psychosocial dimensions of work with coronary heart disease risk factors: a meta-analysis of five United States data bases. *American Journal of Epidemiology.* 129: 483–94.

Reed D *et al.* (1983) Social networks and coronary heart disease among Japanese men in Hawaii. *American Journal of Epidemiology.* 117:384–96.

Reed D *et al.* (1984) Psychosocial processes and general susceptibility to chronic disease. *American Journal of Epidemiology.* 119:356–70.

Reed D *et al.* (1989) Occupational strain and the incidence of coronary heart disease. *American Journal of Epidemiology.* **129**:495–502.

Rosengren A *et al.* (1990) Social influences and cardiovascular risk factors as determinants of plasma fibrinogen concentration in a general population sample of middle aged men. *British Medical Journal.* **300**:634–8.

Rosengren A *et al.* (1991) Self-perceived psychological stress and incidence of coronary artery disease in middle-aged men. *American Journal of Cardiology.* **68**:1171–5.

Rosenman RH *et al.* (1975) Coronary heart disease in the Western Collaborative Group Study: final follow-up experience of 8½ years. *Journal of the American Medical Association.* **233**:872–7.

Salonen JT (1982) Socioeconomic status and risk of cancer, cerebral stroke, and death due to coronary heart disease and any disease: a longitudinal study in eastern Finland. *Journal of Epidemiology and Community Health.* **36**:294–7.

Salonen JT *et al.* (1988) Leisure time and occupational physical activity: risk of death from ischemic heart disease. *American Journal of Epidemiology.* **127**:87–94.

Scherwitz L *et al.* (1991) Cook-Medley hostility scale and subsets: relationship to demographic and psychosocial characteristics in young adults in the Cardia Study. *Psychosomatic Medicine.* **53**:36–49.

Schnall PL *et al.* (1990) The relationship between 'job strain', workplace diastolic blood pressure, and left ventricular mass index. Results of a case-control study. *Journal of the American Medical Association.* **263**:1929–35.

Schoenbach VJ *et al.* (1986) Social ties and mortality in Evans county, Georgia. *American Journal of Epidemiology.* **123**: 577–91.

Seeman TE and Syme SL (1987) Social networks and coronary artery disease: a comparison of the structure and function of social relations as predictors of disease. *Psychosomatic Medicine.* **49**:341–54.

Shekelle RB *et al.* (1983) Hostility, risk of coronary heart disease, and mortality. *Psychosomatic Medicine.* **45**:109–14.

Siegrist J *et al.* (1990) Low status control, high effort at work and ischemic heart disease: prospective evidence from blue-collar men. *Social Science of Medicine.* **31**:1127–34.

Sobolski J *et al.* (1981) Physical activity, physical fitness and cardiovascular diseases: design of a prospective epidemiologic study. *Cardiology.* **67**:38–51.

Theorell T *et al.* (1975) The relationship of disturbing life-changes and emotions to the early development of myocardial infarction and other serious illnesses. *International Journal of Epidemiology.* **4**:281–93.

Theorell T *et al.* (1987) Psychosocial work conditions before myocardial infarction in young men. *International Journal of Cardiology.* **15**:33–46.

Theorell T *et al.* (1990) Slow-reacting immunoglobulin in relation to social support and changes in job strain: a preliminary note. *Psychosomatic Medicine.* **52**:511–16.

Undén AL *et al.* (1991) Cardiovascular effects of social support in the work place: twenty-four-hour ECG monitoring of men and women. *Psychosomatic Medicine.* **53**:50–60.

Welin L *et al.* (1985) Prospective study of social influences on mortality. The study of men born in 1913 and 1923. *The Lancet.* **i**: 915–18.

Williams RB *et al.* (1980) Type A behavior hostility and coronary atherosclerosis. *Psychosomatic Medicine.* **42**:539–49.

Williams RB *et al.* (1992) Prognostic importance of social and economic resources among medically treated patients with angiographically documented coronary artery disease. *Journal of the American Medical Association.* **267**:520–4.

Woodward M *et al.* (1992) Social status and coronary heart disease: results from the Scottish Heart Health Study. *Preventive Medicine.* **21**:136–48.

25

Can we Manipulate Diets?

JACQUI LYNAS AND SIMON THOM

Britons are getting fatter—30% of the adult population are overweight, 60% have a blood cholesterol level above 5.2 mmol/l, and 1% have diabetes, so it would seem that the majority of the population are hungry for some dietary advice.

Practical dietary guidelines for people with diabetes, hyperlipidaemia, obesity and hypertension are becoming similar to those for the general population for healthy eating. Special diets could now be considered the 'trend setters' rather than the exceptions. Diet, together with exercise, weight control, moderation of alcohol intake and stopping smoking, forms a cornerstone in the management of these conditions. In each case, diet enhances the response to drug treatment when this becomes necessary.

Guidelines for a healthy diet

Managing each disease requires some fine dietary tuning to suit the individual concerned, but the following guidelines will act as a sound foundation for all practical advice (WHO, 1990):

- enjoy your food
- eat a variety of different foods
- eat the right amount to be a healthy weight
- eat foods high in starch and fibre content
- do not eat too much fat
- do not eat sugary food too often
- include vitamins and minerals in your diet
- if you drink alcohol, keep within sensible limits.

Overall the changes we are seeking in our current western diet are as recommended by Bingham (1991):

- reduction in total fat, saturated fat and cholesterol
- relative increase in poly- and mono-unsaturated fats
- increase in unrefined carohydrate
- increased vitamin and mineral antioxidant intake
- reduced dietary sodium and increased potassium.

Advice on dietary change must focus on 'what to eat' rather than a long list of 'what not to eat'. Alternatives for dietary management must fulfil the following four criteria: practicality, enjoyment, availability and economy.

Practicality

Although the 'Mediterranean type diet' (Ulbricht and Southgate, 1991) has been heralded as an ideal way to eat and to achieve the above objectives, it must be adapted to suit the British palate. Current practices need to be improved, rather than necessarily introducing foreign ones. Change may often be restricted by the limits of cultural habits.

The Mediterranean diet consists of salads dressed in olive oil, lightly cooked vegetables, fresh fruit, bread, pasta, rice, fish and lean meat. The diet is low in saturated fat and high in complex carbohydrates. The fruit and fresh vegetables provide antioxidant vitamins, trace minerals and potassium. Oily fish is a rich source of n-3 polyunsaturated fatty acids and eicosapentanenoic acid. Olive oil is rich in oleic acid, and the cereals are rich in fibre. The garlic and wine characteristic of Mediterranean meals may also confer additional benefits (Mansell and Reckless, 1991; Rimm et al., 1991).

Simple concepts can be borrowed from the Mediterranean diet: when planning meals, it is sensible to consider the carbohydrate portion first: potatoes, rice, pasta or bread with at least two vegetables or salad. Use a small portion of fish or white meat, followed by fruit rather than the traditional English pudding. Spaghetti bolognaise and pizza are now firm favourites of today's children and these can be made in a well balanced style.

The traditional Mediterranean lifestyle gives more time and importance to the preparation, eating and enjoyment of a formal meal in a family group. This is gradually being eroded in many British families where both parents work and pressures of time enforce quick and easy meals often eaten separately or in transit. Three meals per week are taken outside the home and the western housewife now spends less than an hour in the kitchen per day (Loughridge et al., 1989). Take-away and convenience foods are generally high in fat.

Enjoyment

Flavour is a complex result of taste, smell and texture and it is one of the most important factors influencing food choice. Food must look attractive, interesting and varied, and be fun to prepare. It must taste appealing, give pleasure and satisfy appetite. An alternative diet will not be maintained if it is unpalatable.

Availability

50% of goods are now bought in supermarket chains which carry a huge variety and range of products. This can paradoxically make shopping more expensive: for example only grade I quality fruit and vegetables are sold and there is greater temptation to overspend. Larger stores are now located out of town, leaving the inner cities relatively deprived. The local corner shop may not carry the full range of special products intended for the affluent, health-conscious buyer. However, the 2000 new products per year on the supermarket shelves may not realistically deliver the dietary benefits many of them claim. In these circumstances particularly the consumer needs the help of clear and standardized food labelling.

Economy

The cost of food is a major worry for many families (Terry *et al.*, 1991). Healthy eating is widely regarded as an expensive luxury. Cost is the main barrier to manipulating diet in certain sectors of the community and, as low-income groups carry a greater risk of coronary heart disease, they warrant special attention with advice tailored to their budget (Ammerman *et al.*,1991). Special diets can cost up to 20% more because of increased prices on wholemeal bread, fresh fruit, fish, lean meat, modified spreading fats and low fat products. The elderly, those in low-income groups and students may find it difficult to afford the diet. A family of four on supplementary income benefit may need half of their extra cash to sustain a healthy diet.

If manufactured convenience products are replaced by healthier home cooked food using fresh ingredients, including lean meat, fish and fruit, and if pasta, pulses, bread and rice are used to add bulk to the meal, shopping may be cheaper.

The dietitian

The dietitian is the best qualified person to translate dietary principles into practical recommendations. Dietetic training takes four years before graduation. There are currently 2800 state registered dietitians, of whom 50% are employed by the National Health Service. 350 are specialist 'community dietitians'. General practice is their fastest growing area of activity. Recent changes in primary care have provided funding to employ dietitians, either directly or with 70% reimbursement from the FHSA. Some general practices group together to employ one dietitian working on a sessional basis in each of the clinics. Alternatively, dietetic sessions may be purchased from the local health authority.

30% of GPs are now running dietary clinics as part of 'health promotion programmes', for which they are financially reimbursed. Practice nurses usually run these clinics and can play an important role in giving first-line dietary advice, but they must be offered further training in dietary counselling. As the practice nurse profession develops it is likely that nutrition training will be accredited if not mandatory, and many dietitians already offer such training to all members of the primary care team. Close links between local nutrition and dietetic departments are important, and will improve the standard of management (Francis *et al.*, 1989).

The physician's role

The physician's enthusiasm for dietary and lifestyle measures in disease management is essential in placing emphasis on this approach and supporting the efforts of the dietitian and the rest of the health care team. If lifestyle advice is perceived as only subsidiary to a prescription for pills, the patient is unlikely to listen to the dietitian.

The physician must also be well versed in nutrition and dietetics, because a 'diet sheet' thrust into the hand of a confused patient without a confident and detailed explanation is doomed to fail. This knowledge is often lacking as so little relevant teaching is yet included in medical school curricula (Gray, 1983). Medical students and staff are notably ill informed in this respect, and many express a wish for more teaching on practical aspects of nutrition (Brett *et al.*, 1986). Leaflets and 'diet sheets' are useful only as a reinforcement and reminder of the verbal message.

Shortage of time poses one of the major constraints on the physician's scope to give health promotion advice, but even extending consultation times by a minute in general practice can be effective (Wilson *et al.*, 1992).

The patient, the family and the cook

The dietitian needs to advise the patient in the context of his/her family, and school or work. Often the whole family needs to eat in the same healthy way, and this is most practical for the cook. Whoever does the family shopping and cooking must be present at the dietary interview as their understanding is paramount. Advice must be clear, current and concise. Despite the age of the 'new man' it is still the woman who usually does the shopping: but the more the man is involved, the more positive is his attitude to dietary adjustment.

The family is of utmost importance in supporting and encouraging the patient through the difficult time of changing food habits.

Cooking methods

It is important to discuss the practical issues of cooking methods, as many basic cookery skills have been lost through the rapid growth of manufactured food and the lack of mother-to-daughter teaching at home. Cooking and home economics are no longer widely included as foundation subjects in school curricula. All dietary information must therefore be accompanied by recipe booklets and recommended cook books which include practical and economical dishes which are easy to prepare. Modified versions of familiar dishes enable cooks to gain confidence to alter their own recipes. Cookery demonstrations to facilitate learning by involvement are ideal ways of teaching both principles and practice.

Cooking equipment must be considered. Low-income families may not have a cooker at all, and the cost of buying prepared hot and cold food is appreciably higher. The freezer, the microwave oven and the wok (for stir-frying) afford greater flexibility in food preparation.

Understanding and education

Individuals and families must be strongly motivated to maintain permanent changes in their diet. They need to understand the reasons for dieting and its potential long-term benefits.

Effective dietary counselling takes time. Dietary history must be elicited in detail and advice must be tailored to the individual's requirements, lifestyle and cultural background. Time is required to negotiate mutually agreed targets for weight reduction, blood pressure, and lipid and glucose control, and for the patient to be closely involved in treatment and monitoring. Time must be given for regular follow-up appointments to check understanding and compliance, and to answer questions competently and personally. Observations in diabetic and lipid clinics have demonstrated the positive impact of free patient access to a dietitian and frequent follow-up visits (British Diabetic Association, 1982). Ultimately the one-to-one relationship between the patient and an enthusiastic dietitian sparks motivation and progress.

Schools and work

Dietitians should be advising on the nutritional standards of school meals. School meals were introduced in 1906 to combat malnutrition and subsequently improved in 1944 by the Education Act which introduced minimum nutritional standards. School dinners have influenced dietary habits over many generations. Financial savings in the past decade abolished these standards rather than revising them and forced a significant adverse shift in the dietary pattern of schoolchildren. Many schools employ fewer staff, necessitating the wider use of convenience foods which are typically high in saturated fat and salt. Some health conscious education authorities have been perceptive enough to provide more varied, exciting and healthy choices for the children, with a consequent rise in uptake and revenue. Others have stopped providing school meals altogether with only a sandwich service for children entitled to free school meals.

Apart from the right diet, schoolchildren and teenagers also need nutritional education to influence current food choices in the home and to make them better informed consumers of the future.

Shops and supermarkets

Many dietitians are now employed by supermarket chains as 'corporate nutritionists' to advise on products and product labelling, and to write nutrition literature. Clear labelling must help inform consumer choice and should be clear, consistent and unambiguous. This information should be presented in a standardized format so that rational choices can be made between products to help people follow dietary recommendations. The Coronary Prevention Group has been a vociferous advocate of such a uniform system (O'Connor, 1992).

The works canteen

300 meals per person per year may be taken in the canteen at work and healthy choices must be available. Industry needs advice in this area and large corporations are expressing increasing interest in the health of their work-force. Practical health support on site helps to reduce absenteeism. The work-site is also an ideal place for health screening and dietary intervention programmes (Wilson *et al.*, 1992).

Does the advice work?

There is ample evidence that dietary measures are effective in the prevention and treatment of hypertension (Langford *et al.*, 1985; Stamler *et al.*, 1989). Some doubt the value of reducing cholesterol by dietary measures (Expert Panel, 1988) and argue that the changes necessary are beyond the parameters of the 'step 1 diet', and are therefore unacceptably rigorous and unpalatable (Ramsay *et al.*, 1991). However closer examination of the data shows that most of the effective cholesterol lowering dietary trials were conducted with interventions equivalent to the 'step 1 diet' (Thompson, 1991). These measures are effective in lowering cholesterol (Evans *et al.*, 1972; Hjermann *et al.*, 1981) and without much further effort are effective in causing regression of coronary artery disease (Watts *et al.*, 1992).

Dietary modification with a modest reduction in total fat and cholesterol intake, and an increase in the P:S ratio from 0.7 to 1.2 plus additional antioxidant vitamin intake has been shown to have a striking effect in reducing the rate of recurrent cardiac events, cardiac deaths and total mortality in post-infarction patients (Singh *et al.*, 1992). The debate about cholesterol-reducing diets should focus on the style of the diet rather than whether or not to bother.

Cost-effectiveness

Monthly visits to a dietitian cost in total about £70 per patient per year. This is half the annual cost of the cheapest lipid-lowering medication and less than a quarter of the price of the most expensive drug. A basic-grade dietitian's salary is £13 000. The cost of a single coronary artery bypass operation is £12 000 and rising. If the dietitian has an effective influence on just a few of the hundreds of patients he or she can see in a year, this is enormously cost-effective. Dietitians are a scarce resource and many more are needed.

References

Ammerman AS *et al.* (1991) A brief dietary assessment to guide cholesterol reduction in low income individuals: design and validation. *Journal of the American Dietetic Association.* **91**:1385–90.

Bingham S (1991) Dietary aspects of a health strategy for England. *British Medical Journal*. **303**:353–5.

Brett A *et al.* (1986) Nutritional knowledge of medical staff and students—is present education adequate? *Human Nutrition: Applied Nutrition*. **40A**:217–24.

British Diabetic Association (1982) Dietary recommendations for diabetics for the 1980s. Nutrition subcommittee, British Diabetic Association. *Human Nutrition: Applied Nutrition*. **36A**:378–94.

Expert Panel (1988) Report of the national cholesterol education program expert panel on detection, evaluation and treatment of high blood cholesterol in adults. *Archives of Internal Medicine*. **148**:36–69.

Evans DW *et al.* (1972) Feasibility of long-term plasma cholesterol reduction by diet. *The Lancet*. **i**:172–4.

Francis J *et al.* (1989) Would primary health care workers give appropriate dietary advice after cholesterol screening? *British Medical Journal*. **298**:1620–2.

Gray J (ed.) (1983) *Nutrition in medical education. Report of the British Nutrition Foundation Task Force on human nutrition*. British Nutrition Foundation, London.

Hjermann I *et al.* (1981) Effect of diet and smoking intervention on the incidence of coronary heart disease. Report from the Oslo study group of a randomised study in healthy men. *The Lancet*. **ii**:1303–10.

Langford HG *et al.* (1985) Dietary therapy slows the return of hypertension after stopping prolonged medication. *Journal of the American Medical Association*. **253**:657–64.

Loughridge JM *et al.* (1989) Foods eaten outside the home, nutrient contribution to total diet. *Journal of Human Nutrition and Dietetics*. **2**:361–70.

Mansell P and Reckless JPD (1991) Garlic, effects on serum lipids, blood pressure, coagulation, platelet aggregation and vasodilation. *British Medical Journal*. **303**:379.

O'Connor M (1992) Europe and nutrition: prospects for public health. *British Medical Journal*. **304**:464–8.

Ramsay LE *et al.* (1991) Dietary reduction of serum cholesterol: time to think again. *British Medical Journal*. **303**:953–7.

Rimm EB *et al.* (1991) Prospective study of alcohol consumption and risk of coronary disease in men. *The Lancet*. **338**:464–8.

Singh RB *et al.* (1992) Randomised controlled trial of cardioprotective diet in patients with acute myocardial infarction: results of one year follow up. *British Medical Journal*. **304**:1015–19.

Stamler R *et al.* (1989) Primary prevention of hypertension by nutritional-hygienic means. *Journal of the American Medical Association.* **262**:1801–7.

Terry RD *et al.* (1991) Factors associated with adoption of dietary behaviour to reduce heart disease risk among males. *Journal of Nutrition Education.* **23**:154–9.

Thompson GR (1991) Dietary reduction of serum cholesterol. *British Medical Journal.* **303**:1332.

Ulbricht TLV and Southgate DAT (1991) Coronary heart disease: seven dietary factors. *The Lancet.* **338**:985–92.

Watts GF *et al.* (1992) Effects on coronary artery disease of lipid-lowering diet, or diet plus cholestyramine, in the St Thomas' Atherosclerosis Regression Study (STARS). *The Lancet.* **i**:339–69.

WHO (1990) Diet, nutrition and the prevention of chronic diseases. Report of a WHO Study Group. *WHO Technical Report Series.* **797**.

Wilson A *et al.* (1992) Health promotion in the general practice consultation: a minute makes a difference. *British Medical Journal.* **304**:227–30.

Wilson MG *et al.* (1992) Cost effectiveness of work-site screening and intervention programs. *Journal of Occupational Medicine.* **36**:642–9.

26

Exercise in the Primary Prevention of Coronary Heart Disease

ADRIANNE E HARDMAN

The question 'Does exercise reduce the risk of coronary heart disease?' was first addressed nearly 40 years ago. An obvious starting point was to compare groups of men whose occupation demanded high levels of physical activity with their more sedentary counterparts, for example employees of London Transport (conductors compared with drivers) and postal workers (postmen delivering mail compared with clerks) (Morris *et al.*, 1953) and San Francisco dockworkers (Paffenbarger and Hale, 1975). The dockworkers were followed for 22 years, during which period 11% died from coronary heart disease (CHD). Job assignment was relatively free of selection bias because union rules required all dockworkers to work in physically demanding jobs for at least their first five years of service. Measurements of the energy expenditure of work tasks allowed death rates from this disease to be compared in men with different levels of work activity. The more sedentary workers had 80% excess risk of fatal CHD compared with the men engaged in heavy work, defined as expending more than 35.7 MJ (8500 kcal) per week in occupational work.

As the number of physically demanding occupations diminished it was recognized that inter-individual differences in physical activity would increasingly be attributable to exercise in leisure time. The well established alumni network at Harvard was employed to examine the influence of leisure time physical activity on the incidence of CHD in cohorts of ex-students entering the university between 1916 and 1950 (Paffenbarger *et al.*, 1978). Six- to 10-year follow-up showed that the risk of first heart attack was 64% higher in men who expended fewer than 8.4 MJ (2000 kcal) per week in physical activity than in classmates with higher levels of physical activity (Paffenbarger *et al.*, 1978). Of particular interest is the finding that only alumni who were physically active in middle age were afforded a degree of protection: men who were university athletes in their youth but who became sedentary had the same risk of CHD as men who had never been physically active. This observation, confirmed in a later study of British civil servants (Morris *et al.*, 1990), suggests that only continuing and current exercise is effective. If one assumes that constitutional factors are strong predictors of participation in representative university sport, it also argues against a critical genetic component in the exercise effect.

Studies of English executive grade civil servant office workers found that those who reported taking part in vigorous physical activity in their leisure time on initial survey in 1968–70 had, over the next eight and a half years, an incidence of CHD which was somewhat less than half that of their colleagues who recorded no such vigorous exercise (Morris *et al.*, 1973, 1980). The benefit of vigorous exercise (swimming, jogging, cycling, brisk walking, racket games and other sports) was evident in all subgroups examined: these included men with a family history of CHD, the obese, the short of stature, cigarette smokers and men with severe hypertension and subclinical angina. Moreover, a recent report from the British Regional Heart Study showed no association between serum total cholesterol and increasing physical activity (Shaper and Wannamethee, 1991). In the latter study, although the risk of CHD associated with inactivity was attenuated after adjusting for recognized risk factors, it remained significant. Thus regular exercise appears to confer a lower risk of CHD which is independent of other risk factors.

At least two studies show some evidence of a dose-response relationship: amongst Harvard alumni the risk of fatal and non-fatal heart attacks was reduced as exercise energy expenditure increased from less than 2.1 MJ (500 kcal) to about 12.6 MJ (3000 kcal) per week, with no further reduction thereafter (Paffenbarger *et al.*, 1978). In the British Regional Heart Study heart attack rate decreased with increasing physical activity index (Shaper and Wannamethee, 1991).

Altogether, nearly 50 epidemiological studies have now compared the risk of CHD in physically active men with that exhibited by their sedentary counterparts. No study has found a higher risk of CHD in physically active men. A comprehensive review suggests that regular exercise diminishes the risk of heart attack, such that a sedentary lifestyle carries a median relative risk of 1.9. For the 'better' studies, ie those judged positively with regard to at least two of the following—measure of physical activity, measure of CHD, and epidemiological methods—the relative risk is increased to 2.4 (Powell *et al.*, 1987). Thus 40 years of research carried out in many countries strongly supports the suggestion that regular exercise reduces the risk of CHD in men and that its influence is strong, independent and graded. Too little is known to permit any such conclusions for women.

What is less certain is whether a reduction in risk can be acquired by an exercise regimen which large numbers of people are prepared to follow. This issue needs to be addressed before the potential of exercise to contribute to a preventive strategy against CHD can be properly assessed. The thresholds of activity selected to characterize active men in epidemiological studies have varied greatly: the 'heavy occupational work' which conferred benefit amongst San Francisco dockworkers involved expending more than 35.7 MJ per week in exercise. This is about the energy expended in walking or running in excess of 85 miles per week and an unrealistic goal for leisure time exercise for the average man.

More attainable amounts of exercise have, however, been associated with a lower risk than that seen in sedentary men. Data from the Harvard alumni are presented in terms of total exercise energy expenditure per week and a clear benefit was evident in men expending more than 8.4 MJ per week. Activities contributing to the index employed included blocks walked and stairs climbed as well as sports participation. In contrast, the studies of British civil servants have consistently failed to observe an effect of any criterion amount of exercise, finding an effect only in those men who undertook 'vigorous' exercise, ie a threshold of intensity. This is particularly clear in the second study where a dose-response relationship between frequency of exercise and attack rate of CHD was evident only for vigorous exercise (Morris *et al.*, 1990). One reason for these conflicting findings may be related to the characteristics of the men studied. For example, it is possible that levels of endurance fitness were generally lower amongst the Harvard alumni and that simply doing some exercise, regardless of intensity, conferred some protection. Amongst British men, if the background levels of fitness were higher, the benefit might only be apparent for those who undertook more vigorous exercise.

Further research is necessary before the minimum amount and intensity of exercise needed to confer a lower risk of CHD can be stated with confidence. In the meantime there are aspects of the available evidence that do show that socially acceptable types of exercise in amounts that are attainable in leisure time are sufficient to confer a worthwhile degree of protection against CHD.

First it is necessary to clarify the definition of 'vigorous exercise' employed by Morris *et al.*, (1980, 1990). They defined it as exercise liable to entail peaks of energy expenditure of 31.5 kJ/min (7.5 kcal/min). The term 'vigorous' is well justified in that this level of exercise involves a six fold increase over resting metabolic rate and would be expected to produce and maintain a cardiorespiratory training effect in the population of men involved (American College of Sports Medicine, 1991). However, it is important to note that this energy expenditure suggests an oxygen uptake of about 21 ml/kg/min for a 70 kg man, sufficient to walk at 4.5 mph, an attainable exercise goal for most middle-aged men. This suggests that activities like fast walking and cycling, which can be used for 'getting about', are worthy of examination.

The Harvard alumni study compared total mortality in men with different regular amounts of walking: there was a 21% lower risk of death as distance walked was increased from less than three miles to nine or more miles per week (Paffenbarger *et al.*, 1986). In the British Regional Heart Study even when all men reporting regular sporting activity were excluded, there was a strong inverse relationship between physical activity and the risk of heart attack. Moreover, although regular walking was not associated with risk, those who walked 41–60 minutes a day to and from work (more than one mile each time at a fast pace) showed a decreased risk compared with other men (Shaper and Wannamethee, 1991). Finally, in British civil servants there were particularly low rates of CHD in the men who rated their regular speed of walking as fast (> 4 mph) and in those who did considerable amounts of cycling (Morris *et al.*, 1990). Consequently, exercise need not be very intense or of a sporting nature in order to confer benefit.

Mechanisms of benefit

Randomized, controlled trials of the influence of exercise on the risk of CHD are unlikely to be conducted and consequently a judgement has to be made from available evidence. Many will find this more convincing if the mechanisms of influence can be clarified.

Regular endurance exercise has well documented effects on cardiovascular and metabolic functions. After training there is a bradycardia at rest and at a given exercise intensity which may influence risk because it decreases the work, and therefore the oxygen consumption, of the myocardium. In adults with mild to moderate hypertension, the effect is enhanced by reductions in systolic and diastolic arterial blood pressure of, on average, 13 and 10 mmHg respectively (Seals and Hagberg, 1984). One well controlled study suggests that low-intensity exercise (50% maximal oxygen uptake) may be as or even more effective than high-intensity training (70% maximal oxygen uptake) in this regard (Hagberg et al., 1989).

Adaptations in trained muscle may contribute to the more favourable plasma lipoprotein profile frequently shown in athletes or joggers compared with sedentary controls (Williams et al., 1986). In particular, plasma triglyceride concentration is almost invariably lower and plasma high-density lipoprotein (HDL) cholesterol level higher in the athletes (Haskell, 1986). The results from longitudinal studies are less consistent but many show an increase in HDL cholesterol. It is not clear how much exercise is needed to modify HDL cholesterol but a modest programme of jogging in overweight men (average over one year of 18.9 km or 11.7 miles per week) resulted in a 10.4% increase in HDL cholesterol in relation to controls which was related to total distance run (Wood et al., 1988). Some less structured, unsupervised exercise program-mes have also been successful in modifying lipoprotein metabolism. In men, two hours of jogging per week for four months increased HDL cholesterol (Marti et al., 1990) and about 2.5 hours per week of brisk walking over one year was sufficient to provoke a 27% increase in HDL cholesterol in middle-aged women (Hardman et al., 1989). However, in another Loughborough study, 27 minutes of brisk walking per day over one year failed to influence any of the lipid or lipoprotein variables measured in previously sedentary men (mean age 51 years), despite clear evidence of improved endurance fitness (Stensel et al., 1992). This would be consistent with the observation that, amongst men in the British Regional Heart Study, HDL cholesterol was raised significantly only in the men who were vigorously, rather than moderately, active (Shaper and Wannamethee, 1991).

Changes in lipoprotein metabolism may be due, in part, to the weight loss which sometimes accompanies exercise programmes. Weight loss, presumably reflecting fat loss, appears to augment the exercise effect on HDL cholesterol (Tran and Weltman, 1985), but the proliferation of capillaries in skeletal muscle is probably also important. Lipoprotein lipase, the enzyme responsible for the hydrolysis of triglyceride in lipoproteins, is situated in capillary endothelium. Consequently, increased capillarization accelerates the removal from the circulation of triglyceride-rich lipoproteins, increasing the synthesis of HDL_2 (Keins and Lithell, 1989). This would be consistent with improved reverse cholesterol transport, a mechanism which may explain the decreased atheroma found in the coronary arteries of trained monkeys (compared with untrained monkeys) fed on an atherogenic diet (Kramsch et al., 1981).

Other mechanisms by which regular exercise may decrease the risk of CHD, which are currently less well explored, include an anti-thrombotic effect. To be protective, exercise has to be continuing and current, suggesting an effect on the acute phases of CHD rather than on the chronic build-up of atheroma. This directs attention to the clotting processes and platelet aggregation (Morris et al., 1990) and a recent report shows that fibrinogen levels are lower in men reporting strenuous exercise than in those who took only mild exercise or who did no exercise (Connelly et al., 1992)

Safety of exercise

There is concern that vigorous activity which causes a marked increase in the work of the heart might precipitate an acute episode of myocardial ischaemia. However, the transient increase in risk during an acute bout of exercise has to be considered alongside the long term cardiovascular benefits of exercising regularly.

Siscovick et al. (1984) interviewed the wives of 133 men who suffered primary cardiac arrest and classified the men according to their activity at the time of the arrest and the amount of their habitual vigorous activity. From interviews with the wives of a random sample of healthy men, they then estimated the time that members of the community spent in vigorous activity. Amongst men with low levels of habitual activity, the relative risk of cardiac arrest during exercise compared with at other times was 56. For the men with the highest level of habitual activity the risk during exercise was also elevated, but only by a factor of 5. However, for these men the overall risk of primary cardiac arrest, was only 40% of that of the sedentary men. The important conclusion is that the balance of risks of habitual vigorous exercise is favourable, but this study also shows that unaccustomed strenuous exercise is potentially hazardous for middle-aged or older persons. Advice for such individuals must be to increase progressively, and over a long period, the amount of low-intensity exercise they undertake.

Despite the increased cardiac risk during exercise, death during recreational exercise is uncommon. For example, the incidence in Rhode Island has been estimated as only 4.46 deaths per 100 000 of the male population (exercisers and others) per year (Ragosta et al., 1984). These most frequently occur in individuals with relevant medical histories or recognized risk factors for CHD, and are predominantly due to atherosclerotic heart disease (Ragosta et al., 1984).

Implications for a preventive strategy

Although the two most recent British studies suggest that the relative risk of physical inactivity is over two (Morris *et al.*, 1990; Shaper and Wannamethee, 1991), the median value for studies reviewed in 1987 was 1.9 (Powell *et al.*, 1987)—a value approaching those reported for other major risk factors (Pooling Project Research Group, 1978). This information contributes to the assessment of individual risk and helps the clinician to identify those areas of lifestyle change most likely to modify risk in a particular patient.

From the public health point of view, it is also important to estimate the population-attributable risk which depends not only on the prevalence but also on the strength of a particular factor. Estimating prevalence is not an easy task in respect of physical inactivity: there are uncertainties about the amount and type of exercise needed, and the methods used for collecting data about exercise habits are crude and lack uniformity. Estimates from two sources, Heartbeat Wales (Welsh Heart Programme Directorate, 1987) and the National Fitness Survey (1992) suggest that between 33–70% of British men could decrease their risk of CHD by taking more exercise (Table 26.1). The potential to decrease the incidence of this disease in the population by increasing physical activity levels is therefore considerable. Even more women than men are physically inactive. It is biologically plausible that the relative risk of sedentariness in women is similar to that in men, and therefore there are good reasons for promoting exercise amongst both sexes. Moreover, it is important to remember that the estimate of relative risk presented in Table 26.1 is (1) conservative, and (2) based on comparisons of risk in men undertaking quite modest amounts of exercise with those who are sedentary. The 'active' men

	% with risk factor	Relative risk
Hypertension[1]	15	2.1[4]
High serum cholesterol[2]	26	2.4[5]
Cigarette smoking[3]	17–38	2.5[6]
Physical inactivity	33–57 (Welsh Heart Programme Directorate, 1987) 70 (National Fitness Survey, 1992)	1.9[7]

[1](>160/90 mmHg), [2](>6.5 mmol/l) from studies in four British towns (Mann *et al..*, 1988), [3](15-24/d), [4](systolic blood pressure >150 mmHg versus ≤130 mmHg), [5](>6.9mmol/l versus ≤5.6 mmol/l) from the Coronary Pooling Project Research Group, 1978, [6](≤20 cigarettes/d versus no smoking), [7](Powell *et al.*, 1987).

Table 26.1: Prevalence of risk factors and relative risk for CHD in British men.

are not trained endurance athletes. Some of the exercise reported by active men was recreational sport, but for many—perhaps even the majority— exercise took the form of activities like walking, cycling and climbing stairs.

Conclusion

Currently the emphasis of preventive strategies tends to be on changing behaviour with regard to smoking and diet. This may be, in part, because of the perception that only intense exercise of a sporting nature is likely to be effective. This is not the case. Exercise needs to be frequent and fairly vigorous in relation to individual capacity, and it should constitute a sufficient challenge to cardiovascular and metabolic functions to provoke adaptation. However, for most middle-aged and older persons this can be achieved during socially acceptable endurance activities like brisk walking, cycling, swimming and dancing. A varied programme is probably desirable because it will maximize peripheral adapations of skeletal muscle, whilst keeping the risk of injury low. Bearing in mind the additional benefits of endurance exercise in terms of maintaining or increasing functional capacity, the inclusion of exercise promotion in a preventive strategy against CVD is well justified.

References

American College of Sports Medicine (1991) *Guidelines for exercise testing and prescription*. Lea and Febiger, Philadelphia.

Connelly JB, Cooper JA and Meade TW (1992) Strenuous exercise, plasma fibrinogen and factor VII activity. *British Heart Journal*. 67:351–4.

Hagberg JM *et al.* (1989) Effect of exercise training in 60–69-year-old persons with essential hypertension. *American Journal of Cardiology*. 64:348–53.

Hardman AE *et al.* (1989) Brisk walking and high density lipoprotein cholesterol concentration in formerly sedentary women. *British Medical Journal*. 299:1204–5.

Haskell WL (1986) The influence of exercise training on plasma lipids and lipoproteins in health and disease. In: Astrand P-O and Grimby G (eds) Physical activity in health and disease. *Acta Medica Scandinavica*. Suppl. 711:pp. 25–37.

Keins B and Lithell H (1989) Lipoprotein metabolism influenced by training-induced changes in human skeletal muscle. *Journal of Clinical Investiagation*. 83: 558–64.

Kramsch DM *et al.* (1981) Reduction of coronary atherosclerosis by moderate conditioning exercise in monkeys on an atherogenic diet. *New England Journal of Medicine*. **305**:1483–9.

Mann JI *et al.* (1988) Blood lipid concentrations and other cardiovascular risk factors: distribution, prevalence, and detection in Britain. *British Medical Journal*. **296**:1702–6.

Marti B *et al.* (1990) Effects of long-term, self-monitored exercise on the serum lipoprotein and apolipoprotein profile in middle-aged men. *Atherosclerosis*. **81**:19–31.

Morris JN *et al.* (1953) Coronary heart-disease and physical activity of work. *The Lancet*. **ii**:1053–7, 1111–20.

Morris JN *et al.* (1973) Vigorous exercise in leisure-time and the incidence of coronary heart disease. *The Lancet*. **i**:333–9.

Morris JN *et al.* (1980) Vigorous exercise in leisure-time: protection against coronary heart disease. *The Lancet*. **ii**:1207–10.

Morris JN *et al.* (1990) Exercise in leisure-time: coronary attack and death rates. *British Heart Journal*. **63**:325–34.

National Fitness Survey (1992) *Report*. Health Education Authority and Sports Council, London.

Paffenbarger RS and Hale WE (1975) Work activity and coronary heart mortality. *New England Journal of Medicine*. **292**:545–50.

Paffenbarger RS *et al.* (1978) Physical activity as an index of heart attack risk in college alumni. *American Journal of Epidemiology*. **108**:161–75.

Paffenbarger RS *et al.* (1986) Physical activity, all-cause mortality, and longevity of college alumni. *New England Journal of Medicine*. **314**:605–13.

Pooling Project Research Group (1978) Relationship of blood pressure, serum cholesterol, smoking habit, relative weight and ECG abnormalities to incidence of major coronary events: final report of the Pooling Project. *Journal of Chronic Diseases*. **31**:202–306.

Powell KE *et al.* (1987) Physical activity and the incidence of coronary heart disease. *Annual Review of Public Health*. **8**:253–87.

Ragosta M *et al.* (1984) Death during recreational exercise in the State of Rhode Island. *Medicine and Science in Sports and Exercise*. **16**:207–15.

Seals DR and Hagberg JM (1984) The effect of exercise training on human hypertension: a review. *Medicine and Science in Sports and Exercise*. **16**:207–15.

Shaper AG and Wannamethee G (1991) Physical activity and ischaemic heart disease in middle-aged British men. *British Heart Journal*. **66**:384–94.

Siscovick DS *et al*. (1984) The incidence of primary cardiac arrest during vigorous exercise. *New England Journal of Medicine*. **311**:874–7.

Stensel DJ *et al*. (1992) The influence of brisk walking on endurance fitness in previously sedentary, middle-aged men. *Journal of Physiology*. **446**:123P.

Tran ZV and Weltman A (1985) Differential effects of exercise on serum lipid and lipoprotein levels seen with changes in body weight. A meta-analysis. *Journal of the American Medical Association*. **254**:919–24.

Welsh Heart Programme Directorate (1987) *Exercise for health: health related fitness in Wales*. Heartbeat Report, No. 23.

Williams PT *et al*. (1986) Lipoprotein subfractions of runners and sedentary men. *Metabolism*. **35**:45–52.

Wood PD *et al*. (1988) Changes in plasma lipids and lipoproteins in overweight men during weight loss through dieting as compared with exercise. *New England Journal of Medicine*. **319**:1173–9.

27

Garlic and Prevention of Coronary Heart Disease

JOHN PD RECKLESS

The use of garlic (Allium sativum) for possible health-giving properties has a very long tradition, dating back at least as far as the Codex Ebers, an Egyptian medical papyrus of 1550 BC, where garlic is mentioned in 22 of 800 herbal remedies. Garlic has been advocated for treatment and/or prevention of a wide variety of conditions including heart disease, headache, bites, worms, tumours (Block, 1985), cancer and infections (McElnay and Li Wan Po, 1991). Recent work suggests a possible preventive role in premature atherosclerosis and coronary heart disease (CHD), (Mansell and Reckless, 1991). Effects may occur on plasma lipid levels, on blood pressure, and on fibrinolysis.

Popular interest is currently greatest in Germany, where garlic preparations are the largest selling over-the-counter drugs (Fulder, 1989). The long-recognized principle side effect that may occur with garlic usage is odour, and this was acknowledged by Bottom when instructing his actors to 'eat no onions nor garlic, for we are to utter sweet breath' (*A Midsummer Night's Dream*, Act 4, Scene 2).

Chemistry

The ingredients in garlic which are thought to be active medicinally, and which are also the ingredients responsible for the characteristic odour, are organosulphur compounds, the thiosulphinates, and their breakdown products. The principal active agent in garlic is allicin (Block, 1985). Allicin is formed enzymatically from an odourless precursor, alliin, when cloves are mechanically disrupted. Other biologically active compounds related to allicin, such as ajoene, may also be extracted from fresh garlic. Allicin was first identified as an unstable, odorous sulphurous compound in 1944, and the name was derived from the name of the garlic plant, Allium sativum. The odourless precursor compound alliin was identified in 1948.

The quantities of allicin can vary very greatly, depending on the origin, agriculture and handling of the garlic. In fresh garlic samples, allicin concentration may range from 0.1% to 0.5%. In various dried garlic preparations it has been shown that the allicin content may range from 0.1% to 0.9%, with preparations of Chinese origin being of superior quality. The quantity of allicin that can be released from fresh garlic has been shown to decline greatly over a few weeks at room temperature. In contrast, carefully dried and stored powder preparations of garlic have been shown to retain up to 90% of releasable allicin over five years (Aye, 1989; Müller, 1991).

When fresh garlic is cut or crushed, enzymes such as alliinase act on precursor products such as alliin, to form allicin and other metabolites such as ajoenes. While the precursor compounds in dried garlic are quite stable, allicin and other products of alliinase activity are much less stable after cutting or crushing of garlic. The precise active ingredients from garlic are not defined, although the allicin releasable activity bears some relation to the biological activity, and has been proposed as a marker for product standardization, rather than the total sulphur content of the garlic preparation. Garlic products prepared by maceration in oil have low thiosulphinate contents of 0.02–0.1%, compared to garlic powder tablets, although these also have been shown to have variable contents from 0.02%–0.48% (Aye, 1989; Müller, 1991). One of the reasons for the difficulty in demonstrating the effectiveness of garlic preparations is likely to be this loss of active ingredients during processing (Block, 1985). Carefully dried sliced cloves are satisfactory but extracts or oils prepared using steam distillation or organic solvents may have little activity (Aye, 1989; Müller 1991).

The modes of action of alliin or allicin are not clearly established, but studies have examined the effects on cholesterol biosynthesis (Gebhardt, 1991). Cultured rat hepatocytes, able to synthesize cholesterol from radiolabelled acetate, were cultured with water-soluble extracts of garlic powder, with pure alliin or allicin, or with lovastatin and mevastatin, inhibitors of hydroxymethylglutaryl-Coenzyme A (HMGCoA) reductase. Water-soluble garlic powder extracts significantly reduced cholesterol biosynthesis, with inhibition of HMGCoA reductase, but alliin and allicin were not active (Gebhardt, 1991).

Side-effects

The issue of 'odourless' garlic preparations is complicated by confusion as to whether it is the odour of tablet or recipient that is being described. Some garlic preparations contain no active ingredients and do not smell. Active preparations may themselves be odourless (such as alliin) but if allicin is released on ingestion there must be a substantial chance of a detectable aroma. A number of different catabolic products of alliin metabolism may occur, which may not be biologically active, but being sulphur-containing may still have odour. 'Odour blockers' appear ineffective (Aye, 1989). Other side-effects such as gastrointestinal disturbance, asthma and contact dermatitis are uncommon although a spinal haematoma has been attributed to anti-platelet effects of garlic (Rose *et al.*, 1990).

Garlic and macrovascular disease

Garlic can apparently have beneficial effects on coagulation, platelet aggregation, and vasodilatation. Falls in serum lipids have been shown in normal and hyperlipidaemic rats, and also in man. Fibrinogen may fall (Harenberg *et al.*, 1988; Jung *et al.*, 1989) and an increase in rates of fibrinolysis has been reported (Harenberg *et al.*, 1988). Garlic extract has been shown to reduce acute platelet thrombus formation *in vivo* in stenosed coronary arteries of dogs (DeBoer and Folts, 1989). Synthetic allicin has been shown to inhibit platelet aggregation *in vitro* (Mayeux *et al.*, 1988), by mechanisms which are not clear (Makheja *et al.*, 1979; Apitz-Castro *et al.*, 1983; Makheja and Bailey, 1990). Vasodilator properties of garlic have been demonstrated in human skin vessels (Jung *et al.*, 1990), and also in conjunctival vessels (Wolf *et al.*, 1990). With garlic usage, falls have been demonstrated in haematocrit, in plasma viscosity (Jung *et al.*, 1989) and in blood pressure (Harenberg *et al.*, 1988) Garlic may lead to falls in triglycerides, total and low-density lipoprotein (LDL) cholesterol and a rise in high-density lipoprotein (HDL) cholesterol (Bordia, 1981; Harenberg *et al.*, 1988), by unknown mechanisms, although some studies have been contradictory (Luley *et al.*, 1986).

A 1989 review (Kleijnen *et al.*, 1989) concluded that whereas large doses of fresh garlic (between seven and 28 cloves per day) had beneficial effects on cardiovascular risk factors, data for many commercial preparations were unconvincing, and there was inadequate evidence to recommend garlic supplementation.

Garlic and hyperlipidaemia

Criticisms (Kleijnen *et al.*, 1989) that previous reports may have used inactive products and were poorly designed or open studies, have recently been met by a placebo-controlled, randomized, double-blind, 16-week German study (Mader, 1990). One hundred and fifteen men (58 active treatment) and 146 women (76 active treatment) of mean age 59 years were recruited by 30 general practitioners. A variety of concurrent conditions and drug therapies were present in both groups. Criteria for entry were a cholesterol between 5.2 mmol/l and 7.8 mmol/l, and triglycerides between 2.26 mmol/l and 3.39 mmol/l. Levels of cholesterol and triglycerides were measured in individual laboratories, rather than centrally. With four tablets daily containing 800 mg dried garlic powder ('Kwai' with 1.3% allicin), total serum cholesterol fell by 11.7% from 6.87 mmol/l to 6.07 mmol/l ($P < 0.001$), and serum triglycerides fell by 17% from 2.55 mmol/l to 2.12 mmol/l ($P < 0.001$). The fall in cholesterol was greater when the initial cholesterol was in the range 6.5 to 7.8 mmol/l than when it was less than 6.5 mmol/l. At baseline actual cholesterol levels exceeded 7.8 mmol/l in 17 patients on active and 18 patients on placebo treatment, mean values being 8.35 mmol/l and 8.43 mmol/l respectively. At 16 weeks cholesterol fell to 7.06 mmol/l (P <0.001) and to 7.86 mmol/l (P <0.01) respectively, the difference between the two groups being significant at P < 0.05. A garlic smell was reported (most frequently by spouses) in 21% of individuals receiving active garlic and in 9% of those receiving placebo.

These falls in cholesterol and triglycerides are of a similar order to those seen in other reported open studies.

Garlic and hypertension

In another study (Auer *et al.*, 1990), a similar dosage of 800 mg dried garlic powder ('Kwai' with 1.3% allicin) taken for three months was associated with a significant fall in blood pressure. Auer and colleagues showed a reduction in blood pressure in hypertensive patients from pre-treatment mean values of 171/102 mmHg to 152/89 mmHg. One in eight of the subjects on active treatment reported a garlic odour.

Conclusions

Evidence that garlic reduces cardiovascular risk factors is accumulating but is incomplete. Some garlic preparations, with significant alliin/allicin content, may be useful in treating hyperlipidaemia and hypertension, but no studies yet have been undertaken to show concomitant reductions in either morbidity or mortality from macrovascular disease. Detectable aroma in at least some individuals seems to be an inevitable consequence of ingesting an active garlic product. A late 20th century Bottom might accept that potential benefits of garlic can be offset by the social consequences of uttering without sweet breath.

References

Apitz-Castro R *et al.* (1983) Effects of garlic extract and of three pure components isolated from it on human platelet aggregation, arachidonate metabolism, release reaction, and platelet ultrastructure. *Thrombosis Research.* 32:155–69.

Auer W *et al.* (1990) Hypertension and hyperlipidaemia: garlic helps in mild cases. *British Journal of Clinical Practice.* 44 (Symp. Suppl. 69):3–6.

Aye R-D (1989) Garlic preparations and processing. *Cardiology in Practice.* 10 (Symp. Suppl.):7–8.

Block E (1985) The chemistry of garlic and onions. *Scientific American.* 252:94–9.

Bordia A (1981) Effect of garlic on blood lipids in patients with coronary heart disease. *American Journal of Clinical Nutrition.* 34:2100–3.

DeBoer LWV and Folts JD (1989) Garlic extract prevents acute platelet thrombus formation in stenosed canine coronary arteries. *American Heart Journal*. 117:973–5.

Fulder S (1989) Garlic and the prevention of cardiovascular disease. *Cardiology in Practice*. 7:30–5.

Gebhardt R (1991) Inhibition of cholesterol biosynthesis by a water-soluble garlic extract in primary cultures of rat hepatocytes. *Arzneimittelforschung/Drug Research*. **41** (II):800–4.

Harenberg J *et al.* (1988). Effect of dried garlic on blood coagulation, fibrinolysis, platelet aggregation and serum cholesterol levels in patients with hyperlipoproteinaemia. *Atherosclerosis*. **74**:247–9.

Jung F *et al.* (1989) Akutwirkung eines zusammengesetzten Knoblauchpraparates auf die Fleissfahigkeit des Blutes. *Zeitschrift für Phytotherapie*. 10:87–91.

Jung F *et al.* (1990) Influence of garlic powder on cutaneous microcirculation: a randomised, placebo-controlled, double-blind crossover study in apparently healthy subjects. *British Journal of Clinical Practice*. **44** (Symp. Suppl. 69):30–5.

Kleijnen J *et al.* (1989) Garlic, onions and cardiovascular risk factors. A review of the evidence from human experiments with emphasis on commercially available preparations. *British Journal of Clinical Pharmacology*. **28**:533–44.

Luley C *et al.* (1986) Lack of efficacy of dried garlic in patients with hyperlipoproteinaemia. *Arzneimittelforschung/Drug Research*. **36**:766–8.

Mader FH (1990) Treatment of hyperlipidaemia with garlic-powder tablets. *Arzneimittelforschung/Drug Research*. **40**:3–8.

Makheja AN *et al.* (1979) Inhibition of platelet aggregation and thromboxane synthesis by onion and garlic. *The Lancet*. **i**:781.

Makheja AN and Bailey JM (1990) Antiplatelet constituents of garlic and onion. *Agents and Actions*. **29**:360–3.

Mansell P and Reckless JPD (1991) Garlic: effects on serum lipids, blood pressure, coagulation, platelet aggregation, and vasodilatation. *British Medical Journal*. **303**:379–80.

Mayeux PR *et al.* (1988) The pharmacological effects of allicin, a constituent of garlic oil. *Agents and Actions*. **25**:182–90.

McElnay JC and Li Wan Po A (1991) Dietary supplements (8). Garlic. *The Pharmaceutical Journal*. **March 16**:324–6.

Müller B (1991) Standardisation of garlic preparations. *Cardiology in Practice*. **12** (Symp. Suppl.):4–5.

Rose KD *et al.* (1990) Spontaneous spinal epidural haematoma with associated platelet dysfunction from excessive garlic ingestion: a case report. *Neurosurgery.* 26:880–2.

Wolf S *et al.* (1990) Effect of garlic on conjunctival vessels: a randomised, placebo-controlled, double-blind trial. *British Journal of Clinical Practice.* **44** (Symp. Suppl. 69):36–9.

28

The Hypertension Trials

PETER SEVER

Prospective epidemiological data have shown that an increased risk of cardiovascular disease (CVD) is predicted by increments in both systolic and diastolic blood pressure. This increase in risk is continuous and graded with no evidence for a J-shaped relationship (MacMahon *et al.*, 1990). It is estimated that in middle-aged men, a 20 mmHg higher systolic pressure is associated with a 60% increase in cardiovascular mortality and with a 50% higher all cause mortality over a 10-year period.

Prior to the introduction of drug therapy for severe hypertension, associated morbidity and mortality from stroke, coronary heart disease (CHD), congestive heart failure and renal failure were high. Fifty years ago, the Mayo Clinic reports (Keith *et al.*, 1939) showed that 80% of hypertensive patients who developed papilloedema died within a year, 90% were dead within two years and few remained alive after three years. With the introduction of drug therapy, survival was dramatically improved; in the early study from the Hammersmith Hospital, 50% of treated patients survived two years (Harrison *et al.*, 1959). The introduction of therapy changed not only the associated mortality rates, but also the relative importance of the causes of death, so that congestive heart failure and renal disease were virtually eliminated and stroke was no longer the main cause of death.

The results of the Veterans' Administration Studies (1967, 1970) laid to rest any doubts which may have existed about the advantages of treating moderate (diastolic blood pressure 105–114 mmHg) and severe (diastolic blood pressure ≥ 115 mmHg) levels of blood pressure. Drug treatment reduced strokes, heart failure and other cardiovascular and renal endpoints, but not myocardial infarction (Figure 28.1).

From this and other early trials, a number of observations were made: a greater reduction in morbid events was seen in the higher blood-pressure groups at entry; men fared better than women; the incidence of accelerated phase hypertension was greatly reduced by treatment, and the older patients benefited more than the young. On the whole, however, the limited number of participants in these early trials reduced their power to answer the question as to whether treating blood pressure reduced coronary events.

The benefits of treating hypertension have been extended to the larger population at risk from mild hypertension; this has been confirmed in several

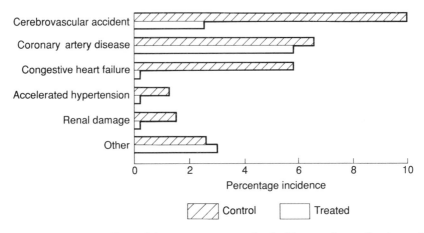

Figure 28.1: The effect of drug treatment on the incidence of complications of hypertension (modified from Veterans' Administration studies, 1970, 1977)

studies. In these patients it was particularly important to demonstrate that the advantages of blood pressure reduction were not counteracted by long-term adverse responses to the antihypertensive drugs. This assessment of risk benefit ratio is particularly important in a group of patients for whom the individual attributable risk is relatively small.

In all the trials that have involved patients with mild hypertension, active treatment has conferred benefits when compared with placebo or, in the case of the Hypertension Detection and Follow-up Programme (HDFP Cooperative Group, 1979, 1982) and the Multiple Risk Factor Intervention Trial (MRFIT Research Group, 1982) the outcome in the special care group was better than those patients who continued with 'usual' medical care.

In the Australian trial (entry diastolic pressures 95–109 mmHg) (Australian National Blood Pressure Management Committee, 1980), active treatment reduced the incidence of stroke. Although fewer cases of fatal ischaemic heart disease (IHD) occurred in the active treatment group, the numbers were small and the difference just failed to achieve statistical significance.

In the Medical Research Council Trial of mild hypertension (diastolic pressure 90–109 mmHg) (MRC Working Party, 1985), stroke rate was again reduced by active treatment but there was no overall reduction in coronary events. The results of subgroup analysis from this trial require cautious interpretation. Comparing the two active regimes, the diuretic was more effective than the beta-blocker in reducing stroke rate. Strokes were reduced in both smokers and non-smokers by the diuretic, but only in non-smokers by propranolol. With the exception of non-smoking males, in whom a modest reduction in coronary events was associated with a beta-blocker, there was no effect of either treatment on coronary morbidity. When overall morbidity was assessed, including silent infarcts diagnosed electrocardiographically, the beta-blocker group fared significantly better than the diuretic or placebo group.

In the HDFP, which also included patients in the mild hypertension category, special treatment conferred additional benefits to usual care, both in respect of stroke prevention and coronary morbidity. However, because neither this study nor the MRFIT were placebo-controlled, no conclusive statement can be made about the definitive benefits of antihypertensive treatment.

The International Prospective Primary Prevention Study in Hypertension (IPPPSH Collaborative Group, 1985) addressed the question of whether the incidence of cardiac and cerebrovascular events could be influenced by the inclusion in an antihypertensive regime of a beta-adrenoceptor blocker (oxprenolol), compared with treatment not containing a beta-blocker. No overall differences were found between treatment groups in total mortality, cardiac events or strokes. However, as in the MRC Trial, subgroup analysis suggested that beta-blockers may confer some benefit in terms of a reduction in cardiac events in non-smoking men.

Another trial, the Heart Attack Primary Prevention Trial in Hypertension (HAPPHY), Wilhelmson et al., (1987) also addressed the question of whether a beta-blocker-based regimen differed from a diuretic-based regimen with regard to the prevention of coronary artery disease in men with mild-moderate hypertension. The outcome of the trial was similar for the two groups and neither regimen preferentially reduced the incidence of hypertensive complications, including CHD. Further analysis failed to confirm the observations (from the MRC and IPPPSH studies) that non-smokers benefited from beta-blockers compared with diuretics with respect to coronary morbidity.

Patients in the HAPPHY trial received one of two beta-blockers, atenolol or metoprolol. Those receiving metoprolol were followed for a slightly longer period and the data were analysed separately (Wikstrand et al., 1988). In the metoprolol-treated group overall mortality was lower than in the thiazide group because of fewer deaths from CHD and stroke. However, the number of end points was small in this subgroup analysis, so these data should be interpreted with caution.

Meta-analysis

In evaluating the potential benefits from drug treatment of hypertension, it is important to remember that individual trials rarely have sufficient power to reliably detect differences between drug and placebo, or between one drug and another, in overall cardiovascular morbidity and mortality. With the exception of stroke, for which the benefits of treatment are consistent, an apparently negative outcome (particularly with respect to CHD) may be explained by this insufficient power to detect a real difference even when one exists.

Collins and colleagues (1990) have pooled data from a number of prospective observational studies (Figures 28.2, 28.3). Their analysis suggests that a prolonged reduction of 6 mmHg in diastolic pressure would lead to 35–40% fewer strokes and 20–25% fewer coronary events. When the results of the

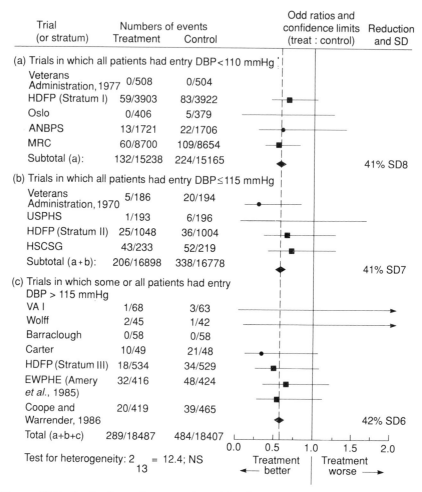

Figure 28.2: Stroke in antihypertensive trials. (Reproduced by permission from Collins *et al.*, 1990.)

intervention trials were analysed, treatment was found to have reduced the risk of stroke by 42% and that of non-fatal myocardial infarction (MI) and CHD death by 14%. This figure rises to 16% if the recent trials in the elderly are included. There is therefore an apparent shortfall in benefit from drug treatment on coronary disease (*see* below).

Trials in the elderly

The results of trials of drug treatment in elderly patients with hypertension are generally consistent with those undertaken in younger subjects (Table 28.1).

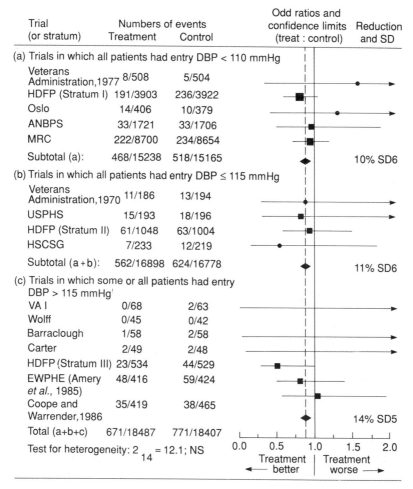

Trial (or stratum)	Numbers of events		Odd ratios and confidence limits (treat : control)	Reduction and SD
	Treatment	Control		
(a) Trials in which all patients had entry DBP < 110 mmHg				
Veterans Administration,1977	8/508	5/504		
HDFP (Stratum I)	191/3903	236/3922		
Oslo	14/406	10/379		
ANBPS	33/1721	33/1706		
MRC	222/8700	234/8654		
Subtotal (a):	468/15238	518/15165		10% SD6
(b) Trials in which all patients had entry DBP ≤ 115 mmHg				
Veterans Administration,1970	11/186	13/194		
USPHS	15/193	18/196		
HDFP (Stratum II)	61/1048	63/1004		
HSCSG	7/233	12/219		
Subtotal (a + b):	562/16898	624/16778		11% SD6
(c) Trials in which some or all patients had entry DBP > 115 mmHg				
VA I	0/68	2/63		
Wolff	0/45	0/42		
Barraclough	1/58	2/58		
Carter	2/49	2/48		
HDFP (Stratum III)	23/534	44/529		
EWPHE (Amery et al., 1985)	48/416	59/424		
Coope and Warrender,1986	35/419	38/465		14% SD5
Total (a+b+c)	671/18487	771/18407		

Test for heterogeneity: $\chi^2_{14} = 12.1$; NS

0.0   0.5   1.0   1.5   2.0
Treatment better ← | → Treatment worse

Figure 28.3: CHD in antihypertensive trials. (Reproduced by permission from Collins *et al.*, 1990.)

However, because the absolute risks of stroke and heart failure associated with high blood pressure are much greater in older subjects, the potential benefits from treatment are considerable.

The percentage reduction in the incidence of strokes in the elderly hypertensive receiving drug treatment is similar to that seen in the young (Report by the Management Committee, 1981; Amery *et al.*, 1985; Coope and Warrender, 1986; Collins *et al.*, 1990; Dahlos *et al.*, 1991; SHEP Cooperative Research Group, 1991; MRC Working Party, 1992). In at least two studies a significant reduction in cardiac mortality has also been observed and in two recent trials there has been a significant reduction in the incidence of coronary events. The cardiovascular benefits of therapy are also seen in isolated systolic hypertension

	EWPHE (Amery et al., 1985)	Australian (Report by the Management Committee, 1981)	Coope and Warrender, 1986	SHEP Cooperative Research Group, 1991	STOP (Dahlof et al., 1991)	MRC Working Party, 1992
Stroke	−36*	−34	−42*	−36*	−47*	−25*
Cardiac	−20	−19	−15	−27*	−13**	−19†
Total cardiovascular	+34*	−24	−23*	−32*	−40*	−17*

*P < 0.05; **myocardial infarction; †IHD.

Table 28.1: Percentage change in event rates for fatal plus non-fatal in the six trials.

in the elderly. In this study and in the MRC trial of treatment of older patients the reduction in coronary events appeared to be linked to therapy with a diuretic-based regimen. Whether there are indeed benefits in terms of reduced coronary events due to diuretics as opposed to beta-blocker regimens remains uncertain.

Although in earlier trials little benefit was seen in patients over 80 years of age, there now appears to be preliminary evidence of benefits in the older elderly (up to 84 years).

Benefits of treatment

The absolute benefits of active treatment of hypertension in reducing the incidence of cardiovascular events are difficult to determine from the trials. It is often stated, for example, based on the MRC trial report (MRC Working Party, 1985) that 850 mild hypertensive patients must be treated for one year to prevent one stroke. This estimate may grossly underestimate the benefits of treatment to ordinary hypertensives (Simpson, 1990) for the following reasons. First, the ranges of blood pressure entry criteria in the MRC and Australian trials were 90–109 mmHg and 95–109 mmHg with mean entry levels of 98 and 100.4 mmHg respectively. However, 'actual' mean blood pressures (those recorded a few weeks post randomization and on placebo) were 91 and 93 mmHg. Presumably the benefits observed in the trials therefore relate to these lower actual blood pressure levels, and thus underestimate benefits which would accrue from lowering blood pressures which are genuinely as high as 98 and 100.4 mmHg, Secondly, the mortality rates in the controls in the MRC and Australian trials were low, in part because of the study exclusion criteria and the healthy volunteer effect, and because most of the volunteers were middle-class patients, who generally enjoy better cardiovascular health. Third, the intention to treat analyses make no allowance for the effects of controls receiving active antihypertensive medication. This inevitably leads to an under-estimate of benefit. Furthermore, because treatment is more likely to be initiated in those controls with highest blood pressures (and hence at greatest risk) and those who stop active treatment are likely to be at least risk by virtue of their blood pressure levels, 'on treatment' analyses do not solve all these problems.

Fourth, because inflexible drug regimens, often using high dosages, are inevitably followed in trials, side-effects are likely to be more prevalent and severe (with implications for compliance) than in everyday clinical practice.

Trial data have also shown that, if left untreated, a significant number of mild hypertensives become moderate hypertensives in a relatively short time, demonstrating the clear benefits of treatment in preventing the progression of hypertension.

These considerations have not usually been incorporated into the often quoted evaluation of benefits in the treatment of mild hypertension but need to be borne in mind in considering the introduction of therapy for patients potentially at risk from hypertension-related CVD.

What of the future? There are two important questions that remain unanswered. Are there genuine differences in outcome dependent on the particular drug used to lower blood pressure? And is the shortfall in coronary prevention due to the overriding effect of cholesterol as a risk factor for coronary artery disease in hypertensive patients?

Two major national organizations are currently addressing these questions and planning large-scale intervention trials which, it is hoped, will resolve these critical issues.

References

Amery A *et al*. (1985) Mortality and morbidity results from the European working party on high blood pressure in the elderly trial. *The Lancet*. i:1349–54.

Australian National Blood Pressure Management Committee (1980) The Australian therapeutic trial in mild hypertension. *The Lancet*. i:1261–7.

Collins R *et al*. (1990) Blood pressure, stroke, and coronary heart disease. Part 2, Short-term reductions in blood pressure: overview of randomised drug trials in their epidemiological context. *The Lancet*. 335:827–38.

Coope J and Warrender TS (1986) Randomised trial of treatment of hypertension in elderly patients in primary care. *British Medical Journal*. 293:1145–51.

Dahlof B *et al*. (1991) Morbidity and mortality in the Swedish Trial in Old Patients with Hypertension (STOP-hypertension). *The Lancet*. 338:1281–5.

Harrison M *et al*. (1959) Results of treatment in malignant hypertension. A seven-year experience in 94 cases. *British Medical Journal*. 2:969–80.

HDFP Cooperative Group (1979) Five-year findings of the Hypertension Detection and Follow-up Program. I. Reduction in mortality in persons with high blood pressure, including mild hypertension. *Journal of the American Medical Association*. 242:2562–71.

HDFP Cooperative Group (1982) The effect of treatment on mortality in 'mild' hypertension. *New England Journal of Medicine*. 307:976–80.

IPPPSH Collaborative Group (1985). Cardiovascular risk and risk factors in a randomised trial of treatment based on the beta–blocker oxprenolol. *Journal of Hypertension*. 3:379–92.

Keith NM *et al*. (1939) Some different types of essential hypertension; their course and prognosis. *American Journal of Medical Science*. 197:332–43.

MacMahon S *et al.* (1990) Blood pressure, stroke, and coronary heart disease: part 1. Prolonged differences in blood pressure: prospective observational studies corrected for the regression dilution bias. *The Lancet.* **335**:765–74.

MRC Working Party (1985) MRC trial of treatment of mild hypertension: principal results. *British Medical Journal.* **291**:97–104.

MRC Working Party (1992) MRC treatment trial of hypertension in older adults: principal results. *British Medical Journal.* **304**:405–12.

MRFIT Research Group (1982) Multiple Risk Factor Intervention Trial: risk factor changes and mortality results. *Journal of the American Medical Association.* **248**:1465–77.

Report by the Management Committee (1981) Treatment of mild hypertension in the elderly. *Medical Journal of Australia.* **2**:398–402.

SHEP Cooperative Research Group (1991) Prevention of stroke by antihypertensive drug treatment in older persons with isolated systolic hypertension. *Journal of the American Medical Association.* **265**:3255–64.

Simpson FO (1990) Fallacies in the interpretation of the large-scale trials of treatment of mild to moderate hypertension. *Journal of Cardiovascular Pharmacology.* **16** (suppl. 7):592–5.

Veterans' Administration Cooperative Study Group on Antihypertensive Agents (1967) Effects of treatment on morbidity in hypertension: results in patients with diastolic pressures averaging 115–129 mmHg. *Journal of the American Medical Association.* **202**:116–22.

Veterans' Administration Cooperative Study Group on Antihypertensive Agents (1970) Effects of treatment on morbidity in hypertension: II. Results in patients with diastolic blood pressure averaging 90 through 114 mmHg. *Journal of the American Medical Association.* **213**:1143–92.

Wikstrand J *et al.* (1988) Primary prevention with metoprolol in patients with hypertension. *Journal of the American Medical Association.* **259**:1976–82.

Wilhelmson L *et al.* (1987) Beta-blockers versus diuretics in hypertensive men: main results from the HAPPHY Trial. *Journal of Hypertension.* **5**:561–74.

29

Hypertension in the Elderly: A Modifiable Risk Factor

JOHN P COX, EOIN O'BRIEN AND KEVIN O'MALLEY

Cardiovascular diseases, notably ischaemic heart disease and cerebrovascular disease, account for the majority of deaths in the elderly. Consequently, prevention of cardiovascular disease (CVD) and its sequelae has become an important priority in the medical care of the elderly (Karvonen, 1988). The main modifiable risk factors for these diseases are hypertension, smoking, hyperlipidaemia and hyperglycaemia. Of these, hypertension has emerged as one of the more important predictors of CVD in the elderly (Kannel and Gordon, 1978).

That blood pressure rises with age has been demonstrated in a number of studies (Amery *et al.*, 1991*a*). Diastolic pressure gradually rises with age in men and women up to the age of 50 years, after which it levels off until after the age of 60, when it falls, while systolic pressure continues to rise until after the age of 70 (Kannel and Gordon, 1978 (Figure 29.1). Thus the prevalence of isolated systolic hypertension (ie where the systolic pressure is elevated in the presence of a normal or low diastolic pressure) increases with age (Kannel *et al.*, 1980) (Figure 29.2).

Insurance studies show a positive relationship between mortality and both systolic and diastolic blood pressure at every age and every level of blood pressure (Law, 1973; Society of Actuaries and Association of Life Insurance Medical Directors of America, 1980). These findings have been confirmed in community based prospective studies (Kannel and Gordon, 1978; Miall and Brennan, 1981). In the Framingham Study the risk of CVD tripled in elderly hypertensive patients (age 65–74) compared with normotensive subjects (Kannel and Gordon, 1978).

Isolated systolic hypertension

Systolic pressure has been shown to be a better predictor of cardiovascular mortality in the elderly than diastolic pressure (Miall, 1982). Moreover, isolated systolic hypertension, variously defined as systolic pressure equal to or greater than 160 mmHg where diastolic pressure is less than 95 mmHg (Dyer *et al.*, 1977) or 90 mmHg (Joint National Committee on Detection, Evaluation and Treatment of High Blood Pressure, 1984), has been shown to be associated with an excess cardiovascular mortality in studies in the elderly where such

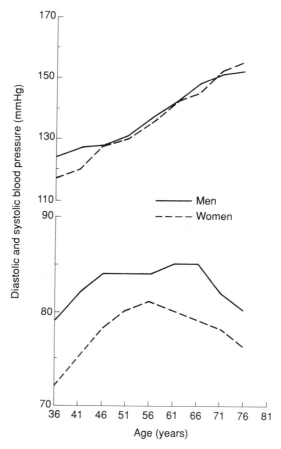

Figure 29.1: Average age trends in blood pressure levels for men and women, based on cohort data on participants in the Framingham Study. (Redrawn from Kannel and Gordon, 1978.)

patients have been specifically identified (Colandrea *et al.*, 1970; Shekelle *et al.*, 1974; Kannel *et al.*, 1980; Forette *et al.*, 1982). In the Framingham Study isolated systolic hypertension (systolic pressure 160 mmHg or greater and diastolic pressure less than 95 mmHg) was associated with a twofold to fivefold greater risk of death from all causes and from CVD in particular, with the risk increasing as steeply in the elderly as in the middle-aged patients studied (Kannel *et al.*, 1980). These data would indicate that isolated systolic hypertension is an important clinical finding in the elderly patient.

Impact of treatment

The results of five major trials of the effects of drug treatment on outcome in elderly patients with hypertension have been reported since 1985. These

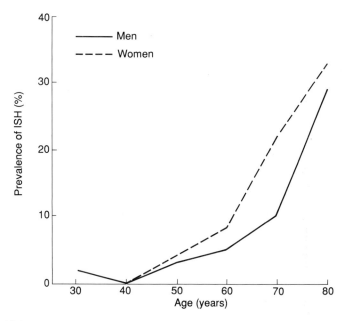

Figure 29.2: Prevalence of isolated systolic hypertension (ISH) by age and sex in 24-year follow-up the Framingham study. (Reproduced from Kannel *et al.*, 1980.)

include the European Working Party on High Blood Pressure in the Elderly (EWPHE) trial (Amery *et al.*, 1985), the Hypertension Trial in Elderly Patients in Primary Care (HEP) (Coope and Warrender, 1986), the Medical Research Council (MRC) trial of treatment of hypertension in older adults (MRC Working Party, 1992), the Systolic Hypertension in the Elderly Program (SHEP) (SHEP Cooperative Research Group, 1991) and the Swedish Trial in Old Patients with Hypertension (STOP-Hypertension) (Dahlof *et al.*, 1991). These studies provide important information on different aspects of the management of elderly patients with hypertension and their findings will be discussed in some detail.

The EWPHE trial was a randomized double-blind placebo-controlled study conducted in patients over the age of 60 (Amery *et al.*, 1985). Entry criteria included both a sitting diastolic blood pressure on placebo treatment in the range 90–119 mmHg and a systolic pressure in the range 160–239 mmHg. Active treatment was with a diuretic (hydrochlorothiazide and triamterine) with methyldopa added if needed for control of blood pressure. The principal findings in this study were a 38% decrease in cardiovascular mortality and a 60% reduction in cardiovascular morbid events in the actively treated group.

In the HEP trial patients aged 60–79 years were randomized to receive active treatment (principally with atenolol and bendrofluazide) or no treatment (Coope and Warrender, 1986). Patients with systolic blood pressure 170 mmHg or above (but less than 280 mmHg) or diastolic pressure 105 mmHg or above (but less than 120 mmHg) were included. In this study, the incidence of fatal stroke was decreased 30% and fatal and non-fatal stroke by 58% with active treatment.

Both of these landmark studies showed a similar beneficial effect on stroke incidence with drug treatment of hypertension. However, apart from a reduction in deaths from myocardial infarction (MI) in the EWPHE trial, neither study showed any reduction in incidence of coronary heart disease (CHD) events with treatment. These findings are similar to those of the major studies carried out in younger patients with mild to moderate hypertension where again the main benefits with treatment were from a reduction in strokes with little effect on CHD events.

Diuretics and outcome

In the MRC trial, a diuretic and beta-blocker were compared (MRC Working Party, 1992). In a single-blind trial, 4396 patients aged 65–74 years with systolic pressures of 160–209 mmHg and mean diastolic blood pressures less than 115 mmHg were randomized to treatment with a diuretic (hydrochlorothiazide 25 mg or 50 mg plus amiloride 2.5 mg or 5 mg daily), a beta-blocker (atenolol 50 mg), or placebo. Mean follow-up was 5.8 years. Compared with the placebo group, actively treated patients had significant reductions in stroke (25%) and all cardiovascular events (17%), findings which were similar to those of the EWPHE and HEP trials. An important finding in this study was that after adjusting for base-line characteristics, the diuretic group had significantly reduced risks of stroke (31%, mainly in non-smokers), coronary events (44%), and all cardiovascular events (35%) compared to those on placebo while the beta-blocker group showed no significant reduction in these end points.

The observed differences between diuretics and beta-blockers in preventing cardiovascular morbidity and mortality in the MRC trial are of interest. These stem primarily from the apparent effectiveness of the diuretic in reducing coronary events and deaths and are contrary to expectations as diuretics have adverse metabolic effects with the potential to negate the beneficial effects of blood pressure reduction on cardiovascular morbidity and mortality.

Increases in lipid levels, primarily in the athrogenic, low-density lipoprotein fraction are associated with diuretic therapy (Weinberger, 1985). However, in the MRC trial, the increases in total cholesterol concentration averaged over the period from three months after entry to the end of follow up were identical and small (0.1 mmol/l) in all three randomized groups. Of greater importance is the fact that the diuretic group experienced a more rapid and greater control of blood pressure compared with the beta-blocker group, and this may have contributed to the differences in effectiveness with regard to coronary events. These findings, therefore, go some way to dispel fears that the metabolic effects of thiazide diuretic treatment attenuate the benefit of blood pressure reduction.

Left ventricular hypertrophy, defined by electrocardiographic (ECG) (Levy, 1988) and echocardiographic criteria (Levy et al., 1990), was an independent predictor of excess risk of cardiovascular mortality and morbidity in elderly subjects in the Framingham Study. While regression in left ventricular hyper-

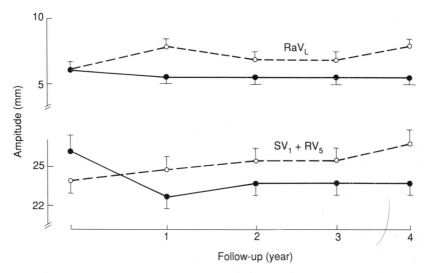

*P < 0.05, **P < 0.01, between placebo and treated patients.

Figure 29.3: Mean (±SE) amplitude of RaV_L and SV1 + RV5 before and after treatment in a four-year cohort of 106 placebo patients (open circles) and 116 treated patients (closed circles). (Reproduced from Van Hoof, 1991.)

trophy after administration of some antihypertensive drugs has been demonstrated in hypertensive patients (Poblete *et al.*, 1973), this has not been the case with thiazide diuretics (Tarazi and Fouad, 1984). However, in a four-year cohort of 222 patients in the EWPHE trial, left ventricular size (as indicated by ECG voltage criteria) was significantly less in the treated than the placebo group (Van Hoof, 1991) (Figure 29.3). The type of treatment (diuretics alone or diuretics plus methyldopa) did not affect ECG voltages. While these findings require confirmation in studies with a larger number of patients, the present evidence augurs well for the use of these agents in this group.

Management of isolated systolic hypertension

The effectiveness of drug treatment in the management of isolated systolic hypertension in the elderly has been addressed in four studies to date. In one of these, the HEP trial, treatment did not significantly reduce death rate in the 23% of patients with isolated systolic hypertension (Coope and Warrender, 1986). In an analysis of data on 247 patients in the EWPHE study with isolated systolic hypertension, while treatment improved cardiovascular mortality and morbidity rates, the difference did not reach statistical significance as the number of patients was insufficient (O'Malley *et al.*, 1988).

In SHEP, 4736 subjects aged 60 years or more with systolic blood pressure between 160 and 219 mmHg and diastolic pressure less than 90 mmHg were randomized to active treatment with low-dose thiazide (chlorthalidone 12.5–25 mg daily) with the addition, if necessary, of atenolol 25–50 mg daily or to treatment with placebo (SHEP Cooperative Research Group, 1991). Patients were followed for an average of 4.5 years. Treatment significantly reduced the incidence of stroke by 36% and of all cardiovascular events by 32%. However, total cardiovascular mortality and deaths from all causes were not significantly reduced.

SHEP demonstrated significant efficacy of active hypertensive drug treatment in preventing stroke in persons aged 60 years and older with isolated systolic hypertension. Moreover, these latter findings were confirmed in the MRC trial (MRC Working Party, 1992), where 45% of patients had a systolic blood pressure between 160 and 219 mmHg and diastolic pressure less than 90 mmHg. While SHEP can be regarded as a landmark study in the management of isolated systolic hypertension in the elderly, these findings should be confirmed or refuted independently in a separate population. We also need further information on the role of the newer compounds, including the calcium antagonists and angiotensin-converting enzyme inhibitors, in the management of this form of hypertension. These issues will be addressed in the Syst-Eur study, a multicentre trial designed by the European Working Party on High Blood Pressure in the Elderly to test the hypothesis that antihypertensive treatment in patients aged 60 or over with isolated systolic hypertension (systolic blood pressure 160–219 mmHg and diastolic pressure less than 95 mmHg), reduces morbidity and mortality from stroke (Amery *et al.*, 1991). In this study, patients are randomized to receive either treatment with nitrendipine, enalapril and hydrochlorothiazide added in a stepwise fashion until systolic blood pressure is controlled, or treatment with matching placebo tablets. Patients will be followed up for five years.

Is there an upper age limit for treatment?

The upper age limit for the drug treatment of hypertension has long been a controversial issue. No benefit could be demonstrated with treatment in patients over the age of 80 years in the EWPHE trial (Amery *et al.*, 1986), although benefits were apparent for this group in SHEP (SHEP Cooperative Research Group, 1991). STOP-Hypertension examined the treatment of diastolic hypertension in the 'very elderly' in a double-blind trial where 1627 patients aged 70–84 years with diastolic blood pressure of at least 90 mmHg were randomized to active treatment with a thiazide diuretic or a beta-blocker, or to placebo, and were followed up for a mean of 25 months (Dahlof *et al.*, 1991). Active treatment was associated with a significant decrease in the incidence of stroke (47%), all cardiovascular events (40%) and total mortality (43%). While STOP-Hypertension confirmed that persistant diastolic hypertension in elderly patients should be treated, and this effect was observed into the ninth decade, these findings only applied to those with relatively severe combined systolic and diastolic hypertension.

Can the elderly hypertensive be overtreated?

Hitherto there has been little evidence to suggest that sustained reduction in blood pressure to normotensive levels with drug therapy is in any way harmful in the elderly. A U-shaped relationship between risk of MI and treated blood pressure has been described in some intervention studies (Cruickshank *et al.*, 1987; Samuelsson *et al.*, 1987). However, data from the HEP trial showed this effect in both the treated and untreated elderly patients (Coope and Warrender, 1987). Moreover, in the EWPHE trial while there was an inverse relationship between mortality and treated diastolic pressure in the actively treated group, there was also a U-shaped relationship between mortality and diastolic pressure in patients taking placebo (Staessen *et al.*, 1989). These findings suggest that the increased mortality in the lower thirds of the actively treated patients in this study may not have been drug induced. Instead, this could possibly have been the expression of a deterioration in general health as suggested by the decreases in body weight and haemoglobin concentration. Thus the relationship between diastolic pressure and mortality is more complex than a linear increase with rising pressure. While it is premature to conclude on the basis of present evidence that reducing blood pressure to the lower part of the normal range is harmful in older patients, it would appear prudent, nonetheless, not to lower blood pressure below 140/80 mmHg with treatment in this group.

Conclusions

Hypertension in elderly patients is a major risk factor for CVD. The main benefit with treatment is a reduction in strokes, a finding which is similar to that of studies carried out in younger patients. Contrary to expectations, diuretics have been shown to be particularly effective in reducing the complications of hypertension in this age group. Active hypertensive drug treatment is also effective in preventing stroke in persons aged 60 years and older with isolated systolic hypertension. However, there is insufficient evidence to recommend starting treatment over the age of 80 unless the blood pressure is greatly raised or complications such as congestive heart failure or angina are present. Finally, while it is premature to conclude on the basis of present evidence that reducing blood pressure to the lower part of the normal range is harmful in older patients, it would appear prudent not to lower blood pressure below 140/80 mmHg with treatment in this group.

References

Amery A *et al.* (1985) Mortality and morbidity results from the European Working Party on High Blood Pressure in the Elderly Trial. *The Lancet.* **i**:1349–54.

Amery A *et al.* (1986) Efficacy of antihypertensive drug treatment according to age, sex, blood pressure, and previous cardiovascular disease in patients over the age of 60. *The Lancet.* **ii**:589–92.

Amery A *et al.* (1991*a*) Isolated systolic hypertension in the elderly: an epidemiologic review. *American Journal of Medicine.* **90** (Suppl. 3A):64–95.

Amery A *et al.* (1991*b*) Syst-Eur. A multicentre trial on the treatment of isolated systolic hypertension in the elderly: objectives, protocol and organisation. *Ageing.* 3:287–302.

Colandrea MA *et al.* (1970). Systolic hypertension in the elderly. An epidemiologic assessment. *Circulation.* **41**:239–45.

Coope J and Warrender TS (1986) Randomised trial of treatment of hypertension in elderly patients in primary care. *British Medical Journal.* **293**:1143–8.

Coope J and Warrender TS (1987) Lowering blood pressure. *The Lancet.* **ii**:518.

Cruickshank JM *et al.* (1987) Benefits and potential harm of lowering high blood pressure. *The Lancet.* **i**:581–4.

Dahlof B *et al.* (1991) Morbidity and mortality in the Swedish Trial in Old Patients with Hypertension (STOP-Hypertension). *The Lancet.* **338**:1281–5.

Dyer AR *et al.* (1977) Hypertension in the elderly. *Medical Clinics of North America.* **61** (3):513–29.

Forette F *et al.* (1982) The prognostic significance of isolated systolic hypertension in the elderly. Results of a ten year longitudinal survey. *Clinical and Experimental Hypertension—Theory and Practice.* **A4**:117–91.

Joint National Committee on Detection, Evaluation and Treatment of High Blood Pressure (1984) *Archives of Internal Medicine.* **144**:1045–57.

Kannel WB and Gordon T (1978) Evaluation of cardiovascular risk in the elderly: the Framingham Study. *Bulletin of the New York Academy of Medicine.* **54**:573–91.

Kannel WB *et al.* (1980) Perspective in systolic hypertension: the Framingham Study. *Circulation.* **61**:1179–82.

Karvonen MJ (1988) Prevention of cardiovascular disease among the elderly. *Bulletin of the World Health Organization.* **66**:7–14.

Levy D (1988) Left ventricular hypertrophy: epidemiological insights from the Framingham study. *Drugs.* **35** (Suppl. 5):1–5.

Levy D *et al.* (1990) Prognostic implications of echocardiographically determined left ventricular mass in the Framingham Heart Study. *New England Journal of Medicine.* **322**:1561–6.

Lew EA (1973) High blood pressure, other risk factors and longevity: the insurance viewpoint. *American Journal of Medicine.* **55**:281–94.

Miall WE and Brennan PJ (1981) Hypertension in the elderly: the South Wales Study. In: *Hypertension in the young and old.* Grune and Stratton, New York. pp. 227–83.

Miall WE (1982) Systolic or diastolic hypertension—which matters most? *Clinical and Experimental Hypertension—Theory and Practice.* A4:1121–31.

MRC Working Party (1992) Medical Research Council trial of treatment of hypertension in older adults: principal results. *British Medical Journal.* **304**:405–12.

O'Malley K *et al.* (1988) Isolated systolic hypertension: data from the European Working Party on Hypertension in the Elderly. *Journal of Hypertension.* **6** (Suppl. 1):S105–8.

Poblete PF *et al.* (1973) Effect of treatment on morbidity in hypertension. Veterans' Administration Cooperative Study on Antihypertensive Agents: effect on the electrocardiogram. *Circulation.* **48**:481–90.

Samuelsson O *et al.* (1987) Cardiovascular morbidity in relation to changes in blood pressure and serum cholesterol levels in treated hypertension: results from the Primary Prevention Trial in Goteborg, Sweden. *Journal of the American Medical Association.* **258**:1768–76.

Shekelle RB *et al.* (1974) Hypertension and risk of stroke in an elderly population. *Stroke.* **5**:71–5.

SHEP Cooperative Research Group (1991) Prevention of stroke by antihypertensive drug treatment in older persons with isolated systolic hypertension. Final results of the systolic hypertension in the elderly program (SHEP). *Journal of the American Medical Association.* **265**:3255–64.

Society of Actuaries and Association of Life Insurance Medical Directors of America (1980) *Blood Pressure Study 1979.* p 197.

Staessen J *et al.* (1989) Relation between mortality and treated blood pressure in elderly patients with hypertension: report of the European Working Party on High Blood Pressure in the Elderly. *British Medical Journal.* **298**:1552–6.

Tarazi RC and Fouad FM (1984) Reversal of cardiac hypertrophy in humans. *Hypertension.* **6** (Suppl. II):140–9.

Van Hoof R (1991) Left ventricular hypertrophy in elderly hypertensive patients: a report from the European Working Party on High Blood Pressure in the Elderly trial. *American Journal of Medicine.* **90** (Suppl. 3A):155–9S.

Weinberger M (1985) Antihypertensive therapy and lipids: evidence, mechanisms and implications. *Archives of Internal Medicine.* **145**:1102–5.

30

Drug Treatment of the Elderly Hypertensive Patient

MJ KENDALL

Three recent trials have demonstrated the benefits of blood pressure reduction in elderly patients (Dahlof *et al.*, 1991; SHEP Cooperative Research Group, 1991; MRC Working Party 1992), confirming the results of earlier studies (Amery *et al.*, 1985; Coope and Warrender, 1986). The impact in this relatively high-risk group of patients is far greater than in younger patients with hypertension. However, care is required in extrapolating results obtained on selected patients admitted to clinical trials, to the general population: and this is particularly true in relation to observations in the management of the elderly. It is now necessary (1) to consider the problems posed when planning any form of drug treatment for elderly individuals, and (2) to review the data from the recent trials and to derive information about the patient population, their cardiovascular risk profile and their response to the treatments given. Thereafter it should be possible to suggest a therapeutic strategy for the drug treatment of elderly hypertensive patients.

Drug treatment of the elderly

Elderly subjects are not only older but they are more likely to suffer from coexisting disorders, and therefore to be on other drugs, than younger groups of patients. The influence of many diseases and of some forms of drug therapy may be far greater than the effects of age itself.

Advancing age

It is possible to conclude that body structures and functions decline with the passing of the years. However, this view is not only gloomy but also oversimplistic and untrue. The capacity to absorb (Kendall, 1970), distribute (Crooks, 1983) and metabolize (Kendall *et al.*, 1981; Rooney *et al.*, 1985) drugs is not materially affected by advancing age. Unfortunately mental function and renal function do deteriorate. The older person is less likely to take their medication regularly (Report of the Royal College of Physicians, 1984), they are less able to eliminate renally excreted drugs (Mawer *et al.*, 1974; Wilkinson, 1983), and they tolerate drugs which impair cerebral functions less well (Castleden *et al.*, 1977). Of these, it is the compliance problem which is most relevant in relation to the treatment of hypertension. When poor eyesight, hearing and manual dexterity are added to memory loss, it is likely that the tablets will not be taken regularly. The situation is made much worse if the patient is already taking a number of other drugs. Thus the advice when treating many elderly patients is keep the treatment as simple as possible and reduce rather than increase the number of different tablets to be taken.

Coexisting disease

There is an extensive literature on the effects that various diseases may have on drug handling in the body (pharmacokinetics) and on the body's response to therapy (pharmacodynamics). When considering the elderly hypertensive, coexisting disease will influence both the decision to treat and the choice of therapy.

When making a decision about treating an elderly hypertensive patient it may be helpful to subdivide the patient population quite arbitrarily into three groups (Table 30.1). The sick elderly, first of all, are those with a poor quality of life and those with a bad prognosis. For these, antihypertensive therapy is almost always inappropriate. They include patients with dementia, malignant disease, other life-threatening disorders such as severe bronchitis and emphysema and those incapacitated by cerebrovascular disease, arthritis or other major disabilities. Secondly, the medically complicated elderly are a large group who may have a reasonable quality of life but who suffer from one of the many disorders common in this age group some of which are listed in the table. In some instances the severity of the coexisting disease or the number of coexisting disorders may argue against making the therapeutic regimen more complicated and may cast doubt on the wisdom of adding long-term disease prevention to measures directed towards severe current medical problems. If a decision is made to treat a patient in this group then the coexisting disease or diseases will

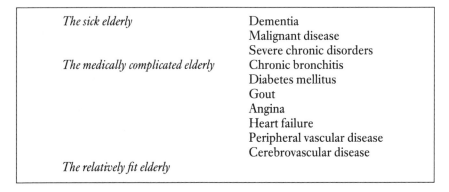

The sick elderly	Dementia
	Malignant disease
	Severe chronic disorders
The medically complicated elderly	Chronic bronchitis
	Diabetes mellitus
	Gout
	Angina
	Heart failure
	Peripheral vascular disease
	Cerebrovascular disease
The relatively fit elderly	

Table 30.1: Subgroups of elderly hypertensives and their diseases.

| Disease | Drugs | |
	Best avoided	Useful
Chronic bronchitis	Beta blockers*	
Diabetes mellitus	Thiazide diuretics	? ACE inhibitors
	Beta blockers*	Alpha blockers
Gout	Thiazide diuretics	
Angina		Calcium antagonists
		Beta-blockers
Heart failure	Beta blockers	ACE inhibitors
		Thiazide diuretics
Peripheral vascular disease	Beta blockers*	? ACE inhibitors
		? Calcium antagonists
Cerebrovascular disease	Alpha blockers†	
	ACE inhibitors†	

* B$_1$ selective beta-blockers may be acceptable
? theoretically beneficial rather than of proven value
† drugs which may cause postural hypotension and falls in cerebral blood flow

Table 30.2: Possible effects of coexisting diseases on choices of antihypertensive therapy.

probably have an influence on the choice of antihypertensive therapy (Table 30.2).

The third group are those relatively fit elderly subjects and it is from this section of the hypertensive population that most of the participants in clinical trials are chosen. Their treatment can therefore be planned in the light of recent trials (Dahlof *et al.*, 1991; SHEP Cooperative Research Group, 1991; MRC Working Party, 1992).

Concomitant therapy

Although having less influence than coexisting disease, the patients' present drug treatment may influence the decision to treat and the choice of therapy. Many elderly individuals take non-steroidal anti-inflammatory drugs for their aches, pains and arthritis. These cause fluid retention and it may be worth trying to replace them with simple analgesics before starting any antihypertensive therapy. Many other potential interactions could be cited. However, the patients' treatment should be reviewed to determine the possible impact of adding additional therapy. A patient on three different drugs may already be having difficulty in taking the right dose at the right time. The addition of a fourth treatment may cause other drugs such as anticoagulants, anticonvulsants or antidiabetic agents to be omitted or taken in overdose with more serious consequences than failing to control mildly raised blood pressure.

Recent trials

As stated above, the patients in trials are a select group. In the SHEP study (SHEP Cooperative Research Group, 1991), 447 921 individuals over 60 years of age were contacted, 11.6% met the inclusion criteria and about 1% of the original group and less than 10% of those initially considered suitable were entered. Females predominated in the trial subjects amounting to 57% in SHEP (SHEP Cooperative Research Group, 1991), 63% in STOP (Dahlof *et al.*, 1991) and 58.2% in the MRC trial (MRC Working Party, 1992).

Tables 30.3–30.5 present the results in an abridged form. They show that strokes are the most common non-fatal event in the elderly and that the treatment dramatically reduces the incidence. Secondly, coronary events including myocardial infarction and sudden death are the most frequent fatal cardiovascular events. Further, sudden and rapid deaths accounted for 91 of the 202 deaths from cardiovascular diseases in the SHEP trial (SHEP Cooperative Research Group, 1991) and 16 of the 58 cardiovascular deaths in the STOP trial (Dahlof *et al.*, 1991). Data on sudden deaths are not given in the MRC trial (MRC Working Party, 1992). In all three trials the incidence of coronary events was lower in the treated groups, but the impact of thiazide treatment in the SHEP trial on sudden and rapid deaths was negligible whilst in the STOP trial—in which beta-blockers and diuretics were used—treatment did reduce the number of sudden deaths.

Plans for treating elderly hypertensives

The sick elderly

In spite of the undeniable benefits of blood pressure reduction, some elderly patients should not be given any antihypertensive therapy. Their prognosis,

	Active therapy	Placebo
Non-fatal events		
Cerebrovascular disease		
Stroke	96	149
TIA	62	82
Total	158	231
Myocardial infarction	50	74
Fatal events		
Stroke	10	14
Coronary artery disease (Total)	59	73
Death within 24 hours	44	47

Table 30.3: Mortality and morbidity in the SHEP trial. Active treatment was chlorthalidone with atenolol added if needed. (Source: SHEP Cooperative Research Group, 1991.)

	Active therapy	Placebo
Non-fatal events		
Stroke	26	41
Myocardial infarction	22	22
Fatal events		
Stroke	4	15
Myocardial infarction	6	8
Sudden death	4	12

Table 30.4: Mortality and morbidity in the STOP Trial. Active treatment was a beta-blocker (atenolol, metoprolol or pindolol) or a thiazide diuretic. (Source: Dahlof *et al.*, 1991.)

	Active therapy	Placebo
Non-fatal events		
Stroke	64	92
Coronary event	43	49
Fatal events		
Stroke	37	42
Myocardial infarction	85	110

Table 30.5: Mortality and morbidity in the MRC (Elderly) Trial. Two active treatment groups (1) atenolol and (2) thiazide diuretic. (Source: MRC Working Party, 1992.)

their quality of life, their other medical problems and the complexity of their current therapy all argue against treating their blood pressure.

The medically complicated elderly

The medically complicated elderly are a large group and many should be offered therapy. Compared with younger hypertensives the frequency with which their other medical problems influence the choice of drug will be very great. In addition, because they are old and have other problems, their treatment regimen should be simple; the risk of adding to their problems by offering drugs which tend to cause side-effects should be minimized, and the consequences of giving a renally excreted drug—particularly one that is long-acting—need to be considered. It is clear that there is no ideal drug, but certain observations can be made.

- Thiazide diuretics and non-selective beta-blockers may be inadvisable in many patients in this group.
- Alpha blockers, the newer agents, should be well tolerated by most patients with coexisting diseases; however, the long-term benefits of improving

lipids have less appeal in the elderly and the short-term adverse effects may be a disadvantage.

- Calcium antagonists usually do not adversely affect coexisting disorders nor interact with other drugs, but the dihydropyridines cause headache and ankle oedema, and verapamil causes constipation. These are disadvantages.
- ACE inhibitors have the theoretical advantages of not adversely affecting other disorders and may have a positive impact in those with heart failure and diabetes. Most are excreted by the renal route and some are relatively long-acting, which are theoretical disadvantages.

From an economical and cost-effective standpoint a low-dose thiazide diuretic could be recommended in many cases. To obtain lower blood pressure with minimal risk of adversely affecting coexisting disorders, an ACE inhibitor (and preferably one which does not accumulate in the old) seems an attractive choice. However, when initiating treatment, to avoid falls and fainting due to first dose hypertension, the patient may need to be kept under observation. Patients with a history of transient ischaemic attacks or those who have recovered from a stroke may be at particular risk.

The fit elderly

The fit elderly group correspond fairly closely to the patients in the trials. Effective blood pressure reduction may be worthwhile up to the age of 84 years (Dahlof et al., 1991). A beneficial effect on fatal and non-fatal strokes can be expected and, based on experience from trials in younger patients, morbidity will improve irrespective of the antihypertensive drug used. However, as in middle-aged hypertensives, to reduce mortality one has to reduce deaths from ischaemic heart disease; and because of the numbers at risk, this means having a positive impact on sudden death (Kannel et al., 1988; Olsson et al., 1991). To date only beta-blockers can be claimed to have an impact on coronary mortality. Diuretics may have an effect (MRC Working Party, 1992); and as for alpha blockers, calcium antagonists and ACE inhibitors, there is inadequate evidence and almost no clinical data available.

Many do not accept that beta-blockers reduce coronary mortality, for two major reasons. First there is the assumption that all beta-blockers are the same. However, the data for lipophilic beta-blockers (metoprolol, timolol and propranolol) is favourable (Kendall and Wikstrand 1991; Kendall, 1992), whereas the data for hydrophilic beta blockers (atenolol, nadolol or satolol) are negative as in the recent MRC (Elderly) Trial (MRC Working Party, 1992), or the studies have not been performed. Lipophilic beta-blockers do have an impact on coronary occlusive disease (Spence et al., 1984; Kaplan et al., 1987) and do reduce the risk of ventricular fibrillation in animal models (Dellsperger et al., 1990; Parker et al., 1990; Ablad et al., 1991). Secondly, in primary prevention trials, the data have been confusing but males in the MRC trial (MRC Working Party, 1992), IPPPSH trial (IPPPSH Collaborative Group, 1985) and HAPPHY Trial (Wikstrand et al., 1988) did better with beta-blocker therapy.

However, the large number of post-infarct studies have shown that beta blockers reduce coronary mortality and sudden death convincingly. The results on timolol (Norwegian Multicentre Study Group, 1981), propanolol (Beta Blocker Heart Attack Trial Research Group, 1982) and metoprolol (Hjalmarson *et al.*, 1981) are well known but the recent overview of metoprolol trials showing a reduction in sudden death rates from 47% of all deaths during the follow-up period to 33% is less well known (Olsson *et al.*, 1992).

For the fit elderly hypertensive, it appears likely that any antihypertensive will reduce the risk of stroke. Thiazide diuretics are not only the simplest and cheapest drugs but also those for which there is good clinical data. However, if the aim is not only to reduce the risk of major disability but to prolong life, then the drug most likely to achieve this is a lipophilic beta-blocker. Although there is a belief that these drugs will be badly tolerated in the elderly, clinical trials do not support this belief (Wilkins and Kendall, 1984; Wikstrand *et al.*, 1986); and in the STOP trial in which 80% of the patients received a beta-blocker, serious adverse effects and drop-outs were not a problem (Dahlof *et al.*, 1991).

Summary

Recent trials have demonstrated that hypertensive elderly patients may benefit from blood pressure reduction. This does not imply that all hypertensives should be treated and that all antihypertensive drugs are equally effective and equally well tolerated. Many elderly patients have serious illnesses and those with hypertension should not have it treated. Most of the other elderly hypertensives have coexisting disorders which will impose restrictions on the choice of drugs. For the fit elderly, the major cause of morbidity will be cerebrovascular disease and the risk of this can be reduced by blood pressure reduction by any antihypertensive regimen. To have a significant impact on mortality it is necessary to have an effect on coronary disease and to date probably only lipophilic beta-blockers could be claimed to do this. These agents are fairly well tolerated in the old, and particularly so if low-dose regimens or slow-release preparations are used.

References

Amery A *et al.* (1985) Mortality and morbidity results from the European Working Party on high blood pressure in the elderly. *The Lancet.* i:1349–54.

Ablad B *et al.* (1991) Role of central nervous beta adrenoceptors in the prevention of ventricular fibrillation through augmentation of vagal tone (Abstract). American College of Cardiology 40th Annual Scientific Session March 3–7. *Journal of the American College of Cardiology.* 17:165A.

Beta Blocker Heart Attack Trial Research Group (1982) A randomized trial of propranolol in patients with acute myocardial infarction. *Journal of the American Medical Association.* **247**:1707–14.

Castleden CM *et al.* (1977) Increased sensitivity to nitrazepam in old age. *British Medical Journal.* **1**:10–12.

Coope J and Warrender TS (1986) Randomised trial of treatment of hypertension in the elderly in primary care. *British Medical Journal.* **293**:1145–51.

Crooks J (1983) Ageing and drug disposition—pharmacodynamics. *Journal of Chronic Diseases.* **36**:85–90.

Dahlof B *et al.* (1991) Morbidity and mortality in the Swedish Trial in Old Patients with Hypertension (STOP-Hypertension). *The Lancet.* **338**:1281–5.

Dellsperger KC *et al.* (1990) Incidence of sudden cardiac death associated with sudden coronary artery occlusion in dogs with hypertension and left ventricular hypertrophy is reduced by chronic beta adrenergic blockade. *Circulation.* **82**:941–50.

Hjalmarson A *et al.* (1981) Effect on mortality of metoprolol in acute myocardial infarction. *The Lancet.* **II**:823–7.

IPPPSH Collaborative Group (1985) Cardiovascular risk and risk factors in a randomised trial of treatment based on the beta blocker exprenolol: the International Prospective Primary Prevention Study in Hypertension (IPPPSH). *Journal of Hypertension.* **3**:379–92.

Kannel WB *et al.* (1988) Hypertension, antihypertensive treatment and sudden coronary death: The Framingham Study. *Hypertension.* **11** (Suppl. II):45–50.

Kaplan J *et al.* (1987) Propranolol inhibits coronary atherosclerosis in behaviourally predisposed monkeys fed on atherogenic diets. *Circulation.* **76**:1364–72.

Kendall MJ (1970) The influence of age on the xylose absorption test. *Gut.* **11**:498–501.

Kendall MJ (1981) The effect of age on pharmacokinetics of metoprolol and its metabolites. *British Journal of Clinical Pharmacology.* **11**:287–94.

Kendall MJ and Wikstrand J (1991) Hypertension and coronary artery disease: impact of beta blockers. *Cardiovascular Risk Factors.* **1**:527–35.

Kendall MJ (1992) Treatment of hypertension in older adults. *British Medical Journal.* **304**:639.

MRC Working Party (1985) MRC trial of treatment of mild hypertension: principal results. *British Medical Journal.* **291**:97–104.

MRC Working Party (1992) Medical Research Council trial of treatment of hypertension in older adults: principal results. *British Medical Journal*. **304**: 405–12.

Mawer GE *et al.* (1974) Prescribing aids for gentamycin. *British Journal of Clinical Pharmacology*. 1:45–50.

Norwegian Multicentre Study Group (1981) Timolol-induced reduction in mortality and reinfarction in patients surviving acute myocardial infarction. *New England Journal of Medicine*. **304**:801–7.

Olsson G *et al.* (1991) Primary prevention of sudden cardiovascular death in hypertensive patients. *American Journal of Hypertension*. 4:151–8.

Olsson G *et al.* (1992) Metoprolol-induced reduction in postinfarction mortality: pooled results from five double-blind randomised trials. *European Heart Journal*. 13:28–32.

Parker GW *et al.* (1990) Central beta adrenergic mechanisms may modulate ischaemic ventricular fibrillation in pigs. *Circulation Research*. **66**:259–70.

Report of the Royal College of Physicians (1984) Medication for the elderly. *Journal of the Royal College of Physicians of London*. 18:7–17.

Rooney L *et al.* (1985) Pharmacokinetics of Pirprofen in young volunteers and elderly patients. *European Journal of Clinical Pharmacology*. **29**:73–7.

SHEP Cooperative Research Group (1991) Prevention of stroke by antihypertensive drug treatment in older persons with isolated systolic hypertension. *Journal of the American Medical Association*. **265**:3255–64.

Spence *et al.* (1984) Haemodynamic modifications of aortic atherosclerosis: effects of propranolol versus hydralazine in hypertensive hyperlipidaemic rabbits. *Atherosclerosis*. **50**:325–33.

Wikstrand J *et al.* (1986) Beta adrenoceptor blocking drugs and the elderly. *Journal of the American Medical Association*. **255**:1304–10.

Wikstrand J *et al.* (1988) Primary prevention with metoprolol in patients with hypertension. Mortality results from the HAPPHY study. *Journal of the American Medical Association*. **259**:1976–82.

Wilkins MR and Kendall MJ (1984) Beta adrenoceptor blocking drugs and the elderly. *Journal of the Royal College of Physicians of London*. 18:42–5.

Wilkinson GR (1983) Drug disposition and renal excretion in the elderly. *Journal of Chronic Diseases*. **36**:91–102.

31

Hypertension in Diabetes and Hyperlipidaemia

NEIL POULTER

'Tailored therapy' is now generally considered to be the ideal way to manage hypertension (Beevers *et al.*, 1991), having replaced stepped-care which was first introduced in 1977 (Joint National Committee, 1977). The essence of tailored therapy is to select the optimal drug compatible with the cardiovascular risk profile of the proposed recipient. Diabetes and hyperlipidaemia are two of the cardiovascular risk factors which are likely to influence drug management (Joint National Committee, 1988), and therefore serum glucose and lipid measurements should form part of the routine assessment of hypertensives.

Increasing evidence is accumulating that hypertension, dyslipidaemia and glucose intolerance appear to 'cluster' in individuals (Zavaroni *et al.*, 1987; McKeigue and Keen, 1992) and form part of the insulin resistance syndrome which is discussed extensively elsewhere in this book (*see* Chapters 5 and 6). In a study of Australian hypertensives, MacMahon and MacDonald (1986) demonstrated that mean serum total cholesterol levels and mean total/HDL ratios were higher in untreated hypertensives than normotensives. Further- more, a study of 2000 English hypertensives from 13 general practices (Poulter *et al.*, 1993) revealed that over 85% had a serum total cholesterol above the ideal level of 5.2 mmol/l, approximately 14% had levels above 7.8 mmol/l (the level above which lipid-lowering drug therapy is recommended), and 5.5% had diabetes.

Because of the high prevalence of hyperlipidaemia and diabetes in hyperten- sives (Poulter *et al.*, 1993) and, when they coexist, their interaction to increase greatly the risk of an adverse cardiovascular event, it is clearly important to pay particular attention to the management of these subgroups of hypertensives.

Hyperlipidaemia

Data from those screened for the Multiple Risk Factor Intervention Trial (MRFIT) (Stamler *et al.*, 1986) show that amongst those labelled 'hyperten- sives' (diastolic blood pressure $\geqslant 90$ mmHg), the effect of increasing levels of serum cholesterol on coronary heart disease (CHD) mortality over six years shows a clear dose-responsive effect irrespective of smoking status (Table 31.1). No trial data specifically on hypertensive hyperlipidaemics are available

Serum cholesterol quintile (mmol/l)	CHD death rates/100	
	DBP <90 mmHg	DBP ≥90 mmHg
Non-smokers		
1. <4.7	1.6	3.7
2. 4.7–5.2	2.5	4.0
3. 5.3–5.6	2.7	5.6
4. 5.7–6.3	3.8	5.6
5. ≥6.4	6.4	10.7
Smokers		
1. <4.7	5.2	6.3
2. 4.7–5.2	5.5	10.0
3. 5.3–5.6	7.3	15.5
4. 5.7–6.3	10.2	16.6
5. ≥6.4	13.3	21.4

Table 31.1: Six-year, age-adjusted CHD death rates by smoking, blood pressure and cholesterol status. MRFIT screenees ($N = 347923$).

to guide us in the optimal management of hypertension in these patients since hyperlipidaemia has usually been an exclusion criterion in the hypertension trials. However the Goteborg Primary Prevention Trial showed that: '*If serum cholesterol levels remained unchanged or even increased, the effect of BP reduction was small, whereas a substantial reduction in both risk factors produced a substantial reduction in cardiovascular disease and CHD morbidity*' (Samuelsson *et al.*, 1987). It would appear then, despite limited trial evidence specifically targeted at this subgroup of hypertensives, that efforts to improve lipid profiles in hypertensives could reasonably be recommended. A general consensus to do so is lacking, however, as evidenced by the non-pharmacological advice included in three recently produced sets of management guidelines from national and international bodies (Joint National Committee, 1988; British Hypertension Society Working Party, 1989; WHO/ISH, 1989). In 1988 the Joint National Committee in the USA routinely recommended reduced saturated fat intake. In 1989 the guidelines produced jointly by WHO and the International Society of Hypertension recommended reducing saturated fat intake if plasma lipids were 'high', but in the same year the British Hypertension Society made no mention of fats in their guidelines. However, in a revised version of the BHS guidelines to be published in 1993, lipid-lowering is likely to be recommended as part of a non-pharmacological 'package'.

With regard to the optimal drug choice for hypertensives with dyslipidaemia, results of a survey of 195 general practitioners (Feher and Lant, 1991) showed that in the presence of 'hyperlipidaemia' (undefined), 30% reported that they would adjust their first-line antihypertensive agents to use 'lipid-neutral' or

Drugs	Total cholesterol	LDL cholesterol	HDL cholesterol	Triglyceride
Thiazides	↑	↑	—	↑
Beta-blockers	—	— ↓ ↑	↓	↑
α_1 inhibitors	↓	↓	↑	↓
ACE inhibitors	—	—	—	—
Ca antagonists	—	—	—	—

Table 31.2: Summary of effects of antihypertensive drugs on serum lipid profile. (↑ increase; ↓ decrease; — no change.)

'lipid-friendly' agents rather than diuretics or beta-blockers. The question as to what level of 'hyperlipidaemia' would precipitate such a change in drug choice remains unanswered.

The theoretical reasons for choosing 'lipid-neutral' or 'lipid-friendly' drugs in the face of hyperlipidaemia are shown in Table 31.2. It is argued that the adverse metabolic effects which diuretics and beta-blockers induce are too small to be of significance, tend to reduce over time, and can be avoided totally by using low doses of these drugs (Berglund and Andersson, 1981; Carlson *et al.*, 1990). However, the size of the adverse effects on lipids which these two drug groups induce are shown in Table 31.3 and should be considered in the context of the findings in one lipid-lowering trial (Lipid Research Clinics Program, 1984) which demonstrated that a 1% fall in total cholesterol is associated with a 2% reduction in risk of a CHD event. The size of this benefit has been subsequently confirmed in a meta-analysis of lipid-lowering trials (Peto *et al.*, 1985). The hypertension trials suggest that diuretics induce an increase in total serum cholesterol of approximately 3%. This is equivalent to a 6% increase in CHD risk which is similar in size to the reported shortfall in CHD event prevention observed in the hypertension trial meta-analyses (Mac-Mahon *et al.*, 1986; Collins *et al.*, 1990). The belief that the induced adverse lipid effects reduce over time is based on trial data. During trials however,

	Total cholesterol	LDL cholesterol	HDL cholesterol	Triglyceride
		% change		
Diuretic	+4	+10	0	+9
Beta-blockers				
non selective	0	0	−7	+29
selective	0	0	−7	+18
ISA	0	0	−2	+13

Table 31.3: Adverse effects on lipids. (Source: Weidman *et al.*, 1985.)

compliance decreases over time and hence so do the associated metabolic effects. There seems little doubt that the use of lower doses of diuretics and beta-blockers reduces the size of the adverse metabolic effects. However, even using very low and not commercially available doses of thiazide along with potassium supplementation, one study demonstrated a fall in serum potassium and a significant rise in serum uric acid and creatinine (Carlsen *et al.*, 1990). Furthermore, the effects on serum HDL and total cholesterol induced by acebutolol (previously considered 'lipid-friendly') and low-dose chlorthalidone respectively after a year in the Treatment of Mild Hypertension Study (1991) were significantly worse than the placebo-treated group. The absolute size of the metabolic side-effects of drugs is best evaluated by measuring the effects consequent on stopping therapy and such a study of diuretic withdrawal demonstrated a 5% decrease in total serum cholesterol (Lithell H, unpublished data).

In summary, the newer anti-hypertensive agents appear to be preferable to diuretics and beta-blockers in terms of their effects on lipid profiles. Unfortunately we do not have long-term morbidity and mortality trial data to evaluate whether these advantages will result in improved prevention of CHD events and equally good prevention of stroke events as those provided by diuretics and beta-blockers. Until we do, it seems reasonable to recommend the newer agents in 'hyperlipidaemia' or 'dyslipidaemia'.

Because the vast majority of hypertensives in the UK have less than ideal lipid profiles, what degree of lipid abnormality is sufficient to merit a modification of antihypertensive agent is controversial. However, in the same way that we are recommended to target our advice and drugs for lipid lowering (Shepherd *et al.*, 1987) amongst 'hyperlipidaemics', a similar flexible approach based on the individual patient's risk profile could be considered for hypertensives with varying degrees of dyslipidaemia. In this way, a hypertensive with another major CHD risk factor such as strong family history or smoking should not receive a drug likely to damage lipids unless the total:high-density lipoprotein (HDL) cholesterol ratio is <4.0. Similarly, for patients with serum triglycerides >2.3 mmol/l, diuretics and beta-blockers should be avoided. In the absence of any other major risk factors the threshold for modifying antihypertensive therapy could be raised to a total:HDL ratio of >5.0.

Diabetes and glucose intolerance

As suggested above, diabetes and glucose intolerance are more common in hypertensives than in normotensives. Furthermore, studies suggest that this situation is worsened in hypertensives receiving 'standard' drug therapy for their hypertension (Bengtsson *et al.*, 1984; McKeigue and Keen, 1992). For any given level of blood pressure the presence of diabetes increases the risk of cardiovascular disease (Pyorila *et al.*, 1984), and this is very clearly reflected in mortality data (Table 31.4). Conversely, the presence of hypertension increases both the macrovascular and microvascular (Knowler *et al.*, 1980) complications of diabetes. Because of the greatly increased risk associated with coexisting

SBP mmHg QUINTILE	DIABETIC		NON-DIABETIC	
	n	Deaths (per 1000)	n	Deaths (per 1000)
<118	616	27(40.0)	69480	644(10.3)
118–124	703	44(54.8)	69296	808(12.8)
125–131	824	54(52.3)	67394	1018(15.8)
132–141	1179	82(57.3)	70029	1456(20.5)
≥142	1841	234(104.0)	66616	2774(36.4)

Table 31.4: Age-adjusted 10-year mortality, by systolic blood pressure (SBP) and history of diabetes mellitus (MRFIT screenee cohort).

hypertension and diabetes, the threshold for intervention on blood pressure should perhaps be lowered. Although this is not universally accepted (Fuller and Stevens, 1991), and there is no trial evidence to support the advice, both the Working Group on Hypertension in Diabetes (1987) and the Working Group on the Management of Patients with Hypertension and High Blood Cholesterol (1990) in the USA, recommended lowering the threshold for drug treatment to 140/90 mmHg and >90 mmHg diastolic respectively. Non-pharmacological intervention should be recommended in the usual way in an effort to improve both hypertension and diabetes control, with weight loss and increased exercise likely to affect both risk factors beneficially.

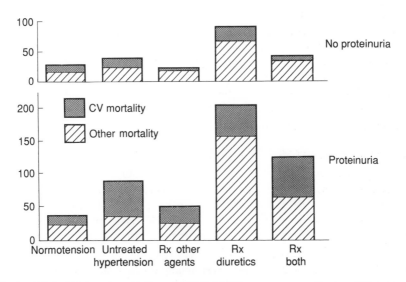

Figure 31.1: Diabetes mortality rates per 1000 person-years. (Source: Warram *et al.*, 1991.)

In the event that non-pharmacological manoeuvres do not control blood pressure adequately, the choice of antihypertensive agent has to be made in the absence of guidance from trial data, because with the exception of a small subgroup in the Hypertension Detection and Follow-up Program Study (1985) no trials of hypertension management in diabetics have been carried out.

Consequently, a judgement as to the optimal management of hypertension in these patients has to be based on other types of data.

One large prospective study carried out over 12 years demonstrated that the risk of developing diabetes amongst hypertensives treated with diuretics, beta-blockers and both diuretics and beta-blockers was increased 3.4, 5.7 and 11.4-fold respectively compared with the risk for normotensives (Bengtsson *et al.*, 1984). A review of deaths associated with anti-hypertensive agents in diabetics irrespective of presence or absence of proteinuria (Warram *et al.*, 1991) strongly suggests that diuretics should not be used for these patients (Figure 31.1). Table 31.5 outlines the special considerations which managing diabetics

	Diuretics	Beta-blockers	α_1 blockers	ACE inhibitors	Calcium antagonists
Nephropathy					
K^+	↓	—	—	↑	—
Renal impairment	—	—	—	?	—
Proteinuria	↓	↓	↓	↓ ↓	↓ ?
Neuropathy					
Impotence	↑ ↑	↑	↓	↑	↑
Orthostatic hypotension	↑	↑	↑ ↑*	—	—
Vascular					
CHD	? ↑	↓	? 0	? +	? +
PVD	↑	↑ ↑	—	—	—
RAS	—	—	—	↑	—
Retinopathy	—	—	—	—	—
Metabolic					
HDL	—	↓**	—/↑ §	—	—
LDL	↑	↑/↓	↓	—	—
Triglycerides	↑	↑	↓	—	—
Glucose	↑	↑	—	—	—(?)
Insulin	↑	↑	↓	↓	—
Obesity	—	↑	—	—	—

Table 31.5: Special considerations for drug treatment of hypertension in diabetics. (↑ increases or worsens; ↓ decreases or improves; — no differential effect; ? uncertain/controversial; * short-acting agents; ** reduces but worsens; § increases but improves.

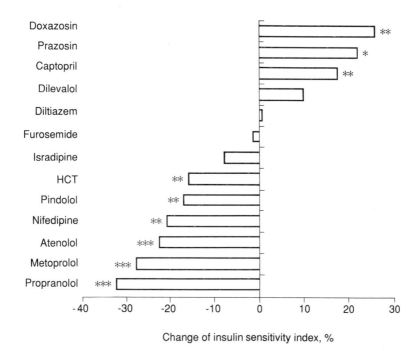

Figure 31.2: Change of insulin sensitivity with drug treatment. (Source: Lithell H, unpublished data.)

requires and the effects which the five major drug groups exert on these variables. The adverse lipid profile classically associated with NIDDM (low HDL-cholesterol and high triglycerides) is worsened by beta-blockers and (as shown in Figure 31.2) beta-blockers and to a lesser extent diuretics worsen insulin sensitivity unlike α_1-blockers and captopril which improve insulin sensitivity (Lithell H, unpublished data). It is clear from this table that ACE inhibitors and selective α_1-blockers appear to have the profile best suited to address these problems.

The prevalence of diabetes is over 5% in white hypertensives (Poulter *et al.*, 1993) but, as suggested by a recent population survey (McKeigue *et al.*, 1991), is likely to be closer to 20% and 15% in South Asian and Afro-Caribbean hypertensives respectively. For this significant proportion of hypertensives, on currently available data (which do not include formal trial evidence), and in keeping with the conclusions of other more extensive reviews (Feher, 1991), the newer antihypertensive agents—particularly ACE inhibitors and selective α_1-blockers—appear to offer major advantages over diuretics and beta-blockers (unless current active CHD co-exists). It also seems reasonable to extend this recommendation to those hypertensives with glucose intolerance since they too are likely to benefit from the advantages of the newer agents and to be adversely affected by the deleterious effects of diuretics and beta-blockers on carbohydrate metabolism, albeit to a lesser extent.

Whilst the newer agents appear more likely to provide greater benefits to these patients, a long-term morbidity and mortality trial to substantiate this 'best-estimate' evaluation is long overdue.

References

Beevers DG *et al.* (1991) In: Hansson L ed. *Clinician's manual on hypertension.* Science Press, London.

Bengtsson C *et al.* (1984) Do antihypertensive drugs precipitate diabetes? *British Medical Journal.* **289**:1495–7.

Berglund G and Andersson O (1981) Beta-blockers or diuretics in hypertension? A six-year follow-up of blood pressure and metabolic side effects. *The Lancet.* i:744–7.

British Hypertension Society Working Party (1989) Treating mild hypertension: agreement from large trials. *British Medical Journal.* **298**:694–8.

Carlsen JE *et al.* (1990) Relation between dose of bendrofluazide, antihypertensive effect, and adverse biochemical effects. *British Medical Journal.* **300**:975–8.

Collins R *et al.* (1990) Blood pressure, stroke, and coronary heart disease, part 2. Short-term reductions in blood pressure: overview of randomised drug trials in their epidemiological context. *The Lancet.* **335**:827–38.

Feher MD (1991) Hypertension in non-insulin dependent diabetes mellitus and its management. *Postgraduate Medical Journal.* **67**:938–46.

Feher MD and Lant AF (1991) Management choices for hypertension with coexistant hypercholesterolaemia. *Journal of the Royal Society of Medicine.* **84**:203–5.

Fuller JH and Stevens LK (1991) Epidemiology of hypertension in diabetic patients and implications for treatment. *Diabetes Care.* **14**(Suppl. 4):8–12.

Hypertension Detection and Follow-up Program Cooperative Group (1985) Mortality findings for stepped-care and referred-care participants in the hypertension detection and follow-up program, stratified by other risk factors. *Preventive Medicine.* **14**:312–35.

Joint National Committee (1977) The Joint National Committee on Detection, Evaluation and Treatment of High Blood Pressure. A cooperative study. *Journal of the American Medical Association.* **237**:255–61.

Joint National Committee (1988) The 1988 Report of the Joint National Committee on Detection, Evaluation, and Treatment of High Blood Pressure. *Archives of Internal Medicine*. **148**:1023–38.

Knowler WC *et al.* (1980) Increased incidence of retinopathy in diabetics with elevated blood pressure. *New England Journal of Medicine*. **302**:645–50.

Lipid Research Clinics Program (1984) The Lipid Research Clinics Coronary Primary Prevention Trial results. II. The relationship of reduction in incidence of coronary heart disease to cholesterol lowering. *Journal of the American Medical Association*. **251**:365–74.

MacMahon SW *et al.* (1986) The effects of drug treatment for hypertension on morbidity and mortality from cardiovascular disease: a review of randomised controlled trials. *Progress in Cardiovascular Disease*. **24**(Suppl. 1):99–118.

MacMahon SW and MacDonald CJ (1986) Antihypertensive treatment and plasma lipoprotein level: the association in data from a population study. *American Journal of Medicine*. **80**(Suppl. 2A):20–47.

McKeigue PM *et al.* (1991) Relation of central obesity and insulin resistance with high diabetes prevalence and cardiovascular risk in South Asians. *The Lancet*. **337**:382–6.

McKeigue PM and Keen H (1992) Diabetes, insulin, ethnicity, and coronary heart disease. In: Marmot MG and Elliot P (eds) *Coronary heart disease epidemiology: from aetiology to public health*. Oxford University Press, Oxford.

Peto R *et al.* (1985) Cholesterol lowering trial results in the epidemiologic context. *Circulation*. **72**(Suppl. 3):45.

Poulter N *et al.* (1993) A survey of coronary risk factors in 2000 hypertensives from English general practices. (In preparation.)

Pyorila K et al. (1984) Hypertension and mortality in diabetic and non-diabetic Finnish men. *Diabetologia*. **27**:322A.

Samuelsson O *et al.* (1987) Cardiovascular morbidity in relation to change in blood pressure and serum cholesterol levels in treated hypertension. *Journal of the American Medical Association*. **258**:1768–76.

Shepherd J *et al.* (1987) Strategies for reducing coronary heart disease and desirable limits for blood lipid concentrations: guidelines of the British Hyperlipidaemia Association. *British Medical Journal*. **295**:1245–6.

Stamler J *et al.* (1986) Is the relationship between serum cholesterol and risk of premature death from coronary heart disease continuous and graded? *Journal of the American Medical Association*. **256**:2823–8.

Treatment of Mild Hypertension Research Group (1991) The Treatment of Mild Hypertension Study. *Archives of Internal Medicine.* **151**:1413–23.

Warram JH *et al.* (1991) Excess mortality associated with diuretic therapy in diabetes mellitus. *Archives of Internal Medicine.* **151**:1350–6.

Weidman P *et al.* (1985) Antihypertensive treatment and serum lipoproteins. *Journal of Hypertension.* **3**:297–306.

WHO/ISH (1989) 1989 guidelines for the management of mild hypertension: memorandum from a WHO/ISH meeting. *Journal of Hypertension.* **7**:689–93.

Working Group on Hypertension in Diabetes (1987) Statement on hypertension in diabetes mellitus: final report. *Archives of Internal Medicine.* **147**:830–42.

Working Group on Management of Patients with Hypertension and High Blood Cholesterol (1990) Working group report on management of patients with hypertension and high blood cholesterol. *NIH Publication* **90–2361**:1–30.

Zavaroni I *et al.* (1987) Evidence that multiple risk factors for coronary artery disease exist in persons with abnormal glucose tolerance. *American Journal of Medicine.* **83**:609–12.

32

Primary and Secondary Prevention Trials of Lipid Lowering

DJ BETTERIDGE

The evidence linking increasing plasma cholesterol concentration to coronary heart disease (CHD) risk is impressive. It derives from prospective population-based studies, comparisons within and across populations, and animal and biochemical studies. In addition, physicians treating lipid disorders are aware of the massive CHD risk of the inherited monogenic disorders of lipoprotein metabolism, particularly familial hypercholesterolaemia (FH). Young individuals with this condition have a 100-fold increased CHD risk without the presence of other risk factors (Scientific Steering Committee, 1991). The genetic defect in FH is at the low-density lipoprotein (LDL) receptor, the activity of which is a major determinant of plasma LDL cholesterol concentrations. It was the study of this condition and the identification of the genetic defect that enabled Brown and Goldstein (1986) to shed so much light on the regulation of cholesterol metabolism. Their work, together with contributions by other groups, has provided a highly plausible mechanism whereby LDL cholesterol interacts with cells of the arterial wall leading to foam cell formation, the early lesion of atherosclerosis.

There is no doubt about the strength of the relationship between LDL cholesterol and CHD. The relationship shows a dose response, increasing LDL cholesterol being associated with increased risk; the relationship is independent of the other major risk factors; data from within populations and between populations has an impressive consistency; the lipid abnormality precedes the development of CHD, and the mechanism whereby LDL cholesterol is involved in atherogenesis is increasingly understood (Steinberg, 1987).

Despite the strength of evidence, what the clinician needs to know is whether LDL cholesterol reduction will delay or prevent the progression of atherosclerosis and reduce CHD risk. In addition, does intervention in an individual with established CHD reduce the risk of reinfarction? These are important questions, bearing in mind that atherogenesis proceeds silently for many decades before the onset of clinical manifestations of the disease. Is it realistic to expect a reduction in CHD risk by intervention to lower LDL cholesterol at a stage when the underlying disease process is likely to be advanced?

Large-scale clinical trials have been conducted to determine whether intervention to lower plasma LDL cholesterol is associated with a decreased risk of CHD. These trials fall into two main groups: the primary prevention trials, which study individuals without overt CHD, and secondary prevention trials, which study individuals with clinically overt disease. The more important trials will be discussed in some detail, together with various meta-analyses of the data that have been peformed. The strengths and weaknesses of the primary prevention trials will be highlighted.

Primary prevention trials

The diet trials

The general impression from early trials of dietary therapy was that CHD prevention by dietary change was a possibility. In the Los Angeles Veterans' Administration Study, 846 men (aged 54–88 years) were studied (Dayton *et al.*, 1969). Approximately one quarter of the men had some evidence of CHD. The intervention group were given a diet with a polyunsaturated:saturated fat ratio of 2:1 compared to a control diet. The trial lasted some eight years, and at the end of the trial period there were fewer cardiovascular endpoints in the intervention group. The beneficial effect was seen in the 'younger' subjects (below 65 years of age). In the Finnish Mental Hospital Study, 700 men and 600 women (aged 34–64 years) were studied (Turpeinen *et al.*, 1979). Again, as in the Los Angeles Veterans' Study, some had evidence of pre-existing disease. The subjects were drawn from two mental hospitals in Helsinki. The protocol involved one hospital taking an experimental diet for a six-year period whilst the other hospital remained on an unchanged control diet. For a further six-year period the diets in the two hospitals were crossed over. The experimental diet was very similar to that used in the Los Angeles Veterans' Study. Interpretation of this trial is difficult because the patient composition of the hospitals changed considerably. However, moderate beneficial effects on CHD were seen particularly in men.

In 1972 Hjermann and colleagues began the Oslo Diet/Anti-smoking Intervention Trial (Hjermann *et al.*, 1981). Over 16 000 men were screened and, of these, 1232 high-risk individuals were recruited for a randomized controlled trial. The total plasma cholesterol level in the men ranged between 7.5 and 9.8 mmol/l and 80% were cigarette smokers. Individual dietary advice was given at the beginning of the trial and then on a six-monthly basis to the intervention group. The dietary advice consisted of a reduction of saturated fat and a slight increase in polyunsaturated fat. For those subjects who were overweight, a reduction in total energy intake was recommended. Individual anti-smoking advice was also given. In the first five years of the study there was an average reduction of 10% in total plasma cholesterol and 20% in fasting plasma triglycerides in the intervention group. Tobacco consumption was 45% less in the intervention group compared to the control group. The main CHD endpoints in this trial were a combination of fatal and non-fatal myocardial infarction and sudden coronary death and after five years there was a 47% reduction in the intervention group. This trial of course consisted of two interventions, one designed to reduce plasma lipids levels and the other to reduce smoking. The authors concluded that the change in cigarette consumption between the two groups accounted for at most 25% of the CHD difference between the two groups. The participants of this trial have been followed up, and at 15 years there is a reduction in overall mortality in addition to a reduction in mortality from CHD.

The evidence from these diet trials does suggest a beneficial effect in reducing coronary risk. Alteration of dietary intake has also been incorporated into several multifactorial trials of CHD reduction where intervention with diet has been just one of the aspects of treatment in the intervention group. These trials are difficult to interpret in relation to the dietary effects as this formed only part of the intervention programme. However, as a generality, the impact on risk factors in the multifactorial studies was small, and often parallel changes were seen in the control group. In the MRFIT trial, for instance, the net difference between the intervention and control groups was only 2% for blood cholesterol (MRFIT Research Group, 1982).

The drug trials

The primary prevention study of the Lipid Research Clinics Program (1984) was a landmark in developing the cholesterol hypothesis. Over 480 000 American men (aged 35–59 years) were screened for hypercholesterolaemia. Of these, 18 000 had serum cholesterol levels above 6.9 mmol/l, which represents the 95th centile for the US population. 3806 of these men were recruited to take part in a double-blind placebo controlled trial of cholesterol reduction using the anion exchange resin cholestyramine at a dose of 24 g/day. All individuals received a moderate cholesterol-lowering diet. The men included in the trial were free of symptomatic coronary disease. The average follow-up of the study was 7.4 years; during this time the overall reduction in total plasma cholesterol was 13.4%, while for LDL cholesterol it was 20.3%. The difference between the cholestyramine and the placebo group was 8.5% for total cholesterol and 12.6% for LDL cholesterol. These differences were less than predicted by the investigators which was mainly due to poor compliance with the study medication. In fact, at the end of the trial, some 27% of the participants were not taking the drug which means that the overall effect was diluted. Despite the small differences between the actively-treated group and the placebo-treated group, there was a significant difference in the major endpoint of the study, number of definite CHD deaths together with non-fatal myocardial infarctions. In the cholestyramine group there were 155 events compared with 187 events in the placebo group. This represents a 19% reduction in risk made up of a 24% reduction in definite CHD death and a 19% reduction in definite non-fatal myocardial infarction. The beneficial effects of treatment were further emphasized by the secondary CHD endpoints which included those individuals developing a positive exercise test or angina as defined by the Rose questionnaire, those requiring coronary bypass surgery or developing congestive heart failure. In all these categories there was a reduction in incidence similar to the reduction seen in the major primary endpoint of the study. It is of interest that, when the authors looked at the cumulative incidence of CHD, the treatment group did not begin to diverge from the control group until approximately two years into the trial (Lipid Research Clinics Program, 1984).

A total of 4081 asymptomatic middle-aged men aged 40–55 years with primary hyperlipidaemia (non high-density lipoprotein [HDL] cholesterol >5.2 mmol/l) were recruited for the Helsinki Heart Study (Frick et al., 1987). All participants in the study were encouraged to give up cigarette smoking, to take up appropriate exercise and to take a cholesterol-lowering diet. In addition, gemfibrozil, a fibric acid derivative was given to half of the trial subjects on a double-blind randomized basis. After five years there was a 34% reduction in the incidence of CHD endpoints. The Helsinki Study is particularly important as an earlier primary prevention trial using the first of the fibrate drugs, clofibrate (Oliver et al., 1978; Committee of Principal Investigators, 1984) had demonstrated that cholesterol lowering was associated with a reduction in cardiac events but an excess of adverse effects (mainly gallbladder disease and gastrointestinal cancer) were observed which appeared to be attributable to the drug. This diverted attention from the finding of reduced CHD. It is of interest that a re-analysis of the WHO trial results has recently been published in *The Lancet* and, when the results were analysed on an intention-to-treat basis, there was no significant increase in cancer deaths during this trial. However there still remained a significant increase in all-cause mortality and all causes of death except ischaemic heart disease (Heady et al., 1992).

Unanswered questions

To those interested in lipid disorders, the primary prevention trials have confirmed the cholesterol hypothesis; and, taken together with the weight of other evidence, they have pointed to a causal relationship between LDL cholesterol and CHD. On this basis, various consensus committees have published guidelines on the identification and treatment of hyperlipidaemia (Consensus Conference, 1985; Shepherd et al., 1987; European Atherosclerosis Society, 1987; National Cholesterol Education Program, 1988), the most recent being the new guidelines of the European Atherosclerosis Society (1992). However, many physicians remain uneasy about the general applicability of these guidelines. The majority of trials have been in middle-aged men and there has been much discussion about whether the trial results can be extrapolated to men of different ages and to women. Furthermore some commentators have concentrated on the finding that the trials have had a bigger impact on non-fatal myocardial infarction than fatal myocardial infarction and sudden cardiac death. Perhaps most concern has arisen from the possible adverse effects of cholesterol lowering.

There is no doubt that the primary prevention trials have not shown a reduction in all-cause mortality. Even when meta-analyses of the primary prevention trials are performed there is no reduction in all-cause mortality and even a slight excess of non-cardiac deaths. However, what many fail to recognize is that these trials were designed primarily to examine effects on CHD and did not have the statistical power to examine non-cardiac deaths. It is of interest that the most sound and comprehensive meta-analysis performed on 19 trials of diet and specific lipid-lowering drugs showed not only a reduction in non-fatal and fatal CHD events but also a trend to lower overall mortality with increasing cholesterol lowering (Holme, 1990).

The picture has been confused by selective meta-analyses which have examined only a few of the available trials, and the conclusions of these have pointed to excess deaths due to suicide or injury. These meta-analyses need to be interpreted with extreme caution as they chose to analyse only a minority of the trials, at least one of which was not a bona fide primary prevention trial (Muldoon *et al.*, 1990; Davey Smith and Pekkanen, 1992). A further meta-analysis published recently included old trials where oestrogen and D-thyroxine were used to lower cholesterol (Ravnskov, 1992). It is difficult to apply this meta-analysis to current practice as these toxic agents have long since been removed from the therapy of lipid disorders with the advent of more appropriate therapeutic agents.

An important issue to have arisen from the more selective meta-analyses has been the possibility that cholesterol lowering is associated with an increase in violent death. This led to outrageous headlines in the lay press, such as 'Murder linked to lipid drugs'. Prompted by the slight (non-significant) increase in accidents and violence in the recent two major primary prevention trials using drugs, Wysowski and Gross (1990) from the FDA looked critically at these deaths to determine whether cholesterol-lowering drugs could be causally linked. There were two homicides in these studies but it is important to point out that the trial participants were victims rather than perpetrators. The authors examined the suicidal and accidental deaths in great detail and their conclusion was that *'when drop-outs and known risk factors for these deaths such as alcohol intoxication and psychiatric histories are considered little evidence remains to support the hypothesis that cholesterol-lowering drugs are causally associated with death due to homicides, suicides and accidents in these trials'.* Critics of the cholesterol hypothesis have pointed to various epidemiological studies that have shown associations between low cholesterol levels and non-cardiac deaths across a wide spectrum of disease classification. These data have been discussed in a recent overview (Jacobs *et al.*, 1992). However, this association does not point to a causal relationship and in the author's view does not have any bearing on reducing cholesterol in the prevention of CHD.

In the author's view the primary prevention trials have confirmed the cholesterol hypothesis. In view of some of the unanswered questions, however, it would seem prudent to target cholesterol screening and treatment to those at highest risk where the benefits of treatment are likely to outweigh any possible adverse effects. The identification and treatment of hypercholesterolaemia should be an important part of the management of those individuals with other risk factors for coronary disease such as hypertension and diabetes and in those with a strong family history of premature coronary artery disease. Individuals with genetic hyperlipidaemias including familial hypercholesterolaemia and familial combined hyperlipidaemia are known to be at high risk and deserve aggressive treatment.

Secondary prevention trials

There is no doubt that the modification of lipid risk factors in those with established coronary disease has been neglected (Cohen *et al.*, 1991). Many physicians have failed to appreciate the strong relationship between LDL cholesterol and the risk of subsequent reinfarction (Pekkanen *et al.*, 1990). Furthermore, a meta-analysis of the secondary prevention trials has shown that not only is cholesterol lowering associated with a significant reduction of fatal and non-fatal infarction but there is no increase in cancer deaths and no significant increase in non-cardiovascular, non-cancer events (Roussow *et al.*, 1990, 1991). This important analysis of the secondary prevention trials points to the importance of the identification and aggressive treatment of lipid abnormalities in those with pre-existing disease. In this group of individuals the great majority of deaths will be attributable to cardiovascular causes (80%), and intervention with cholesterol-lowering therapy is likely to be highly cost-effective. Despite this, only a small proportion of patients with existing clinical coronary disease are actively treated for lipid risk factors.

In view of the strong relationship between LDL cholesterol and risk of further coronary events in those with established disease and the results of the secondary prevention trials taken together with information from the athero-sclerosis regression trials, it has been suggested that the current goals of therapy for those with established disease may not be appropriate. LaRosa and Cleeman (1992) have argued that a more appropriate therapeutic goal in terms of LDL cholesterol for those with established disease should be 100 mg/dl or 2.5 mmol/l.

The need for further trials

Some believe that there will be continuing debate and confusion about the identification and treatment of hypercholesterolaemia until a trial is performed which has sufficient statistical power to determine whether cholesterol lowering is associated with not only a reduction in coronary events but a reduction in overall mortality. It has been argued that despite the fact that current primary and secondary prevention trials employ much more effective therapy, they will still not have the statistical power to answer the all-cause mortality question unless larger numbers are investigated (Collins *et al.*, 1992). Furthermore, the role of hypertriglyceridaemia and HDL cholesterol in atherogenesis needs to be further examined by appropriate primary and secondary prevention trials. Although there is some evidence of the protective effect of increasing HDL cholesterol from the Helsinki trial (Manninen *et al.*, 1988), there has been as yet no trial designed specifically to look at this question. Similarly with plasma triglycerides, although there is some evidence particularly from the Stockholm Secondary Prevention Trial (Carlson and Rosenhammer, 1988) that triglyceride lowering is beneficial, further trials need to be performed in this area. An obvious population group to study would be those with non-insulin-dependent diabetes where the principal lipid abnormality is hypertriglyceridaemia often associated with low HDL cholesterol.

Conclusions

On current evidence, what is the appropriate action for the physician interested in treating lipid disorders? It is the author's opinion that, in those individuals without clinical vascular disease, attention should be focused on those at highest risk; those with a strong family history of coronary disease, those with genetic hyperlipidaemias, and those with other major risk factors such as hypertension and diabetes. Those with established vascular disease should be treated aggressively and the goal of therapy should be much tighter in view of the overwhelming evidence of benefit in this group of individuals.

References

Brown MS and Goldstein JL (1986) A receptor-mediated pathway for cholesterol homeostasis. *Science.* **232**:34–47.

Carlson LA and Rosenhammer G (1988) Reduction of mortality in the Stockholm Ischaemic Heart Disease Secondary Prevention Study by combined treatment with clofibrate and nicotinic acid. *Acta Medica Scandinavica.* **223**:405–18.

Cohen MV *et al.* (1991) Low rate of treatment of hypercholesterolaemia by cardiologists in patients with suspected and proven coronary heart disease. *Circulation.* **83**:1294–304.

Collins R *et al.* (1992) Cholesterol and total mortality: need for larger trials. *British Medical Journal.* **304**:168–9.

Committee of Principal Investigators (1984) WHO co-operative trial of primary prevention of ischaemic heart disease with clofibrate to lower serum cholesterol. Trial mortality follow up. *The Lancet.* **ii**:600–4.

Consensus Conference (1985) Lowering blood cholesterol to prevent heart disease. *Journal of the American Medical Association.* **153**:2080–6.

Davey Smith G and Pekkanen J (1992) Should there be a moratorium on the use of cholesterol lowering drugs? *British Medical Journal.* **304**:431—4.

Dayton, S *et al.* (1969) A controlled clinical trial of a diet high in unsaturated fat in preventing complications of atherosclerosis. *Circulation.* **40** (Suppl. 2):1–63.

European Atherosclerosis Society (1987) Strategies for the prevention of coronary heart disease, a policy statement of the European Atherosclerosis Society. *European Heart Journal.* **8**:77–88.

European Atherosclerosis Society (1992) Prevention of coronary heart disease: scientific background and new clinical guidelines: recommendations of the European Atherosclerosis Society prepared by the International Task Force for Prevention of Coronary Heart Disease. *Nutrition and Metabolism in Cardiovascular Disease.* **2**:113–56.

Frick MH *et al.* (1987) Helsinki Heart Study: primary prevention trial with gemfibrozil in middle-aged men with dyslipidemia. *New England Journal of Medicine.* **317**:1237–45.

Heady JA (1992) WHO clofibrate/cholesterol trial: clarifications. *The Lancet.* **340**:1405–6.

Hjermann J *et al.* (1981) Effect of diet and smoking intervention on the incidence of coronary heart disease: a report from the Oslo Study Group of a randomised trial in healthy men. *The Lancet.* **ii**:1303–10.

Holme I (1990) An analysis of randomized trials evaluating the effect of cholesterol reduction on total mortality and coronary heart disease incidence. *Circulation.* **82**:1916–24.

Jacobs D *et al.* (1992) Report of the conference of low blood cholesterol: mortality associations. *Circulation.* **86**:1046–60.

LaRosa JC and Cleeman JI (1992) Cholesterol lowering as a treatment for established coronary heart disease. *Circulation.* **85**:1229–35.

Lipid Research Clinics Program (1984) The Lipid Research Clinics Coronary Primary Prevention Trial results: I. Reduction in incidence of coronary heart disease. *Journal of the American Medical Association.* **251**:351–64.

Manninen V *et al.* (1988) Lipid alterations and decline in the incidence of coronary heart disease in the Helsinki Heart Study. *Journal of the American Medical Association.* **260**:641–51.

MRFIT Research Group (1982) Multiple Risk Factor Intervention Trial: risk factor changes and mortality results. *Journal of the American Medical Association.* **248**:1465–77.

Muldoon MF (1990) Lowering cholesterol concentrations and mortality: a quantitative review of primary prevention trials. *British Medical Journal.* **301**:309–14.

National Cholesterol Education Program (1988) Report of the expert panel on detection, evaluation and treatment of high blood cholesterol in adults. *Archives of Internal Medicine.* **148**:36–69.

Oliver MF *et al.* (1978) A co-operative trial in the primary prevention of ischaemic heart disease using clofibrate: a report from the Committee of Principal Investigators. *British Heart Journal.* **40**:1069–118.

Pekkanen J *et al.* (1990). Ten year mortality from cardiovascular disease in relation to cholesterol level among men with and without pre-existing cardiovascular disease. *New England Journal of Medicine.* **322**:1700–7.

Ravnskov U (1992) Cholesterol lowering trials in coronary heart disease: frequency of citation and outcome. *British Medical Journal.* **305**:15–19.

Rossouw JE *et al.* (1990) The value of lowering cholesterol after myocardial infarction. *New England Journal of Medicine.* **323**:1112–9.

Rossouw JE *et al.* (1991) Deaths from injury, violence and suicide in secondary prevention trials of cholesterol lowering. *New England Journal of Medicine.* **325**:1813.

Scientific Steering Committee on behalf of Simon Broome Register Group (1991) Risk of fatal coronary heart disease in familial hypercholesterolaemia. *British Medical Journal.* **303**:892–6.

Shepherd J *et al.* (1987) Strategies for reducing coronary heart disease and desirable limits for blood lipid concentrations: guidelines of the British Hyperlipidaemia Association. *British Medical Journal.* **295**:1245–6. .

Steinberg D (1987) Lipoproteins and the pathogenesis of atherosclerosis. *Circulation.* **76**:508–14.

Turpeinen O *et al.* (1979) Dietary prevention of coronary heart disease: the Finnish Mental Hospitals Study. *International Journal of Epidemiology.* **8**:99–118.

Wysowski DK and Gross TP (1990) Deaths due to accidents and violence in two recent trials of cholesterol-lowering drugs. *Archives of Internal Medicine.* **150**: 2169–72.

33

Regression of Coronary Artery Disease

GILBERT R THOMPSON

It has been hypothesized that progression of coronary artery disease (CAD) is correlated most strongly with the prevailing concentration of low-density lipoprotein (LDL) cholesterol whereas regression is more closely related to the level of high-density lipoprotein (HDL) cholesterol (Barth and Arntzenius, 1991). The possible mechanisms underlying these relationships have been examined by Davies *et al.* (1991), including the role of oxidized LDL in foam-cell formation and the potential ability of HDL to act as a vehicle for transporting mobilized cholesterol out of lesions. These authors, as well as Waters and Lesperance (1991), recently reviewed the findings of six of the seven randomized, controlled trials of lipid lowering therapy involving serial coronary angiography which have been published since 1984. The seventh of these trials, listed in Table 33.1, is the St Thomas' Hospital Atherosclerosis Regression Study (STARS) which has only just been published (Watts *et al.*, 1992).

Space constraints preclude detailed consideration of all these trials but a brief résumé of some of their salient findings is pertinent. The Type II Intervention Trial showed less progression of CAD in cholestyramine-treated subjects but no increase in regression (Brensike *et al.*, 1984). The Cholesterol-Lowering Atherosclerosis Study (CLAS) I and II demonstrated that colestipol and nicotinic acid in combination induced regression of existing lesions in native vessels but not in saphenous vein grafts, although the rate of appearance of new lesions in grafts was reduced (Blankenhorn *et al.*, 1987; Cashin-Hemphill et al., 1990). The Program on the Surgical Control of Hyperlipidemia (POSCH) showed that cholesterol reduction over 10 years by partial ileal bypass resulted in highly significant reductions in cardiovascular events and in the need for cardiological interventions (Buchwald *et al.*, 1990). The Familial Atherosclerosis Treatment Study (FATS) showed that drug combinations which predominantly lowered LDL (colestipol and lovastatin) or raised HDL (colestipol and nicotinic acid) were equally effective in arresting progression and inducing regression of CAD (Brown *et al.*, 1990). This trial also showed that the extent of regression with treatment was greatest on vessels which were initially more than 50% stenosed. The University of California at San Francisco Specialized Center of Research (UCSF SCOR) trial involved both male and female patients with familial hypercholesterolaemia, some of whom

1	NHLBI Type II Intervention Trial (Brensike *et al.*, 1984)
2	CLAS I and II (Blankenhorn *et al.*, 1987; Cashin-Hemphill *et al.*, 1990)
3	POSCH (Buchwald *et al.*, 1990)
4	FATS (Brown *et al.*, 1990)
5	UCSF SCOR Intervention Trial (Kane *et al.*, 1990)
6	Lifestyle Heart Trial (Ornish *et al.*, 1990)
7	STARS (Watts *et al.*, 1992)

Table 33.1: Randomized lipid-lowering regression trials. (NHLBI, National Heart, Lung and Blood Institute; CLAS, Cholesterol-Lowering Atherosclerosis Study. For other abbreviations, see text.)

were treated with triple drug therapy (colestipol, nicotinic acid and lovastatin). Treatment reduced the frequency of progression and increased the frequency of regression, these changes seemingly being more marked in females (Kane *et al.*, 1990). The Lifestyle Heart Trial provided evidence that multifactorial intervention with a very low-fat diet, increased exercise and stress reduction measures could lead to angiographic improvement over as short a period as 12–18 months (Ornish *et al.*, 1990). A more detailed appraisal of these trials is contained in the reviews cited previously (Davies *et al.*, 1991; Waters and Lesperance, 1991), with the exception of the recently published STARS (Watts *et al.*, 1992).

The STARS involved 90 men aged more than 66 years old, with CHD, and mean total cholesterol ≥ 7.2 mmol/l, who were randomly allocated to receive either usual care, a low-fat diet or diet plus cholestyramine. Quantitative coronary angiography was performed before and after an average of 39 months. Although the majority of lesions were relatively mild, only 8% being more than 50% stenosed, benefit from treatment was most marked in the worst affected segments. Both diet alone and diet plus cholestyramine resulted in significant reductions in the percentage of patients showing progression and increases in the percentage of patients showing regression, compared with the usual care group. Surprisingly these patient-based criteria improved to a similar extent in diet-treated patients and those treated with both diet and cholestyramine, despite a marked discrepancy in LDL cholesterol between the two treatment groups. However lesion–based criteria, such as mean luminal diameter, improved more markedly in patients treated with diet and cholestyramine, these changes being correlated with changes in LDL cholesterol and the LDL:HDL cholesterol ratio. These results show that a reasonably strict cholesterol-lowering diet (fat 27%, polyunsaturated: saturated fat [P:S] ratio approximately 1, with cholesterol 100 mg and fibre 3.6 g per 1000 calories) had beneficial effects on coronary heart disease (CHD) in patients with moderate hypercholesterolaemia but suggest that cholestyramine conferred little additional advantage.

Table 33.2 summarizes differences between patients in the control and treatment groups in the five trials which used lipid-lowering drugs. There was

Trial	LDL cholesterol $\Delta\%$	HDL cholesterol $\Delta\%$	P $\Delta\%$	R $\Delta\%$
Type II (Ch)	−20	+6	−17	0
CLAS (Co + NA)	−36	+35	−22	+14
FATS (L + Co)	−39	+11	−25	+21
(NA + Co)	−25	+38	−21	+28
UCSF (Co + NA ± L)	−28	+28	−21	+20
STARS (Diet)	−13	0	−31	+34
(Diet + Ch)	−33	−4	−34	+29
Mean change	−28	+16	−24	+21

CH, cholestyramine; Co, colestipol; NA, nicotinic acid; L, lovastatin; P, progression; R, regression; $\Delta\%$, % change.

Table 33.2: Differences between patients in treatment and control groups in five angiographic trials of lipid-lowering therapy.

considerable variation in the changes in LDL and HDL achieved, depending upon the nature of the treatment involved, but on average a 28% greater reduction in LDL cholesterol and a 10% greater increase in HDL cholesterol in treated versus controls resulted in a 24% reduction in patients whose lesions progressed and a 21% increase in those whose lesions regressed. Overall CAD was arrested or reversed in 45% of the patients on treatment.

Table 33.3 shows the mean concentrations of LDL and HDL cholesterol and calculated HDL:LDL ratios in the three trials which provided data on changes in percentage diameter stenosis of lesions. Stenosis increased in all control groups, and decreased in all treatment groups. On average a 3.7% increase in percentage diameter stenosis occurred in controls in whom LDL cholesterol, HDL cholesterol and the HDL:LDL ratio were 4.32, 1.19 mmol/l and 0.276, respectively, whereas a decrease in percentage diameter stenosis of 1.1% was evident at corresponding values of 3.23, 1.16 mmol/l and 0.364 in patients on treatment. Thus within the context of these three trials, a reduction in LDL cholesterol to between 3.0–3.5 mmol/l (apart from the diet group in STARS) was associated with angiographic improvement whereas levels greater than 4 mmol/l were associated with worsening of lesions.

Significant reductions in CHD events were noted not only in POSCH but also in FATS and STARS, suggesting stabilization of lesions. The possibility that this reflected changes in the composition of lesions is supported at the anecdotal level by studies of a hypercholesterolaemic patient who died after 6½ years of lipid-lowering therapy (Koga and Iwata, 1991). Histological studies of his coronary arteries revealed that lesions shown to have regressed angiographically during life consisted largely of fibrous tissue when examined post-mortem.

Trial	LDL cholesterol	HDL cholesterol	HDL:LDL ratio	$\Delta\%$ Diameter stenosis
	mmol/l			
FATS (Brown *et al.*, 1990)				
Placebo + Co	4.20	1.04	0.248	2.0
L + Co	2.77	1.06	0.383	−0.3
NA + Co	3.34	1.42	0.425	−1.1
STARS (Watts *et al.*, 1992)				
Usual care	4.67	1.21	0.259	5.6
Diet	4.19	1.14	0.272	−0.5
Diet + Ch	3.37	1.19	0.353	−1.5
Lifestyle (Ornish *et al.*, 1990)				
Usual diet	4.1	1.31	0.320	3.4
Experimental diet	2.5	0.97	0.388	−2.2
All controls	4.32	1.19	0.276	3.7
All treatments	3.23	1.16	0.364	−1.1

Ch, cholestyramine; Co, colestipol; NA, nicotinic acid; L, lovastatin; $\Delta\%$, percentage change.

Table 33.3: Effects of treatment on lipids and angiographic change in three trials using computer-assisted analysis.

References

Barth JD and Arntzenius AC (1991) Progression and regression of atherosclerosis, what roles for LDL cholesterol and HDL cholesterol: a perspective. *European Heart Journal.* **12**:952–7.

Blankenhorn DH *et al.* (1987) Beneficial effects of combined colestipol-niacin therapy on coronary atherosclerosis and coronary venous bypass grafts. *Journal of the American Medical Association.* **257**:3233–40.

Brensike JF *et al.* (1984) Effects of therapy with cholestyramine on progression of coronary atherosclerosis: results of the NHLBI type II coronary intervention study. *Circulation.* **69**:313–24.

Brown G *et al.* (1990) Regression of coronary heart disease as a result of intensive lipid-lowering therapy in men with high levels of apolipoprotein B. *New England Journal of Medicine.* **323**:1289–98.

Buchwald H *et al.* (1990) Effect of partial ileal bypass surgery on mortality and morbidity from coronary heart disease in patients with hypercholesterolemia. *New England Journal of Medicine.* **323**:946–55.

Cashin-Hemphill L *et al.* (1990) Beneficial effects of colestipol-niacin on coronary atherosclerosis. A 4-year follow-up. *Journal of the American Medical Association.* **264**:3013–17.

Davies MJ *et al.* (1991) Atherosclerosis: inhibition or regression as therapeutic possibilities. *British Heart Journal.* **65**:302–10.

Kane JP *et al.* (1990) Regression of coronary atherosclerosis during treatment of familial hypercholesterolemia with combined drug regimens. *Journal of the American Medical Association.* **264**:3007–12.

Koga N and Iwata Y (1991) Pathological and angiographic regression of coronary atherosclerosis by LDL apheresis in a patient with familial hypercholesterolemia. *Atherosclerosis.* **90**:9–21.

Ornish D *et al.* (1990) Can lifestyle changes reverse coronary heart disease? *The Lancet.* **336**:129–33.

Waters D and Lesperance J (1991) Regression of coronary atherosclerosis: an achievable goal? Review of results from recent clinical trials. *American Journal of Medicine.* **91** (Suppl. 18):10–17S.

Watts GF *et al.* (1992) Effects on coronary artery disease of lipid-lowering diet, or diet plus cholestyramine, in the St Thomas' Atherosclerosis Regression Study (STARS). *The Lancet.* **339**:563–9.

34

The Economics of Cholesterol Lowering

JOHN PD RECKLESS

In developed countries there are considerable variations in absolute and relative health-care costs. In 1987, the absolute spending on health care was 2.7 times more in the United States, and nearly 1.5 times more in France and West Germany, than that in the United Kingdom. Per capita spending in 1987 was £1236 ($2051) in the USA, £666 ($1105) in France, £658 ($1093) in West Germany and £551 ($915) in Japan, compared to £457 ($758) in the United Kingdom*. In relative terms, expenditure on health care in the USA, Sweden, France, West Germany, Japan and the UK was respectively 11.2%, 9.3%, 8.6%, 8.0%, 6.9% and 6.1% of gross national product. Over the last 10–20 years, health-care expenditure has been increasing disproportionately and taking a greater proportion of gross national product, but this increase has been less marked in the UK than in most Western countries (Reinhardt, 1988).

Rational decisions about health care provision need to consider cost, because the potential for diagnosis and treatment will always be greater than the available human and financial resources. In future, costs of medical care will need to be measured and the relative benefits of different treatments assessed. Costs include not just direct costs of a health-care programme but also the concept of *opportunity cost* which, following the use of a resource, is the cost or sacrifice of the alternative programme benefits consequently forgone.

Economic measures

Cost-benefit analysis compares treatment costs with consequent savings such as hospital costs avoided. This was developed into *cost-effectiveness* analysis, comparing the costs and benefits of different types of treatment, to maximize the benefits for a group of patients with a particular condition, using the minimum of resources most appropriately. *Cost-utility* analysis was developed to take account of the comfort and well being of the patients and also their potential financial contribution within the community. Measures of *quality of life* have been developed, and a *quality adjusted life year* (QALY) measures both quality and quantity of life gained from a health-care intervention. Such economic measures are being introduced as a requirement for drug licensing in Australia.

---

*These calculations were worked out when the £/$ ratio was approximately 1.66.

Economic considerations for hypertension treatment

Cost-utility analyses (Stason and Weinstein, 1977; Edelson *et al.*, 1990; Reckless, 1990*a*) have considered whether hypertension treatment pays for itself, how efficient a use of resources it may be, and how resources can be allocated between screening or improving treatment compliance. Cost-effectiveness varies with gender, age at treatment initiation, pre-treatment blood pressure and duration of treatment. Edelson *et al.* (1990) considered blood pressure lowering, side-effect profiles and price, and over 20 years, costs per life-year saved were found to be $10 900, $16 400, $31 600, $61 900 and $72 100 for propranolol, hydrochlorothiazide, nifedipine, prazosin and captopril. Analyses were 60–80% more favourable for smokers.

Hyperlipidaemia and coronary heart disease

Animal, biochemical, epidemiological, genetic and human intervention studies have established a causal relationship between serum (and lipoprotein) cholesterol levels and atherosclerosis. Coronary heart disease (CHD) risk relates to the overall risk-factor profile with smoking, hypertension, raised blood lipids and diabetes mellitus as the four principal factors.

In 361 662 American men aged 35–57 years, screened for the Multiple Risk Factor Intervention Trial (Martin *et al.*, 1986) and followed for six years, mortality from CHD increased progressively above a plasma cholesterol of 4.7 mmol/l (20th centile), and the relative risk above the 85th centile (6.5 mmol/l) was high at 3.8. Many other epidemiological observations, such as those in Framingham (Gordon *et al.*, 1977), are consistent.

Recent intervention studies of cholesterol lowering strongly support this relationship between cholesterol and CHD. The LRC Coronary Primary Prevention Trial (Lipid Research Clinics Program, 1984) showed a 20% reduction in CHD incidence for a 10% cholesterol fall, effects being proportional to the compliance with the medication, the anion exchange resin cholestyramine. In the Helsinki Heart Study (Frick *et al.*, 1987; Manninen *et al.*, 1988), the fibric acid derivative gemfibrozil led to falls in plasma and low-density lipoprotein (LDL) cholesterol, a rise in high-density lipoprotein (HDL) cholesterol, and a 34% reduction in CHD.

In these studies (Gordon *et al.*, 1977; Lipid Research Clinics Program, 1984; Martin *et al.*, 1986; Frick *et al.*, 1987; Manninen *et al.*, 1988), a 1% change in cholesterol was associated with a 2% change in CHD. Allowing for mathematical considerations of regression towards the mean in these and other data, it has been suggested (Peto *et al.*, 1985) that the ratio should be 30% CHD change for 10% cholesterol change. In other populations (in Japan and China), the positive relationship between cholesterol and CHD is present for levels of cholesterol of 3.0 mmol/l upwards.

Hyperlipidaemia is common in the UK, mean levels of cholesterol being about 5.9 mmol/l. Unfortunately it is not possible to identify all those with hypercholesterolaemia even if there is evidence of clinical CHD, family history of premature CHD, stigmata of hyperlipidaemia, obesity, diabetes and hypertension. In particular, many individuals will be missed who have severe, often genetic, hypercholesterolaemia which will not respond adequately to population dietary modification and will require individual attention to prevent or delay CHD.

Modest reductions in CHD deaths have become apparent in the UK since 1978, mainly in males in the 45–64 years age range, but these reductions have been smaller than in other developed countries with previously high rates of CHD (Office of Health Economics, 1990). Northern Ireland, Scotland, Ireland and England and Wales occupied four of the six highest places for age-standardized mortality in 1981, emphasizing the urgent need to tackle the CHD problem.

Cost-utility considerations for hyperlipidaemia

In any CHD prevention programme, only a proportion of those at risk will actually develop CHD. A proportion will be treated who would not have developed CHD, and a proportion who are treated will still develop CHD. The intention is to reduce the numbers affected and/or delay the onset. History, symptoms and signs may reveal some individuals with significant hypercholesterolaemia, but a substantial proportion of those at particular risk will not be so identified unless screened (Mann et al., 1988). While the whole population may be screened, not everyone will require a subsequent intervention: but, because of high risk-factor prevalence in Western populations, many will. Cholesterol levels are sufficiently elevated in the population, and dietary fat (especially saturated fat) intake is sufficiently high, to make a dietary modification appropriate for most individuals. Advocating dietary change without cholesterol measurement involves giving advice to individuals who do not need it and who may not benefit, removing the potential motivation of knowing a cholesterol level, and failing to detect high-risk individuals and major genetic hyperlipidaemias.

Two strategies for CHD prevention, the population strategy and the high-risk or individual strategy, should be looked upon as complementary rather than as alternatives. The population strategy recognizes that many people in North American and European countries have one or more risk factors, and involves educating the whole community to adopt a healthier lifestyle, with improved diet, less smoking and more exercise. The individual strategy seeks to identify people at particularly high risk of CHD, using clinical and laboratory examinations. Of course a successful population strategy will reduce the number of people at high risk requiring individual care, although not the cost of identifying them.

It is essential that drug treatment is used relatively sparingly for individuals at high CHD risk, because of potential side-effects of medication, effort involved in long-term treatment, and overall cost to the individual and/or community of long-term medication. A fixed cholesterol concentration for the introduction of drug treatment is not appropriate, but one should consider the potential risk to a given individual that his level of cholesterol poses in the light of his overall risk factor status. Various economic analyses have made assumptions on drug treatment by assessing how many individuals in different cholesterol ranges (6.5–7.8 mmol/l and > 7.8 mmol/l) will receive lipid lowering drug therapy. It is clear from sensitivity analyses in the economic assessments that cost/utility ratios vary dramatically, and that drug usage rates of 3–5% of the population assumed to calculate the QALY costs are considerable overestimates of likely or appropriate use in our present state of knowledge. Choosing individuals with existing CHD, multiple risk factors and severe single gene disorders will maximize benefits, limit drug usage rates and the overall cost, and give economic performances better than those published. To do this, doctors must be trained to understand the interrelationships of multiple risk factors, and to intervene on all, and not just on single, modifiable risk factors.

In the UK, cost-utility estimates have been made for an opportunistic screening policy (rather than mass screening) for adults of working age, relying on individuals routinely visiting the primary health-care team over five years (Reckless, 1990*b*; SMAC, 1990). Non-attenders include higher-risk individuals, but it is more cost-effective to approach those not screened towards the end of a screening programme rather than to attempt mass screening. Expenses related to screening, counselling and dietary management account for less than 25% of total costs, the major cost being drug usage. Critical consideration must therefore be given to drug choice and effectiveness, drug price, and particularly to the choice of patients treated.

During a visit to the primary health-care team, individuals can be offered brief CHD risk-factor assessment and counselling, including cholesterol estimation. Costs of blood sampling, cholesterol testing, and counselling time were also estimated. The frequency of subsequent measurement and counselling will depend on an individual's initial cholesterol level. Triglyceride and HDL-cholesterol will need to be measured in some individuals.

Those with other significant risk factors will need to be counselled for longer, partly by a doctor but mostly by a nurse. Some will require specialist dietetic support, and a small percentage with the most severe and least responsive hyperlipidaemia—often with complicating medical problems—will need to be referred to the out-patients department of a hospital.

The simplest form of intervention for serum cholesterol is a reduced fat, low cholesterol diet with weight control, which is all that is required for the great majority of the population with cholesterol levels that are higher than are desirable.

Drug therapy is rarely required for individuals presenting with a cholesterol level below 6.5 mmol/l. Allowing for other risks, at most perhaps 5–10% of those with an initial cholesterol level of 6.5–7.8 mmol/l will need drug therapy, as will about 40–50% of those with an initial cholesterol of more than 7.8 mmol/l. In practice, the numbers will be considerably lower. The costs could vary between £120 and £600 per year's drug supply. The bile acid sequestrants and the fibrates have been first-line treatment, but potent and well tolerated inhibitors of cholesterol synthesis—pravastatin and simvastatin—are likely to be increasingly used, particularly for people with major genetic hyperlipi-daemias such as familial hypercholesterolaemia.

The overall costs for the 29 million adults in England and Wales aged 20–65 years would amount to about £8 each per year, or £235 million overall.

Presence of clinical CHD increases cost-effectiveness as the risk of further CHD events is high. Those with the most severe risk-factor level, and particularly those with multiple factors, are likely to benefit most. Most studies have considered the effects of a single intervention, but intervention on all modifiable factors is necessary in clinical practice, and for the best cost-benefit. The cost-benefit ratio over a 10-year period, for instance, will be poorer for younger than older people because the former have a lower risk of CHD. Lifetime cost-benefit ratios are more appropriate and will show less discrepancy between young and old, but corporate health-care payers think and budget over shorter time spans. At any given age, females have a lower CHD risk than males, and therefore will present poorer cost-utility values. On purely economic grounds it may be cheaper to delay risk-factor treatment until the fifth decade, on the basis that two thirds of the benefit of effective cholesterol lowering (for example) may be evident within two or three years of intervention. To a lesser extent, costs may rise somewhat per year of treatment in the seventh and eighth decades of age, as the predictive power of cholesterol is reduced with competing causes of mortality.

Broad estimates have been made of the costs of intervention for hypercholesterolaemia. Using the efficacy of cholestyramine in the Lipid Research Clinics Program (1984), and a multivariate logistic function from the Framingham Heart Study (McGee, 1977), Oster and Epstein (1987) calculated the cost per life year saved to be between £30 000 and £60 000. Individual spontaneous implementation of a dietary policy was calculated to be a saving, and not a cost, per person per annum of £140 (late 1970s costs) (Berwick et al., 1980). Relative costs, and sensitivity analyses from estimates in Europe are shown in Table 34.1 (from Reckless, 1990b), and Table 34.2 (from SMAC, 1990).

Estimates of cholesterol lowering have previously been based on major double-blind placebo-controlled studies, but drug usage in clinical practice is adjusted to individual patient need and response. Estimates of costs have considered potential reduction in total or LDL cholesterol, but not changes in triglycerides or HDL cholesterol, and this is also true for drug effects. Recent drugs are more potent and easier to take, and the degree of cholesterol lowering is easier to predict. With increasing use, and patent changes with time, relative drug costs can be expected to fall. All these changes may improve the cost-utility comparisons.

Age	Treatment	Males	Females	All
20–39	Diet + drugs	4710	26980	7980
	Diet only	1010	5790	1710
	Drugs added	26500	152670	45170
40–64	Diet + drugs	185	545	280
	Diet only	40	120	60
	Drugs added	1050	3080	1550
20–64	Diet + drugs	370	1090	550
	Diet only	80	235	120
	Drugs added	2080	6130	3060

Table 34.1: Costs of a cholesterol screening and treatment programme, in £ sterling per QALY. (Source: Reckless, 1990*b*.)

Treatment	Males	Females	All
Diet + drugs	1957	6521	2979
Diet only	44	605	176
Diet + drugs + personal CHD	223		
Diet + drugs + no CHD history	2598		
Diet + drugs at half rate + no CHD	1481		
Diet + drugs at quarter rate + no CHD	831		
Diet + drugs, smokers	1176		
Diet + drugs, non-smokers	2849		
Diet + drugs, hypertensive	1133		
Diet + drugs, normotensive	2500		
Diet + drugs, hypertensive, smoker	712		
Diet + drugs, normotensive, non-smoker	4076		

Table 34.2: Cost of a cholesterol screening and treatment programme for those aged between 40 and 69 years (in £ sterling per QALY). Hypertension is defined as diastolic blood pressure > 90 mmHg. Drug usage rates have been calculated on hospital lipid clinic experience, where patients have been selected to be at higher risk. Rather than the rate of 4% for usage here, in practice primary health-care rates would not be expected to reach 1%. (Data from SMAC, 1990.)

Note: 'Diet + drugs' refers to the overall management programme, while 'Drugs added' refers to the incremental cost of adding drug therapy in selected individuals, to the overall 'diet only' management costs.

As the variation in figures for costs per life year saved indicates, major changes in costs can occur with apparently modest changes in the necessary assumptions. Thus the QALY costs should be looked upon as a rough guide, not as a precise instrument. They do allow sensitivity analyses, to help give economic support to clinical treatment guidelines, and they do form a basis on which cost-utility ratios can be compared for prevention versus treatment of CHD, and between programmes of prevention against different diseases.

Summary

- An opportunistic screening programme by the primary health-care team is more cost-effective than a mass screening programme.
- Ideally all adults should have had a cholesterol measurement.
- Dietary counselling should be offered.
- Drug treatment should be preceded by multiple lipid measurements and full dietary management.
- Where logistic or other considerations limit initial cholesterol screening programmes, preference should be given to individuals with known CHD, those with a family history of premature CHD or of hyperlipidaemia, those with other known CHD risk factors, to older rather than younger persons, and to males before females.
- Screening should be for all risk factors.
- Intervention should be on all modifiable risk factors, not just on one of them.
- Drug usage for hypercholesterolaemia should follow consideration of an individual's overall CHD risk, and not just a single factor.

References

Berwick DM *et al.* (1980) *Cholesterol, children and heart disease: an analysis of alternatives.* Oxford University Press, New York.

Edelson JT *et al.* (1990) Long term cost-effectiveness of various initial monotherapies for mild to moderate hypertension. *Journal of the American Medical Association.* **263**:407–13.

Frick MH *et al.* (1987) Helsinki Heart Study: primary prevention trial with gemfibrozil in middle aged men with dyslipidemia. *New England Journal of Medicine.* **317**:1237–45.

Gordon T *et al.* (1977) The prediction of coronary heart disease by high density and other lipoproteins: an historical perspective. In: Rifkind B and Levy R (eds) *Hyperlipidemia—diagnosis and therapy.* Grune and Stratton, New York. pp.71–8.

Lipid Research Clinics Program (1984) The Lipid Research Clinics Coronary Primary Prevention Trial Results I and II. *Journal of the American Medical Association.* **251**:351–74.

Mann JI *et al.* (1988) Blood lipid concentrations and other cardiovascular risk factors: distribution, prevalence and detection in Britain. *British Medical Journal.* **296**:1702–6.

Manninen V *et al.* (1988) Lipid alterations and decline in the incidence of coronary heart disease in the Helsinki Heart Study. *Journal of the American Medical Association.* **260**:641–51.

Martin MJ *et al.* (1986) Serum cholesterol, blood pressure and mortality: implications from a cohort of 361,662 men. *The Lancet.* **ii**:933–6.

McGee DL (1977) Probability of developing certain cardiovascular diseases in eight years at specified values of some characteristics. In: Kannel WB and Gordon T (eds) *The Framingham Study: an epidemiological investigation of cardiovascular disease, section 28. US Department of Health, Education and Welfare publication (NIH) 77–1247.* Public Health Service, Bethesda, Maryland.

Office of Health Economics (1990) *Coronary heart disease – the need for action.* Office of Health Economics, London. pp.1–40.

Oster G and Epstein AM (1987) Cost-effectiveness of antihyperlipidemic therapy in the prevention of coronary heart disease. The case for cholestyramine. *Journal of the American Medical Association.* **258**:2381–7.

Peto R *et al.* (1985) Cholesterol-lowering trials in their epidemiological context. *Circulation.* **75**(suppl.2):451.

Reckless JPD (1990*a*) The economics of cholesterol lowering. *Bailliere's Clinical Endocrinology and Metabolism.* **4**:947–72.

Reckless JPD (1990*b*) Cost-effectiveness of clinical care for hyperlipidaemia. In: Lewis B and Assmann G (eds) *The social and economic contexts of coronary prevention.* Current Medical Literature, London. pp.94–103.

Reinhardt UE (1988) Perspectives: an economist. *Health Affairs (Millwood).* **7**: 96–103.

SMAC (Standing Medical Advisory Committee) (1990) *Blood cholesterol testing and the cost-effectiveness of opportunistic cholesterol testing. Report to the Secretary of State for Health.* Department of Health, London.

Stason WB and Weinstein MC (1977) Allocation of resources to manage hypertension. *New England Journal of Medicine.* **296**:732–9.

35

Treatment of Cardiac Arrhythmias Following Myocardial Infarction

ANDREAS LOAIZA AND RONALD WF CAMPBELL

Cardiac arrhythmias have long excited attention, particularly in the context of myocardial infarction (MI). The acute phase of MI is almost always complicated by some type of ventricular arrhythmias (Campbell et al., 1981). Until relatively recently, these have been energetically treated by anti-arrhythmic drugs. Despite encouraging reports that suppression of these arrhythmias was possible (Darby et al., 1972; Lie et al., 1974; Dunn et al., 1984), and despite the observation that ventricular fibrillation rates could be reduced by prophylactic lignocaine (Koster and Dunning, 1985), there is no evidence that either morbidity or mortality are improved by such a strategy. Thus, in recent years, much less anti-arrhythmic therapy has been used in coronary care units.

Arrhythmias are also a common feature in the late phase and post-hospital phase of infarction (Darby et al., 1972). With increased usage of ambulatory monitoring and exercise testing, ventricular arrhythmias in particular are increasingly recognized. Many of these arrhythmias (frequent ventricular ectopic beats [VEB], ventricular tachycardia [VT], etc) are associated with an adverse late prognosis (Darby et al., 1972). Studies using Class I anti-arrhythmic therapy, prescribed either to patients with manifest arrhythmias or alternatively to general high-risk survivors of infarction, have not improved prognosis (Bastian et al., 1980; Chamberlain et al., 1980; Gottlieb et al., 1987; Cardiac Arrhythmia Pilot Study [CAPS] Investigators, 1988); indeed there is growing evidence that these drugs may increase mortality risks (Cardiac Arrhythmia Suppression Trial [CAST] Investigators, 1989; Cardiac Arrhythmia Suppression Trial [CAST II] Investigators; 1992; Teo et al., 1990.)

Thus arrhythmia management following MI is in a state of flux. Asymptomatic but prognostically significant arrhythmias are detected, but the optimal medical response to their recognition is unknown. Furthermore, there is a reluctance to use Class I anti-arrhythmic drugs even for symptomatic ventricular tachyarrhythmias, although this was not the scenario examined in post-infarction studies that defined possible harm from the use of Class I agents.

Arrhythmias post-MI may be either manifest or latent. Manifest arrhythmias may be symptomatic or asymptomatic and optimal treatment may be decided on that basis. Latent arrhythmias, by definition, are yet to occur. There are no symptoms until the arrhythmia occurs. This type of arrhythmia is difficult to manage, not least because predictions of future occurrence are unreliable.

Manifest ventricular arrhythmias following MI

All phases of MI are complicated by manifest arrhythmias (Figure 35.1). Those seen in the earliest hours of the event reflect the short-lived electrical instability of acute ischaemia and the subsequent process of infarction (Campbell *et al.*, 1981). Any problem that they pose usually is contained by the passage of time. There is no evidence that acute treatment is beneficial and indeed it may be detrimental (Koster and Dunning, 1985). By contrast, late-phase arrhythmias may be a permanent legacy of the infarct and have implications for both prognosis and management (Darby *et al.*, 1972).

Manifest ventricular tachycardia

This poses the least controversial problem. *Sustained* monomorphic VT post-MI is serious, associated with a poor prognosis and likely to be recurrent, and should be treated with therapy shown to be effective at an electrophysiological study (Waller *et al.*, 1987). Although there has been great debate about the virtues of electrophysiological studies, it is in this context that the most persuasive aspects of benefit are seen. Prognosis and arrhythmia recurrence rates for those post-infarct individuals with sustained monomorphic VT which can be shown to be suppressed at electrophysiological study are significantly better than that for those patients in whom no effective anti-arrhythmic drug is found. Any other management strategy is suboptimal. Empiric prescription of drugs such as amiodarone and sotalol have been proposed and they do offer a degree of efficacy but the benefits appear less than that which may be obtained with therapy defined as effective at electrophysiology study. When no

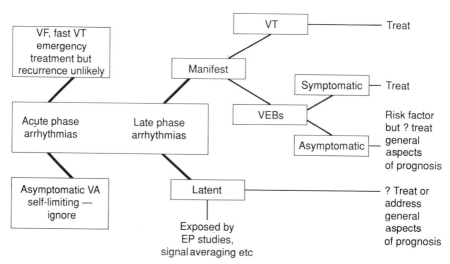

Figure 35.1: Ventricular arrhymias associated with myocardial infarction.

effective anti-arrhythmic drug is found, patients with sustained monomorphic VT should be considered for alternative management strategies including antiarrhythmic surgery (Bourke *et al.*, 1990*a*), a curative procedure albeit with an important mortality risk, or they may be candidates for an implantable cardioverter defibrillator (ICD), an expensive and palliative option (Campbell, 1990). There is a continuing debate on the relative merits of surgery, ICDs and drug therapy. Each has a role to play. No randomized comparative studies have been performed, nor is it likely that they will be, given that each management offers different outcomes and different risks.

Manifest ventricular ectopic beats

The treatment of post-infarction VEBs is a vexed issue. Those that cause intolerable symptoms demand treatment, which should be with the safest effective therapy. In this context, beta-blockers should be considered the agents of first choice. If beta-blockers fail, then a highly specific sodium channel-blocking drug such as mexiletine may be worthy of consideration. Mexiletine produces unwanted gastrointestinal and CNS effects in a moderate proportion of patients, but its cardiac toxicity is very low (Campbell, 1987).

Ventricular ectopic beats which are asymptomatic and infrequent (less than 10 per hour) can safely be ignored. Asymptomatic but frequent ventricular ectopic beats, however, indicate an adverse prognosis (Darby *et al.*, 1972). Their suppression by Class I anti-arrhythmic drugs has not improved prognosis (Bastian *et al.*, 1980; Chamberlain *et al.*, 1980; Gottlieb *et al.*, 1987; Cardiac Arrhythmia Pilot Study [CAPS] Investigators, 1988; Cardiac Arrhythmia Suppression Trial [CAST] Investigators, 1989; Cardiac Arrhythmia Suppression Trial [CAST II] Investigators, 1992) but their optimal therapy is unknown. Preliminary studies using amiodarone suggest that prognostic benefits might accrue (Burkart *et al.*, 1990), and there is also evidence that beta-blockers may offer benefit (Olsson and Rehnqvist, 1986). Subgroup analysis in one study suggested that the benefits of beta-blocker might relate to an anti-arrhythmic effect as evidenced by reduced ventricular ectopic beats (Olsson and Rehnqvist, 1986).

Latent ventricular arrhythmias

Several techniques are used to define patients at high risk of developing arrhythmias following infarction.

Signal averaging defines that some of the necessary components for re-entry are present. Signal-averaging abnormalities are associated with a risk of developing ventricular tachycardia but the specificity and the sensitivity of the technique is insufficient to prompt intervention (Kuchar *et al.*, 1987). In addition, signal-averaged abnormalities are not modified by anti-arrhythmic strategies in a way that might predict future benefits.

Programmed electrical stimulation of the heart can reveal patients in whom spontaneous ventricular tachycardia is likely. If sustained monomorphic VT is induced at the study, the risk of later recurrence is high (Wellens *et al.*, 1974) and there is growing evidence to support that electrophysiologically guided therapy might be appropriate. Less well defined electrophysiological study end-points (eg non-sustained VT) pose particular problems, but studies currently underway should shed light on clinical management.

The role of ischaemia in arrhythmia expression

Many of the tests employed to investigate manifest or latent arrhythmias seek evidence of an established re-entrant substrate. Thus signal averaging detects areas of delayed conduction whilst invasive electrophysiological studies supply trigger phenomena to the substrate, the presence of which is exposed by the development of a sustained arrhythmia. But late post-infarction, ventricular arrhythmias may be the consequence of new active ischaemia rather than the result of activation of an established substrate. A history of prior angina or induction of an arrhythmia by exercise testing, particularly if there have been pre-existing ST changes, should raise suspicions that the primary problem requiring management is the coronary blood supply and that the arrhythmia is merely a consequence of reversible ischaemia. In support of the hypothesis that ischaemia is pivotal in many important post-infarction ventricular arrhythmias is the evidence of benefits from revascularization procedures (Kelly *et al.*, 1990).

Specialist arrhythmia management

There is great disillusionment with drug therapy for the control and prophylaxis of ventricular arrhythmias post-MI. Class I arrhythmic agents have been damned by the Cardiac Arrhythmia Suppression Trials (1989, 1992) but that is not to deny them a place for the control of symptomatic ventricular arrhythmias particularly ventricular tachycardia. Moreover, beta-blockers are anti-arrhythmic agents and their benefits in acute and late phase infarction are not in dispute: indeed, if anything, they could be used more enthusiastically than at present. Pilot studies of amiodarone suggest that this agent may have much to offer, although it would be wise to await the outcome of current studies before endorsing a routine management role for this compound, particularly in view of its side-effect profile.

Drugs will remain the mainstay of arrhythmia treatment for the foreseeable future, but other treatment modalities are of importance in the post-infarct arrhythmia patient. Surgery (anti-arrhythmic or anti-ischaemic) and implantable devices have an important role in ventricular tachyarrhythmia control.

They are expensive and not without associated morbidity and mortality, but are appropriate for carefully selected high-risk patients.

The complex nature of post-infarction arrhythmias means that individual patients are managed according to their particular personal needs. However, we are still woefully short of information. Perhaps most pressing is the need to understand the contribution of ischaemia to arrhythmogenesis and sudden death and to better define the anti-arrhythmic importance of revascularization procedures. The results of late revascularization are impressive (Kelly *et al.*, 1990), but there is evidence that early revascularization during acute infarction by thrombolytic therapy can dramatically change the electrophysiological mileau and the structure of the infarct, to produce fewer patients with substrates for re-entrant ventricular tachycardia (Bourke *et al.*, 1990*b*).

References

Bastian BC *et al.* (1980) A prospective randomized trial of tocainide in patients following myocardial infarction. *American Heart Journal*. **100**:1017–22.

Bourke JP *et al.* (1990*a*) Surgery for control of recurrent life-threatening ventricular tachyarrhythmias within two months of myocardial infarction. *Journal of the American College of Cardiology*. **16**:42–8.

Bourke JP *et al.* (1990*b*) Reduction in incidence of inducible ventricular tachycardia after myocardial infarction by treatment with streptokinase during infarct evolution. *Journal of the American College of Cardiology*. **16**:1703–1710.

Burkart FF *et al.* (1990) Effect of antiarrhythmic therapy on mortality in survivors of myocardial infarction with asymptomatic complex ventricular arrhythmias: Basel Antiarrhythmic Study of Infarct Survival (BASIS). *Journal of the American College of Cardiology*. **16**:1711–18.

Campbell RWF *et al.* (1981) Ventricular arrhythmias in first 12 hours of acute myocardial infarction. Natural history study. *British Heart Journal*. **46**:351–7.

Campbell RWF (1987) Mexiletine. *New England Journal of Medicine*. **316**:29–34.

Campbell RWF (1990) Life at a price—the implantable defibrillator. *British Heart Journal*. **64**:171–3.

Cardiac Arrhythmia Pilot Study (CAPS) Investigators (1988) Effect of encainide, flecainide, imipramine and moricizine on ventricular arrhythmias during the year after acute myocardial infarction. *American Journal of Cardiology*. **61**:501–9.

Cardiac Arrhythmia Suppression Trial (CAST) Investigators (1989) Preliminary report: effect of encainide and flecainide on mortality in a randomized trial of arrhythmia suppression after myocardial infarction. *New England Journal of Medicine.* **321**:406–12.

Cardiac Arrhythmia Suppression Trial [CAST II] Investigators (1992) Effect of the antiarrhythmic agent moricizine on survival after myocardial infarction. *New England Journal of Medicine.* **327**:227–33.

Chamberlain DA *et al.* (1980) Oral mexiletine in high-risk patients after myocardial infarction. *The Lancet.* **ii**:1324–7.

Darby S *et al.* (1972) Trial of combined intramuscular and intravenous lignocaine in prophylaxis of ventricular tachyarrhythmias. *The Lancet.* **i**:817–19.

Dunn HM *et al.* (1984) Prophylactic lidocaine in the early phase of suspected myocardial infarction. *American Heart Journal.* **110**:353–62.

Gottlieb SH *et al.* (1987) Prophylactic antiarrhythmic therapy of high risk survivors of myocardial infarction: lower mortality at 1 month but not at 1 year. *Circulation.* **75**:792–9.

Kelly P *et al.* (1990) Surgical coronary revascularization in survivors of prehospital cardiac arrest: its effect on inducible ventricular arrhythmias and long-term survival. *Journal of the American College of Cardiology.* **15**:267–73.

Koster RW and Dunning AJ (1985) Intramuscular lidocaine for prevention of lethal arrhythmias in the prehospitalization phase of acute myocardial infarction. *New England Journal of Medicine.* **313**:1105–10.

Kuchar DL *et al.* (1987) Prediction of serious arrhythmic events after myocardial infarction: signal-averaged electrocardiogram, Holter monitoring and radionuclide ventriculography. *Journal of the American College of Cardiology.* **9**:531–8.

Lie KI *et al.* (1974) Lidocaine in the prevention of primary ventricular fibrillation. *New England Journal of Medicine.* **29**:1324–6.

Olsson G and Rehnqvist N (1986) Evaluation of antiarrhythmic effects of metoprolol treatment after acute myocardial infarction: relationship between treatment responses and survival during a three-year follow-up. *European Heart Journal.* **7**:312–19.

Teo K *et al.* (1990) Effect of antiarrhythmic drug therapy on mortality following myocardial infarction. *Circulation.* **82** (Suppl III):197.

Waller TJ *et al.* (1987) Reduction in sudden death and total mortality by antiarrhythmic therapy evaluated by electrophysiologic drug testing: criteria of efficacy in patients with sustained ventricular tachyarrhythmia. *Journal of the American College of Cardiology.* **10**:83–89.

Wellens HJJ *et al.* (1974) Further observations on ventricular tachycardia as studied by electrical stimulation of the heart. *Circulation.* **49**:647–53.

Index

oat bran, 216, 217
obesity, 20, 153–60
  android, 37
  fat intake and, 119
  insulin resistance and, 49–50, 156
  in South Asians, 58–9
  socio-economic status and, 236
  in women, 37–8
oestrogen replacement, 42–4
oleic acid, 123–4
Oslo Study, 167, 316–17
OXCHECK Study, 71, 72, 74, 76

passive smoking, 168
pentoxifylline, 194
physical activity *see* exercise
pipe smoking, 19, 163
placental size, 32–3
plasminogen activator inhibitor 1, 51
Pooling Project, 72
POSCH, 325–8
potassium intake, 145–51
  sodium/potassium ratio, 21
prazosin, 332
prevastatin, 335
prevention of CHD, 68
  dietary salt reduction, 147
  dietitian's role, 253, 256
  ethnic considerations, 68
  fibrinogen reduction, 194
  publicity/educational materials, 77
  screening programmes, 71–80
  see also cholesterol-lowering
psychosocial factors, 231–50
publicity materials, 77
Puerto Rican Study, 82

Quatelet's Index, 153

Rancho Bernardo Study, 82, 87
Reflotron analyser, 72, 76
resources *see* cost; funding
rheology, 201–13
rheumatoid arthritis, 191
rice bran, 216
risk scores, 72–5, 194

salt (dietary), 7, 145–51

ethnic differences, 68
  sodium/potassium ratio, 21
school meals, 255
screening, 71–80, 226, 334
  Birmingham Factory Screening
    Project, 65–8
  National Lipid Screening Project,
    17
senile dementia, 95
Seralyser, 76
Seven Countries Study, 1, 13
  cholesterol data, 16
  fat intake data, 119, 120
  obesity data, 153–5
  smoking data, 154, 161
sex differences in CHD, 37–8
  in elderly, 96
Shaper score, 73
SHEP trial, 84, 89–90, 278–82,
  286–91, 295–8
simvastatin, 335
smoking, 18–19, 161–9
  atherosclerosis and, 171–83
  coffee consumption and, 216
  educational factors and, 233, 235
  in elderly, 81–5, 93, 163
  ethnic differences, 55, 66, 161
  falling rates, 4–5, 161
  fibrinogen levels and, 185, 189–91,
    194, 202
  haematological effects, 206–9
    blood viscosity, 201, 202, 205
  job strain and, 241
  obesity and, 155
  Oslo Trial, 316–17
  passive, 168
  plasma fibrinogen and, 185
  Seven Countries Study data, 154,
    161
social class, 1–3
  smoking and, 161
social factors, 231–8
sodium intake, 145–51
  sodium/potassium ratio, 21
sotalol, 340
stanozolol, 194
STARS, 325–8
STOP-Hypertension trial, 278–82,
  286–91, 298

stress, 240–5
stroke, 1
   blood viscosity and, 205
   in elderly, 298
   ethnic differences, 63–8
   fibrinogen and, 187
   hypertension and, 275–81
   risk reduction, 89–90
   smoking and, 164
   sodium/potassium intake, 145–51
   Whitehall Study, 155
syndrome X, 31–2, 33, 305, 308–12
Syst-Eur study, 290

Tangier disease, 131
thiazide diuretics *see* diuretics
ticlopidine, 194
tobacco *see* smoking
triglycerides *see* lipid metabolism
Tromso Heart Study, 233

ultrasound, intravascular, 115

vegetables, 139–44, 148–9
Veterans' Administration Studies,
   275, 316
viral infections, 191
Vision analyser, 76
vitamin A, 139–44
vitamin C, 139–44
vitamin E, 139–44, 178

weight
   at one year, 27–8, 30
   birthweight, 27–35
   smoking and, 155
   weight loss/fluctuations, 157
   see also obesity
wheat bran, 216
Whitehall Study, 155, 167, 231, 233
wine, 252
women, 37–46
   exercise and CHD risks, 260, 264
   older women, 82, 91, 96
   smoking data, 161–2, 209
works canteen, 256